Biological Barriers in Behavioral Medicine

THE PLENUM SERIES IN BEHAVIORAL PSYCHOPHYSIOLOGY

Series Editor:
William J. Ray, *Pennsylvania State University, University Park, Pennsylvania*

BIOLOGICAL BARRIERS IN BEHAVIORAL MEDICINE
Edited by Wolfgang Linden

PHYSIOLOGY AND BEHAVIOR THERAPY
Conceptual Guidelines for the Clinician
James G. Hollandsworth, Jr.

Biological Barriers in Behavioral Medicine

Edited by
Wolfgang Linden
University of British Columbia
Vancouver, British Columbia, Canada

Plenum Press • New York and London

Library of Congress Cataloging in Publication Data

Biological barriers in behavioral medicine / edited by Wolfgang Linden.
p. cm.—(The Plenum series in behavioral psychophysiology)
Includes bibliographies and index.
ISBN-13: 978-1-4684-5376-8 e-ISBN-13: 978-1-4684-5374-4
DOI: 10.1007/978-1-4684-5374-4
1. Medicine, Psychosomatic. 2. Behavior therapy. 3. Medicine and psychology. I. Linden, Wolfgang. II. Series. [DNLM: 1. Behavioral Medicine. 2. Biological Psychiatry. 3. Psychophysiology. WM 100 B6144]
RC49.B488 1988 87-36137
616.08—dc19 CIP

Softcover reprint of the hardcover 1st edition 1988
A Division of Plenum Publishing Corporation
233 Spring Street, New York, N.Y. 10013

To Isabelle
who knows no barriers

Contributors

J. Allan Best, Department of Health Studies, University of Waterloo, Waterloo, Ontario

T.D. Borkovec, Department of Psychology, Pennsylvania State University, University Park, Pennsylvania

Kelly D. Brownell, Department of Psychiatry, University of Pennsylvania School of Medicine, Philadelphia, Pennsylvania

Margaret A. Chesney, Department of Behavioral Medicine, Stanford Research Institute, Menlo Park, California

Kenneth D. Craig, Department of Psychology, University of British Columbia, Vancouver, British Columbia

Michele Craske, Center for Stress and Anxiety Disorders, State University of New York at Albany, Albany, New York

Thomas L. Creer, Department of Psychology, Ohio University, Athens, Ohio

Nanette M. Frautschi, Outpatient Behavioral Medicine, Southern California Permanente Medical Group, Los Angeles, California

Ruth V. E. Grunau, Department of Psychology, University of British Columbia, Vancouver, British Columbia

Susan A. Kirkland, Department of Health Studies, University of Waterloo, Waterloo, Ontario

David M. Lawson, Department of Psychology, Shaughnessy Hospital, Vancouver, British Columbia

Edward Lichtenstein, Department of Psychology, University of Oregon, and Oregon Research Institute, Eugene, Oregon

Wolfgang Linden, Department of Psychology, University of British Columbia, Vancouver, British Columbia

G. Alan Marlatt, Department of Psychology, University of Washington, Seattle, Washington

David E. Mills, Department of Health Studies, University of Waterloo, Waterloo, Ontario

Harry S. Shabsin, Division of Digestive Diseases, Francis Scott Key Medical Center, and Johns Hopkins University School of Medicine, Baltimore, Maryland

P.H. Van Oot, Department of Psychology, Pennsylvania State University, University Park, Pennsylvania

Patricia E. Wainwright, Department of Health Studies, University of Waterloo, Waterloo, Ontario

Donna Romano White, Centre for Research in Human Development, Concordia University, Montreal, Québec

Norman M. White, Department of Psychology, McGill University, Montreal, Québec

William E. Whitehead, Division of Digestive Diseases, Francis Scott Key Medical Center, and Johns Hopkins University School of Medicine, Baltimore, Maryland

G. Terence Wilson, Department of Psychology, Rutgers University, New Brunswick, New Jersey

Foreword

A "New Looking Glass" for Behavioral Medicine

In 1984, John Briggs, a science writer and specialist in interdisciplinary studies teaching at the New School for Social Research, and F. David Peat, a physicist who was for many years a fellow with the National Research Council of Canada, published a book about the revolutions that were taking place in physics, mathematics, chemistry, biology, and neurophysiology and about the scientists whose new theories were changing our understanding about the nature of the universe. The title of their book was *Looking Glass Universe*, after Lewis Carroll's classic story of Alice and her friends, *Through the Looking Glass*. Briggs and Peat's book is a well-written, challenging volume about human beings and how they think about old problems in new and sometimes startling ways.

I mention Briggs and Peat's book only partially because I happen to have a personal interest in the potential applications of new ways of looking at and thinking about nature and data derived from modern physics and systems theory for health psychology and behavioral medicine (e.g., Schwartz, 1984). In a letter Wolfgang Linden wrote to me on January 23, 1987, he shared with me (at my request) his rough thoughts about his personal goals for this book. I have paraphrased his thoughts below not only because I happen to agree with his overall assessment of the volume at hand, but also because of the implications of his bold, well-chosen words (quoted below) for theories, research, and practice in the emerging biobehavioral-biopsychosocial views of health and illness.

1. Instead of focusing on specific treatments or syndromes individually, the book and its underlying concepts are intended to serve as a "new looking glass for old problems."

2. The layout of the book consists of a general introduction to the overall concepts, detailed applications of the "new looking glass" procedure to different disorders, and a final chapter that attempts to integrate commonalities across chapters and provides suggestions for use in clinical applications.
3. The individual chapters, written in most cases by known experts serve similarly as reflectors of particular specialties at closer range.
4. This book should have a long half-life because it is not meant just to provide literature updates but also to lay the groundwork for a "new perspective."

There have been many books published to date in the areas of health psychology and behavioral medicine. However, only a small percentage of these books have attempted to propose new ways of looking at and thinking about health and illness and have done so in an integrated and scholarly manner. As with any edited book, some chapters in this collection follow the editor's mission more closely than others. In this particular book, the theme of biological barriers is to various degrees and in various ways addressed in each of the chapters. The reader will decide how successfully integrated and useful a given chapter is and how well it fits within the volume as a whole.

As Linden points out in the preface, the title of the volume seems on first glance to convey a critical if not a negative impression about health psychology and behavioral medicine. Biological barriers, by definition, imply limits. However, it is worth noting that one way to look at and think about a biological system (or any system) is to define a system as a set of limits. To create a system is to configure a unique set of limits in a particular, newly organized way. To understand biological barriers is to understand biological mechanisms. To understand biological mechanisms is to understand biological limits. To understand biological limits is to understand biological systems. And to understand biological systems is to understand the capacity for systemic self-regulation and hence for self-healing.

If this looks circular it is understandable, since it reflects the view through a new looking glass. Our ability to discover new looking glasses that improve our ability to organize, explain, and predict new phenomena is a fundamental goal of science. Metaphorically speaking, we must try new glasses and see what we can see. Linden's looking glass focuses on the view linking self-regulation theory with biological barriers and biological potentials across multiple disorders. Whether these particular glasses improve our vision or not is a question for future basic and clinical research to determine.

GARY E. SCHWARTZ

Department of Psychology
Yale University
New Haven, Connecticut

References

Briggs, John, & Peat, F. David. (1984). *Looking glass universe.* New York: Simon and Schuster Cornerstone Library.

Schwartz, G. E. (1984). Psychobiology and health: A new synthesis. In C. J. Scheirer & B. L. Hammonds (Eds.), *Psychology in health: Master lecture series* (Vol. 3). Washington, DC: American Psychological Association.

Preface

The title of this volume appears to forecast a critical if not negative perspective on behavioral medicine. The critical component is fully intended, however, with the ultimate purpose of being constructive and progressive. The intention of the book is to stress those biological mechanisms that behavioral interventions attempt to influence and that at the same time define the very limitations of behavioral medicine. In the eyes of many health professionals, behavioral medicine is an exciting, relatively new field with tremendous potential for the improvement of general medical care and preventive efforts, and the large number of journal and book publications which have shown explosive growth over the last decade reflect this promise. Many of the initial promises for prevention and treatment, however, have failed to be replicable for populations other than those first studied; some of the findings do not generalize to other settings; and certain treatment results simply do not last beyond active intervention periods. All these observations dampen, of course, the initial enthusiasm for this new approach.

I believe that the development of behavioral medicine closely resembles in many respects the development of behavioral therapy some 20 to 30 years earlier. In both instances, a new technology and perspective became available which permitted well-controlled research on etiology and empirical, replicable intervention studies; also, both orientations have been rapidly accepted by practicing health professionals. However, after initially overwhelming enthusiasm, behavior therapy was observed to possess limitations and the literature has witnessed a fair number of rather critical evaluations of the behavioral movement. For example, Aubrey Yates's *Theory and Practice in Behavior Therapy* is representative of such critical, yet constructive, appraisals of the limits of applied behavior theory. It is the intention of the present text to replicate and provoke a similarly critical discussion of advances in behavioral medicine. Herein, the various contributors delineate the ways in which failure and shortcomings of particular behavioral approaches to medical problems can be attributed to biological limitations that may be so powerful that they can override the impact of psychological and behavioral interventions. The particular example that has been most influential in nurturing my curiosity about self-regulatory mechanisms has been the concept of set point in obesity research whereby many dieters, therapists, and researchers could finally explain their frustrations with continuous failures to lose weight or to maintain weight loss. Our purpose here is to investigate the psychobiology of prevalent biopsychosocial disorders and phenomena in the search for compensatory, self-regulatory mechanisms like "set points" that are likely to counteract the success of behavioral interventions. Again, the main objective is to be critical but constructive by contrasting present treatment approaches and their underlying rationales with the biological mechanisms governing the etiology and maintenance of given disorders and by analyzing the specific suitability in each case. I believe that a text of this nature is of interest not only to practitioners but also to academic specialists whose work brings them to the interface of medicine and psychology. This includes a variety of medical specialists, for example in internal medicine, cardiology, endocrinology, gastroenterology, and family practice, as well as clinical and health psychologists, nurses, rehabilitation specialists, health educators, and policymakers in the field of health care and prevention.

The sequence of topics is somewhat arbitrary but has nevertheless three broad inherent categories. The first chapters deal with disorders traditionally considered to be addictions in which the high likelihood of failing with behavioral treatment has long been an essential ingredient of the disorder's conceptualization. The next group of chapters represents either health risk factors or medical disorders that the *Diagnostic and Statistical Manual of Mental Disorders* (third edition, revised) would classify as "Psychological factors affecting physical condition" (Code 316.00). In the third broad category, the discussion of biological mechanisms in pain cuts across various disorders since pain is not a unique property of a single disorder but a shared feature of many. Finally, the concluding chapter on preventing relapse summarizes in one conceptual framework many of the previously raised issues. The choice of topics implies no claim of being comprehensive; many other areas deserve similar attention. And, of course, as an editor I would feel amply rewarded if the concepts and perspectives represented throughout this text generated sufficient interest to be applied to other domains not covered here.

I am very grateful to all the authors who have lent their expertise to this investigation of self-regulatory mechanisms. I would also like to thank Mr. James Frankish, Miss Heather M. McEachern, and Miss Holly Austin for their critical reading of the manuscripts and Miss Liz McCririck for her efforts in transforming my scribbles and mumbles into neat-looking book chapters.

Appreciation is expressed to W. B. Saunders Co., Philadelphia, W. H. Freeman and Co., New York, and Plenum Press, New York, for their permission to reprint some of the figures in this volume. Particular gratitude is due to the American Psychological Association for permitting us to reprint Brownell, Marlatt, Lichtenstein, and Wilson's chapter, which initially appeared in the *American Psychologist*.

Last, but certainly not least, I would like to thank editors Robert Jystad and Eliot Werner at Plenum Press who masterfully and patiently helped to overcome the barriers to publishing this text.

WOLFGANG LINDEN

Vancouver, B.C.

Reference

Yates, Aubrey. (1975). *Theory and practice in behavior therapy*. New York: Wiley Interscience.

Contents

CHAPTER 1

Self-Regulation Theory in Behavioral Medicine

An Introduction

Wolfgang Linden

This chapter has five objectives:

1. To discuss briefly the scientific and historical trends that have led to the rise of behavioral medicine.
2. To outline the role that theory (in particular, self-regulation theory; Schwartz, 1977, 1979, 1983) plays in its development.
3. To discuss the potential and the limitations of self-regulation theory.
4. To use the modified health belief model (Feuerstein & Linden, 1984) to illustrate the complex interactions of social, behavioral, and biological self-regulatory mechanisms that account for many forms of medical illness.
5. To delineate from this discussion the objective of the present book, that is, to provide an in-depth analysis of how closely current treatment rationales reflect and integrate available knowledge of underlying biological self-regulatory mechanisms which may effectively function as barriers to short-term treatment success and/or to the maintenance of initially positive outcome.

Wolfgang Linden • Department of Psychology, University of British Columbia, Vancouver, British Columbia, Canada V6T 1Y7.

Historical Developments

A perspective on health and illness that focuses on both psychological and biological factors has existed for thousands of years. Socrates recognized that soma and psyche interacted as contributors to health and illness. The concept of soma represented what is considered today the empirical approach to medicine whereas the psyche reflected its more esoteric aspects. Despite this early emphasis on the interaction of mind and body, most conceptualizations of illness have been dominated by a traditional medical model with its reductionist principles that focuses solely on the biological aspects of disease.

The 2nd and 3rd decade of this century witnessed a revival of a more comprehensive approach to illness with the development of psychosomatic medicine (cf. Cannon, 1936). Much was learned through the psychosomatic approach, but a number of factors have limited the value of its contribution to our basic understanding of the psychobiological aspects of illness. The almost exclusive use of a psychodynamic framework for understanding the mechanisms by which psychological factors contributed to illness was one such limitation. Although psychodynamic principles permit explanations at one level of analysis, they are limited by virtue of the inability to validate certain internal constructs and also by the fact that clinical procedures resulting from such theory have resulted in only limited treatment success with somatic disturbances (Kellner, 1975). The second problem with the psychosomatic approach relates to its focus on the psychological factors associated with, rather than predictive of, a given illness. This orientation does not permit specification of the etiological role of psychological factors in illness. Despite these limitations, it should be noted that the traditional psychosomatic approach significantly contributed to our understanding of a number of areas, particularly the biochemistry and psychophysiology of stress and certain stress-related disorders (cf. Weiner, 1977).

A major breakthrough for the field of behavioral medicine can be attributed to Miller's work (1969), wherein it was discovered that a number of autonomic functions are clearly more open to environmental input and voluntary change than had previously been assumed. This insight was the "starter's shot" for the rapid development of biofeedback, a procedure that uses visual or auditory display of autonomic activity and has since helped many patients in dealing with a variety of autonomic dysfunctions. Adding to many early studies, there was a further breakthrough in biofeedback when Schwartz documented that there may be voluntary fractionation and patterning in physiological responses (1975, 1976). Studies on patterning indicated that a variety of functions previously believed to be regulated by the same biological system possess in fact separate regulatory systems, such as systolic and diastolic blood pressure. Given the separate regulation of such activity, it has been possible to teach increases in one function while at the same time decreasing activity levels in another. Although biofeedback has added valuable technology and important empirical findings, the movement was initially criticized by traditional clinicians and theoreticians as being overly technical and atheoretical. Only recently have researchers begun systematically to evaluate what cognitive-behavioral strategies subjects use to alter physiological functions voluntarily (e.g., Levenson & Ditto, 1981). One decade later, when the domains of health psychology and behavioral medicine surfaced (Schwartz & Weiss, 1978), biofeedback appeared to have found an appropriate conceptual framework. What today is conceptualized as behavioral medicine has been developed by researchers and clinicians from a variety of disciplines who were dissatisfied with both the pure technology of biofeedback and the traditional psychosomatic approach. The common focus of this group was to promote interdisciplinary research on the etiology, prevention, and treatment of physical illness. The "movement" currently referred to as behavioral medicine has been defined as:

> The field concerned with the development of behavioral science knowledge and techniques relevant to the understanding of physical health and illness and the application of this knowledge and these techniques to prevention, diagnosis, treatment, and rehabilitation. Psychoses, neurosis, and substance abuse are included only and so far as they contribute to physical disorders as an endpoint. (Schwartz & Weiss, 1978, p. 250)

At this juncture, the field does not appear to be bound by current theoretical or disciplinary limitations; rather, it represents an integrative approach to health and illness, one that is illustrated throughout this book. The fact that behavioral medicine is ascribed to by practitioners and researchers from many different domains represents considerable challenge and an unusual opportunity. Although issues of territoriality have yet to be resolved among the different health professions, the collaboration of various disciplines, methodologies, and theoretical approaches permits a wide, comprehensive approach to problems and challenges researchers to seek conceptual formulations beyond previous boundaries. Within this theoretical framework, the systems and cybernetics approach has taken an important place. Again, Schwartz (1977, 1979, 1983) has been a major proponent of this view and the cybernetic model of health and illness is often linked with his name. The systems–cybernetics approach can be considered a response to the criticism that biofeedback as a precursor to behavioral medicine was largely atheoretical and established a fairly comprehensive, yet seemingly simple model which attempts to explain the interaction between environmental demands and various body system responses. Figure 1 presents a highly simplified but conceptually useful way of linking environmental stimuli (Stage 1) to changes in the central nervous system (Stage 2) and their expression in the peripheral organ (Stage 3).

Of particular importance to Schwartz's concept of "the brain as a health care system" is the existence of a negative feedback system (Stage 4), which returns body messages to the brain (Stage 2). It is the existence of these negative feedback loops that makes it possible for the brain to monitor the state of its peripheral organs and thereby to maintain stable functioning of the body (Cannon, 1963) and itself. This homeostatic model has been prevalent for a number of decades and is useful in explaining a number of biological functions. However, the model is inappropriate since total homeostasis presumes closed feedback loops such that information from the environment has no port of entry into this system. A system based on totally closed feedback loops cannot explain disregulation within biological systems that is presumably due to envi-

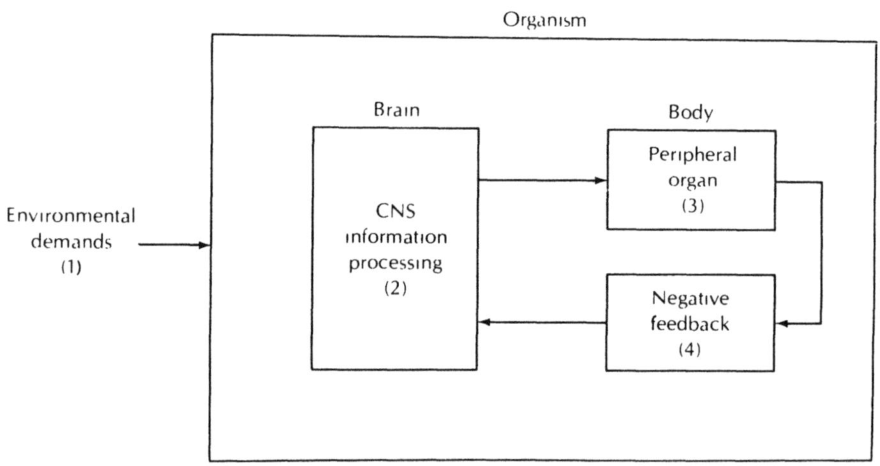

Figure 1. Simplified block diagram depicting (1) environmental demands influencing (2) the brain's regulation of (3) peripheral organs and (4) negative feedback from the periphery back to the brain. Disregulation can be initiated at each of these stages. Biofeedback (Stage 5) is a parallel feedback loop to Stage 4, detecting the activity of the peripheral organ (Stage 3) and converting it into environmental (Stage 1) input that can be used by the brain (Stage 2) to increase self-regulation. From *Psychopathology: Experimental Models* (p. 281), 1977, by J. D. Maser and M. E. P. Seligman (Eds.), New York: W. H. Freeman. Copyright 1977 by W. H. Freeman and Company. Reprinted by permission.

ronmental stress. This novel and somewhat disturbing implication of the position on disregulation taken by Schwartz (1977) questions the logic and the ultimate utility of the traditional medical model which ignores Stage 1 and Stage 2 variables as important components of health and illness. The strict medical model implies the use of direct biological intervention (pharmacological or surgical) to treat injury or disease. The disregulation model, in contrast, predicts that because of incomplete diagnosis and treatment of disregulation the strict medical model may inadvertently lead to the perpetuation of disregulation, not only in bodily disease but in human social behavior as well (Schwartz, 1977).

The basic premise of the disregulation model is that the brain has primary responsibility for maintaining the health of itself and of the body, and that it succeeds in this task by altering or regulating itself to meet the needs of specific organs. Because the body, as with any complex physical device, can work effectively only within certain tolerances, the brain must adjust itself to bring the disregulation back to balance. As Schwartz (1977) points out, disregulation can be initiated and perpetuated at four stages. Often, the disregulation is initiated by exogenous stimulus demands (Stage 1) and the brain responds to them (Stage 2). If the brain is exposed to environmental conditions that ultimately lead to the breakdown of a given organ system (Stage 3) and a functional disorder develops, appropriate internal feedback loops are activated (Stage 4), many of which generate feedback through pain messages. This negative stimulus triggers corrective action in the brain. Even if such higher centers are busy attending to other stimuli and fail to recognize the breakdown of a particular organ, at some point the organ will generate sufficient negative feedback (if the loop is intact) to redirect the brain. Anyone who has experienced a really strong stomachache caused by overeating is aware of negative feedback and its commanding of attention that subsequently may lead to a change in behavior. However, certain disorders, like elevated blood pressure, do not have a known protective mechanism that activates conscious symptoms of pain and distress; such disorders are particularly difficult to treat because of a lack of immediate motivation for change and the lack of success feedback (Feuerstein & Linden, 1984; Linden, 1984).

The fundamental question becomes one of the correct response of the brain to the internal stimulation. From a psychobiological perspective, the brain should either make modifications in the outside environment, leave the environment, or modify its interactions. Consequently, the pain of the disturbed stomach keeps behavior in check by regulating of eating patterns.

However useful this may appear, typical patients would rather not change their life-style or their environment, the two factors (Stages 1 and

2) that together augment or cause the bodily dysfunction in the first place (Schwartz, 1977). One can argue that humans choose instead to modify Stage 3 or Stage 4, or both, directly, by intrinsic biological intervention. According to the disregulation model, if the negative feedback mechanisms are removed artifically (for example, by taking a pain killer), the brain is free to continue behaving in maladaptive ways that ultimately may become deleterious to the maintenance of health. Lacking the stabilizing impact of negative regulation, the brain becomes increasingly useless relative to its own "healing powers."

Schwartz (1977) used a simple stomachache to illustrate this point. Modern society strongly reinforces the practice of taking drugs to eliminate the stomachaches caused by the brain's disregulation, that is, allowing overeating despite signals of discomfort. Antacid commercials of a few years ago exemplify this habit. For example, they depict an obese man stuffing himself with apple pies or spaghetti. When an actually functional stomachache follows, the obvious conclusion should be that the stomach and the rest of the body were not meant to be fed in that manner. The man's stomache represents the biological feedback mechanism necessary to keep him from abusing his body further. Instead, what is communicated is "Eat, eat, and if you get a stomachache don't change your environment or behavior since you may eliminate your discomfort by taking a pill which is a lot easier."

Simple antacids are a mild drug, and they do not always work. When they do not, other stronger medication is often described to lessen the pain. When the organ becomes so abused that, for example, an ulcer develops and internal bleeding occurs, does the person listen to his or her stomach then and radically change his or her external environment and/or behavior? Often times, no. What a person does instead is go to a surgeon for repair. Medical science is now developing newer and finer means of bypassing many normal and adaptive feedback mechanisms. A patient can have a vagotomy and totally eliminate the brain's ability to regulate the stomach neurally. And if this trend in modern medicine continues, people can look forward to the day when, if their stomachs continue to be bothersome, they can simply go to their local surgeon and obtain an artificial stomach.

At this point the brain would no longer be constrained by the needs of a natural stomach and would no longer serve as a natural health care system. According to the disregulation model, this brain would be free to continue and even to expand upon the inappropriate disregulation initially causing the problem. Whereas the stomach is only one organ, modern medicine is using this strategy for all systems of the body. Modern culture often reinforces the idea that if the brain and body cannot cope with the external environment, they will simply have to undergo medical alteration to adjust. According to the disregulation model, this prospect, when carried to its extreme, would have serious consequences for the survival of the human species as we now know it. Schwartz (1977) warns any reader of his elaboration on self-regulation theory against falsely believing that all biomedical interventions are inappropriate. On the contrary, a psychobiological perspective emphasizing self-regulation and disregulation helps to indicate under what specific conditions biomedical intervention is adaptive. The point is that one is not to succumb to the overly simplistic conclusion that the correction of Stages 3 and 4 of disregulation through biomedical interventions should be the sole approach to treatment. Instead, to keep the health and behavior of the human species intact, it may be necessary to accept limitations of the body as it is, even though this may require more active self-regulation on the part of the brain. A psychobiological perspective on biofeedback and behavioral medicine could play an extraordinary important role in this development.

Potential of the Self-Regulation Theory

Self-regulation theory is certainly useful in trying to understand the operating mechanism of biofeedback and can also be used to understand how environmental demands can translate into bodily changes which require adaptation on the part of organ systems. In deviating from previous, purely homeostatic models, the self-regulation model represents a theory of disregulation based on a conceptualization of the inherent feedback system as an open loop that can be accessed through various channels by the environment. Although Figure 1 illustrates the general principle of self-regulation, it is of course difficult to display any theory involving more than two dimensions in such a figure. Given that body systems are highly complex and interactive, one needs to conceptualize self-regulation and disregulation as models with a number of interacting dimensions. In particular, it appears that negative and positive feedback loops serve only one objective, namely, that of achieving self-regulation, a process in which the brain plays a central mediating role. The figure cannot reflect the infinite number of potential interactions that can be categorized as serving at least two, albeit opposing, functions: It is possible that change in one system, for example, as brought about by biofeedback, may be complemented by subsequent change in other systems that will then perpetuate and stabilize the change initially seen in the intended target system. But it is also theoretically possible that change in one system (whether brought about by cognitive change or biofeedback or by any environmental input) may trigger processes in other systems that have opposing effects such that change initiated or attempted in the target system will be counteracted by one or a series of other body systems. For example, it has been observed that once regulation in a particular body systems has occurred, this may lead to disregulation in other systems which may henceforth impede maintained self-regulation because of anatomical or physiological limitations. For example, it has been established that in the case of chronically high blood pressure there is damage to artery walls such that ultimately anatomical changes secondary to the original problem will maintain the disorder and impede any self-regulation process. Also, it has been argued that excessive weight loss through repeated caloric restriction may result in an effect opposing the intended one such that the metabolic rate drops and makes a maintenance of weight reduction even less likely (Rodin, 1981; see also Chapter 3).

The Modified Health Belief Model

The observation that voluntary change and attempts to reestablish self-regulation may be limited by biological constraints has been underlined by Feuerstein and Linden (1984), who have taken the original health belief model (Becker & Maiman, 1975) and expanded it to explain why prevention and treatment efforts in behavioral medicine have often been less successful that expected or hoped for. The original health belief model proposes a set of variables that determine compliance with health care recommendations and permit predictions about the reduction or elimination of health risk behavior. Becker and Maiman (1975) defined compliance as the patient's acceptance of recommended health behavior. According to the model, the initiation of preventive health action is usually triggered by environmental cues, such as newspaper or magazine articles; advice from family members, friends, or health professionals; and mass media campaigns (Becker & Maiman, 1975). A major stumbling block to preventive health action is that many signs or symptoms do not receive much attention by the individual because they are not associated with significant discomfort. In the case of certain coronary heart disease risk factors, for example, the symptoms are often not perceived (elevated blood pressure or high serum cholesterol levels) or if unpleasant effects are experienced, either there is no specificity or there is no patent result in a continuous or recurrent pain or discomfort (smoking, inactivity, obesity, and the Type A behavior pattern). A review of the empirical literature on the health belief model (Becker, Haefner, Kasl, Kirscht, Maiman, & Rosenstock, 1978) provided empirical support for the hypothesized influence of the four variables within the model: (a) perceived susceptibility to a given illness, (b) perceived severity of such illness, (c) perceived benefits of preventive health action, and (d) perceived barriers in establishing preventive health actions. This empirical set of predictors can be utilized to determine the likelihood of preventive action with respect to any health risk factor. Although Becker *et al.* have provided a good deal of empirical evidence indicating that these factors have predictive power with respect to health behavior, Feuerstein and Linden (1984) have suggested that the risk factor literature as available today warrants the inclusion of an additional parameter in Becker and Maiman's model (1975). Becker and Maiman included and focused primarily on psychological aspects of effective health action but did not address the psychobiological interactions that may characterize a given illness and its contributing risk factors. The literature suggests that the development and maintenance of many risk factors imply complicated psychobiological mechanisms that may either facilitate or hinder the maintenance of health risk behavior. Obesity, for example, has been described as at least partially being maintained by a homeostatic, autonomic physiological mechanism that is not easily influenced by psychological factors (Rodin, 1981; see also Chapter 3). Other risk factors may be maintained through concomitant psychobiological mechanisms such as tension reduction after smoking or attenuated distress through elevations in blood pressure (Dworkin, Filewich, Miller & Craigmyle, 1979). The existence of such counteractive psychobiological mechanisms can be integrated into the Becker and Maiman (1975) model by diferentiating those variables hypothesized to effect the initiation of positive health actions from those variables that may counteract the maintenance of these health actions once initiated. The extended model (Feuerstein & Linden, 1984) is illustrated in Figure 2.

The extended model overlaps with Becker and Maiman's model by incorporating identical variables to predict the likelihood of preventive action for the initiation of new healthy behaviors. However, it extends the health belief model by including the possible counteractive effects of psychobiological, self-regulatory mechanisms that may interfere with health behavior maintenance. Consideration of biological self-regulatory mechanisms appears to be important because only continuous change (that is, modification of life-style) will effectively reduce many health risks. With respect to the demonstrated failure in the maintenance of many health behaviors over substantial periods of time, it may be that the sum of all positive health beliefs does not outweigh the impact of existing

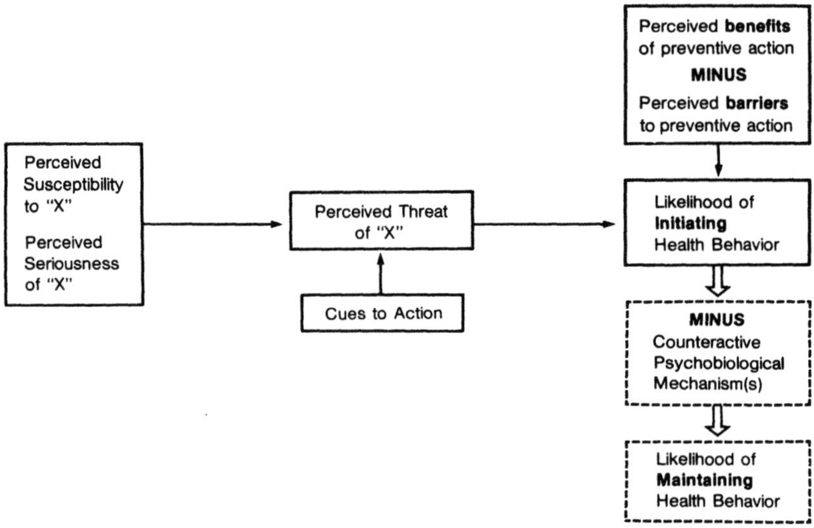

Figure 2. Block diagram of the modified health belief model. From M. Feuerstein and W. Linden, 1984, p. 834. Reprinted by permission.

counteractive psychobiological mechanisms that influence the individual's behavior.

At this point in the discussion it may be advisable to attempt an integration of both Schwartz's self-regulation model with its inherent implications and limitations and the extended health belief model (Feuerstein & Linden, 1984). The integration of these two models provides the theoretical rationale for the present book in that extensive analyses of underlying biological mechanisms are undertaken for a variety of disorders that are focal in behavioral medicine; the emphasis within these analyses is on biological self-regulatory systems. Each chapter outlines complex interacting systems and attempts to answer the question whether any one of these systems may possibly be counteractive with any other. Most interesting in this context is the identification of regulatory systems that during the course of the disorder shift from open loops (permitting disregulation) to closed loops and that maintain themselves at levels that may appear adaptive within the limited system under observation but are also known to be maladaptive from a larger multisystem perspective. If any such systems can be identified, it is strikingly evident that there are multiple implications for treatment. Above all, it is necessary to contrast existing treatment rationales with their functionality, given the existing psychobiological self-regulatory systems. Regulatory mechanisms are highlighted that make psychological or behavioral intervention difficult due to their inherent self-stabilizing interactive nature that a particular treatment rationale may not account for. On the basis of this review of the literature, each chapter of the book is structured primarily to address three key issues. First, the chapters review the present outcome literature and attempt to assess how successful psychological treatments have actually been. Within this discussion of treatment outcome, rationales for the choice of a particular treatment is underlined. In a second step, a review of biological regulating mechanisms for various disorders is provided and the existence of self-regulation mechanisms and interactions with other systems will be highlighted. Finally, the third step is a synthesis whereby each chapter attempts to contrast the biological regulation underlying a particular disorder with the presently used treatment rationales. It is thereby determined whether treatment success or failure as prevalent in the literature can be explained by a poor match between the inherent psychobiology and the prevalent treatment approach. If possible, each contributor points out cases wherein previous conceptualizations of treatment are sufficient and only procedural changes are necessary to maximize treatment outcome; it is also noted where there may be mismatches between biological regulation principles and the rationale of presently used treatment steps. These syntheses have as an objective the provision of new challenges and higher degrees of freedom for the development of more coherent links between treatment rationale and the true biological dysfunction underlying the disorder.

References

Becker, M. H., & Maiman, L. A. (1975). Sociobehavioral determinants of compliance with health and medical care recommendations. *Medical Care, 13*, 10–24.

Becker, M. H., Haefner, D. P., Kasl, S. U., Kirscht, J. P., Maiman, L. A., & Rosenstock, I. M. (1978). Selected psychosocial models and correlates of individual health-related behaviors. *Medical Care, 15* (Suppl.), 27–47.

Cannon, W. B. (1963). *Wisdom of the body*. New York: Norton.

Dworkin, B. R., Filewich, R. J., Miller, N. E., & Craigmyle, N. (1979). Baroreceptor activation reduces reactivity to noxious stimulation: Implications for hypertension. *Science, 205*, 1299–1301.

Feuerstein, M., & Linden, W. (1984). Psychobiological aspects of health and disease. In H. E. Adams & P. B. Sutker (Eds.), *Comprehensive handbook of psychopathology*. New York: Plenum Press.

Keller, R. (1975). Psychotherapy in psychosomatic disorders: A survey of controlled studies. *Archives of General Psychiatry, 32,* 1021–1028.

Levenson, R. W., & Ditto, W. B. (1981). Individual differences in ability to control heart rate: Personality, strategy, physiological, and other variables. *Psychophysiology, 18,* 91–100.

Linden, W. (1984). *Psychological perspectives of essential hypertension: Etiology, maintenance, and treatment.* Basel/New York: S. Karger.

Miller, N. E. (1969). Learning of visceral and glandular responses. *Sciences, 163,* 434–445.

Rodin, J. (1981). Current status of the internal–external hypothesis for obesity. *American Psychologist, 30,* 361–372.

Schwartz, G. E. (1975). Biofeedback, self-regulation and the patterning of physiological processes. *American Scientist, 63,* 314–324.

Schwartz, G. E. (1976). Self-regulation of response patterning: Implications for psychophysiological research and therapy. *Biofeedback and Self-Regulation, 1,* 7–30.

Schwartz, G. E. (1977). Psychosomatic disorders and biofeedback: A psychobiological model of disregulation. In J. D. Maser & M. E. P. Seligman (Eds.), *Psychopathology: Experimental models.* San Francisco: Freeman.

Schwartz, G. E. (1979). Disregulation and systems theory: A biobehavioral framework for biofeedback and behavioral medicine. In N. Birbaumer & H. D. Kimmel (Eds.), *Biofeedback and self-regulation.* Hillsdale, NJ: Lawrence Erlbaum.

Schwartz, G. E. (1983). Disregulation theory and disease: Applications to the repression/cerebral disconnection/cardiovascular disorder hypothesis. *International Review of Applied Psychology, 32,* 95–118.

Schwartz, G. E., & Weiss, S. M. (1978). Behavioral medicine revisited: An amended definition. *Journal of Behavioral Medicine, 1,* 249–251.

Weiner, H. (1977). *The psychobiology of human disease.* New York: Elsevier.

CHAPTER 2

Biological Barriers in the Treatment of Alcoholism

David M. Lawson and Michelle Craske

For more than 20 years, a controversy has raged between the proponents of two conflicting models of alcoholism. One model, typically referred to as the traditional or disease model (Pattison, Sobell, & Sobell, 1977) assumes that alcoholism is a progressive, irreversible disease which may cause the abstaining alcoholic to experience an irresistible craving for alcohol and the indulgent alcoholic to lose control over alcohol consumption. The etiology of alcoholism, according to this model, is physiological and/or genetic in origin. In contrast, the behavioral model assumes that alcohol consumption is a socially acquired, learned pattern of behavior which occurs as a function of antecedent and consequent events. Such events include situational or environmental factors as well as the alcoholic's cognitive and affective states.

The controversy has unfortunately polarized views of clinicians and researchers alike. The effect of this polarization has been that those who adhere to a traditional view have continued to neglect the role of environmental, cognitive, and affective determinants of abusive drinking, whereas adherents of the behavioral model have neglected the role of physiological variables. The objective of this chapter is twofold: to reexamine the evidence for the role of physiological variables in the maintenance of abusive drinking habits and to consider how the efficacy of

David M. Lawson • Department of Psychology, Shaughnessy Hospital, Vancouver, British Columbia, Canada V6H 3N1. *Michelle Craske* • Center for Stress and Anxiety Disorders, State University of New York at Albany, Albany, New York 12203

behavioral treatments might be enhanced by explicitly taking into account the effect of physiological determinants of alcohol consumption.

To preface these issues, we will present a brief overview of the rationale and efficacy of current behavioral techniques used in the treatment of alcoholism.

Behavioral Treatments for Alcoholism

A wide variety of techniques has been implemented in behavioral treatment programs for alcohol abuse. No single treatment, however, is generally considered the treatment of choice, nor is it the case that treatment consists of a single technique. Rather, abusive drinking is regarded as being functionally related to a range of potential controlling variables, and treatment programs typically include techniques that are specific to each variable class involved. Using the assessment model developed by Goldfried and Sprafkin (1974), the range of potential controlling variables can be divided into four general classes: stimulus antecedents, organismic variables, response variables, and consequences. In this section, the rationale underlying techniques that focus specifically on each of these classes of controlling factors will be briefly described.

It has long been recognized that among the most influential *stimulus antecedents* of abusive drinking are the sight, smell, and taste of alcoholic beverages. In fact, it is not at all uncommon for alcohol abusers to report a subjective craving for alcohol merely upon presentation of these stimuli. Two behavioral techniques, chemical aversion and cue-exposure response prevention, are used specifically for the purpose of reducing the effect of alcohol-related stimuli.

In chemical aversion, alcoholics are injected with an emetic drug and subsequently presented with bottles and glasses of their preferred alcoholic beverages which they are encouraged to smell and to taste. The presentation of these alcohol-related stimuli is timed as nearly as possible to coincide with the onset of drug-induced nausea. This procedure, which is usually repeated five times over a period of 10 days, is based on a classical conditioning paradigm in which the emetic and its subsequent effects are conceptualized as unconditioned stimulus and unconditioned response, respectively. By repeated association of the alcohol cues with the onset of nausea, it is assumed that the former will eventually elicit the latter and that the abusive drinker will acquire an aversion to alcohol. Although abstinence rates one year following chemical aversion average between 50% and 60% and are among the highest reported for any treatment, there have been no controlled outcome evaluations in which chemical aversion has been compared to a no-treatment control group (Miller, 1982).

Cue-exposure response prevention, like chemical aversion, is intended to diminish the influence of alcohol cues on drinking behavior. Unlike chemical aversion, however, its effectiveness does not depend on the acquisition of a conditioned aversive response. Instead, the craving elicited by alcohol and the abusive drinking that typically follows are conceptualized as aspects of an obsessive-compulsive disorder. As in the treatment of other compulsive behaviors, the abusive drinker is exposed at length not only to the sight and smell of preferred alcoholic beverages but also to the interoceptive cues resulting from the consumption of a "priming" dose of alcohol itself. During the period of exposure, which lasts 45 minutes, the alcohol abuser is strongly encouraged to resist the urge to continue drinking and, presumably as a result of extinction, experiences a gradual reduction in the intensity of craving. Although cue-exposure response prevention has only recently been used in the treatment of alcoholism, preliminary data regarding its effectiveness are encouraging. After six inpatient treatment sessions, for example, exposure to the effects of a priming dose followed by the presentation of additional alcohol has been shown to have minimal effects on craving (Rankin, Hodgson, & Stockwell, 1983).

The second general class of potentially relevant variables in the functional analysis of abusive drinking are the *organismic variables*, including cognitive, affective, and physiological factors. Proponents of both the traditional and behavioral models of alcoholism have long recognized the importance of many of these factors, and it is customary for both types of treatment program to include components to address problems arising from depression, poor nutrition, inadequate health care, and misconceptions regarding the physiological and behavioral effects of alcohol. More recently, however, increasing attention has been paid by behavioral clinicians to the role of cognitive variables, particularly as they contribute to relapse.

Marlatt (1985), whose cognitive-behavioral analysis of the relapse process best exemplifies work in this area, refers to three interrelated cognitive processes that are assumed to mediate the effect of the external environment on the resumption of abusive drinking. First is the alcoholic's appraisal of his or her coping skills with regard to situations previously associated with abusive drinking. Successful coping without resort to alcohol is assumed to enhance the alcoholic's self-efficacy, thereby reducing the likelihood of relapse. The second cognitive process concerns the alcoholic's expectations regarding the effects of alcohol. To the extent that these expectations are positive, the likelihood of relapse increases. Finally, in the event a drink is taken, the alcoholic's attribution of the cause to either personal or situational factors will also determine the likelihood of a complete relapse.

Relapse prevention programs based on Marlatt's cognitive-behavioral analysis include numerous techniques that focus specifically on each of these cognitive processes. Efficacy enhancement techniques include skills training, not only to enable the alcoholic to cope with high-risk situations but also to provide an opportunity for the alcoholic to experience mastery in areas not directly related to alcohol abuse. To reduce the influence of positive expectations of alcohol, abusive drinkers are instructed, among other things, about the differential effects of increasing and decreasing blood alcohol levels and the influence of environmental effects on the experience of craving. Cognitive restructuring is also used to aid the alcoholic in reattributing the cause of an initial drink to specific, controllable situational factors rather than to personal, stable ones and in viewing such a relapse as an opportunity for skill acquisition rather than the beginning of an inevitable binge. Marlatt has also proposed the programmed relapse technique, in which the alcoholic actually consumes a drink, as a further means of enhancing perceptions of personal control and responsibility and to provide an opportunity for the alcoholic to experience and to cope with the resultant cognitive and affective reactions, which Marlatt calls the "abstinence violation effect." Despite the strongly empirical foundation of Marlatt's relapse prevention model, the efficacy of programs incorporating the range of treatment procedures suggested by it remains to be demonstrated.

The third general class of controlling variables in a behavioral analysis focuses upon *response characteristics* including not only the frequency, amplitude, and duration of specific target behaviors but also the availability of alternative responses in the client's behavioral repertoire. According to the behavioral model, abusive drinking can be conceptualized as a maladaptive coping response which occurs in part because alternative, more adaptive responses have not been acquired. By conducting a detailed assessment of the circumstances in which abusive drinking occurs, the clinician develops hypotheses concerning specific response deficits which are then assessed more directly.

A wide range of coping skills deficits has been identified among alcoholics and specific training in these skills has been incorporated in their treatment. Recognizing that the most ubiquitous such deficit is the relative inability of abusive drinkers to decline a proffered drink. Foy, Miller, Eisler, and O'Toole (1976) developed a drink-refusal training program in which the therapist and client role-play specific situations wherein the client is pressured to drink. Assertiveness training procedures are also used in the behavioral treatment of alcoholics to remediate deficits in other areas such as refusing unreasonable requests, responding to criticism, and requesting changes in the behavior of others. Marital discord may also be functionally related to abusive drinking, in which case, marital therapy is the vehicle by which deficient social skills are acquired. Perhaps the most generally applicable skills training program used in the treatment of alcohol abuse is problem solving, which Chaney, O'Leary, and Marlatt (1978) used with participants in their program to develop coping responses to a range of problem situations. In general, programs that develop alternative coping skills for situations associated with alcohol consumption tend to produce successful treatment outcomes.

Undoubtedly, the most controversial alternative response training procedures are those intended to produce moderate drinking outcomes. In the behavioral self-control training program of Miller and Munoz (1982), for example, problem drinkers are taught a variety of self-management techniques, such as self-monitoring, goal setting, self-reinforcement, and drink spacing, specifically with the objective of teaching controlled drinking. In an extensive review of the outcome research on controlled drinking treatment programs, including Miller's own behavioral self-control training, Miller and Hester (1980) reported that between 60% and 70% of problem drinkers were consistently classified as abstinent, controlled, or improved at 1-year follow-up.

The fourth class of variables that exerts a controlling influence on behavior is *consequences*. With respect to abusive drinking, any changes in the external environmental or in the drinker's physiological, cognitive, or affective state that occur following the consumption of alcohol may act as reinforcers to increase the probability of subsequent abusive drinkig episodes. Accordingly, behavioral treatment programs often attempt to rearrange these contingencies to ensure that abusive drinking either goes unreinforced or is punished.

Two procedures have been included in behaviorally oriented treatment programs to counteract the relatively immediate subjective and physiological consequences of alcohol consumption. The first is administration of disulfiram, a drug that is ingested daily by carefully screened alcohol abusers and causes a very unpleasant reaction characterized by vasodilation, hypotension, nausea, and vomiting within a short time after alcohol ingestion (Kwentus & Major, 1979). To ensure compliance with the administration of disulfiram, specific training procedures have been developed to teach the alcohol abuser to take the medication at a predetermined time and place and in the presence of a spouse, friend, or employer. Under these conditions, disulfiram has been shown to produce near total sobriety among married or cohabitating alcohol abusers at 6-month follow-up (Azrin, Sisson, Meyers, & Godley, 1982).

In the second procedure, covert sensitization, patients are first relaxed and then instructed to imagine as vividly as possible a succession of drinking scenes in which they become nauseated and vomit immediately after consuming alcohol. The guided imagery includes detailed descriptions not only of the patient's desire for alcohol and the sensory and motor components of drinking but also of the onset of nausea and vomitig. The procedure is repeated with the suggestion regarding nausea occurring progressively earlier in the drinking sequence and suggestions of relief occurring immediately following the selection of a nonalcoholic beverage or engagement in an activity unrelated to drinking (Elkins, 1980). Although treatment outcomes following covert sensitization have been variable, the abstinence rates are comparable to those following chemical aversion (Miller, 1982).

A variety of contingency management procedures has also been used in behavioral treatment programs to minimize the reinforcing consequences of alcohol consumption. In a case study, for example, Peter Miller (1972) successfully implemented a behavioral contract which specified a monetary fine and withdrawal of spousal attention in the event the participating male alcohol abuser exceeded self-imposed drinking limits. When he drank in moderation, however, he was rewarded by increased attention and affection from his spouse. In the community reinforcement approach developed by Hunt and Azrin (1973), access by alcohol abusers to vocational, family, and social reinforcers was first increased, then made contingent upon abstinence. For example, patients were given paid memberships to a self-supporting social club and were encouraged to participate in activities such as card games, dances, bingo games, and picnics. Any member who gave any indication that he had been drinking before arriving at the club, however, was turned away. According to Bigelow, Stiltzer, Griffiths, and Liebson (1981), specific behavioral contingencies that ensure reinforcement of abstinence and punishment of drinking are among the most effective techiques available.

Biological Factors Associated with Alcohol Abuse

It can be seen from the preceding review that behavioral techniques used in the treatment of alcohol abuse are based almost exclusively upon empirical findings of experimental psychology, in the areas of conditioning and learning in particular. There is, however, a large body of research on biological factors associated with alcohol abuse which has important implications for the treatment of alcoholics but which to a large extent has been overlooked by behaviorally oriented clinicians. In this section, a selective review will be presented of the biological factors that, if neglected, are most likely to limit the effectiveness of behavioral interventions.

Neuropsychological Deficits

The neuropsychological deficits associated with alcoholism have been examined extensively in animal and human subjects. Unfortunately, research with humans is limited often by methodological problems, such as failure to consider the concomitant effects of psychoactive medication and head injury, or failure to determine the length of time since alcohol ingestion (Eckardt & Ryback, 1981). Despite these limitations, however, it is generally agreed that the chronic abuse of alcohol can produce brain damage because alcohol is neurotoxic and causes specific neuropathological changes (Tarter & Alterman, 1984).

It has been estimated that 50–70% of chronic alcoholics are cognitively impaired (Eckardt & Ryback, 1981; Miller & Saucedo, 1983). Neuropsychological assessment has consistently revealed deficiencies in memory, perception, motor performance, abstraction, learning, and problem solving. Mild to moderate brain damage is usually indicated (Eckhardt & Ryback, 1981). The structural changes that accompany neuropsychological performance deficits include cerebral atrophy, EEG abnormalities, and ventricular enlargement (Miller & Saucedo, 1983; Tarter & Alterman, 1984).

Complications arising from alcohol abuse can produce additional cognitive impairments. Wernicke–Korsakoff syndrome, for example, is characterized by initial global confusion followed by amnesic deficit. Thiamine replacement treatment removes the associated muscular and visual disturbances within a few days, but the memory deficit associated with Wernicke–Korsakoff syndrome is slow to recover and incomplete in 80% of cases (Carlen & Wilkinson, 1983; Hemmingsen, Kramp, & Rafaelsen, 1983).

In addition to these neuropsychological deficits, there is evidence to suggest that alcohol produces a dissociative effect which impairs the alcohol abuser's recall while sober of events that occurred during periods of intoxication (Mello, 1983). Recall of a drinking episode may, in fact, be more consistent with predrinking expectations of alcohol's effects than with the actual experience of intoxication. Moreover, to the extent that expectations regarding alcohol's effects are generally positive whereas the actual effects are often aversive, this dissociative effect may interfere with the punitive effect of the aversive consequences of abusive drinking. In fact, in the absence of disconfirmation, widely held positive beliefs regarding the effects of alcohol often appear to act as incentives for the resumption of abusive drinking.

Many aspects of neuropsychological performance recover with abstinence. Quite dramatic improvment, that parallels the recession of withdrawal synptoms, is noted between the 1st and 3rd week. This occurs because the central nervous system is believed to be in a state of hyperactivity during acute withdrawal, and therefore the consequent lack of concentration and agitation impair performance (Eckardt & Ryback, 1981). The subsequent 6 to 12 weeks generally evidence continued improvements in some areas of functioning. The extent of recovery depends on age, initial level of impairment, and neuropsychological function. Younger and less seriously impaired alcoholics show better recovery than older, more impaired alcoholics (Miller & Saucedo, 1983). Memory functions recover more slowly, especially in older patients; and the memory improvements that do occur generally take at least 3 to 6 months (Page, 1983).

Tolerance and Dependence

It is widely assumed that the relatively immediate pharmacological effects of alcohol maintain alcohol consumption through both positive and negative reinforcement mechanisms. Positively reinforcing consequences of alcohol may include relaxation, sociability, and euphoria (Cappell & LeBlanc, 1983; Mellow, 1983), whereas the negatively reinforcing consequences include relief from aversive states such as frustration and anxiety and withdrawal symptoms. Although positively and negatively reinforcing consequences may be influenced by set and expectation, it is clear that they are also pharmacologically determined (Cappell & LeBlanc, 1983).

It is evident, however, that the pharmacological effects of a fixed dosage of alcohol diminish after repeated use with the result that abusive drinkers increase their consumption. This change in the pattern of drinking denotes the development of tolerance and cannot be adequately explained by an operant model. There is, however, evidence to support a classical conditioning model of alcohol tolerance and withdrawal which, unlike most models of drug dependence, recognizes the conditioned physiological effects of exposure to the environment in which alcohol consumption occurs.

According to the classical conditioning model of tolerance (Siegel, 1983), the drug itself constitutes an unconditioned stimulus and its central effects constitute the unconditioned response. Environmental stimuli that predictably precede these effects, such as drug preparation procedures, constitute the conditioned stimulus. Unlike Pavlov's findings, in which repeated association of the conditioned stimulus and unconditioned stimulus elicited a conditioned response which was a facsimile of the unconditioned response, recent research has shown that the direction of conditioned drug responses may be either the same or opposite to the unconditioned response. When the conditioned drug response occurs in the same direction as the drug itself, the pharmacological effect of the drug is augmented and the individual is said to have become sensitized to it. When the conditioned response is in the direction opposite to that elicited by the drug, the pharmacological effects of the drug are attenuated and the individual taking the drug is said to have acquired a tolerance for its effects.

Although most of the evidence in support of a classical conditioning model of drug tolerance has come from animal research with opiates, there is some evidence to suggest that tolerance to the effects of alcohol in humans can be explained in part by the development of conditioned responses which elicit physiological changes in a direction opposite to the effects of alcohol. In research conducted by Lightfoot (19 ; cited in Siegel, 1983), social drinkers consumed beer in sufficient quantities to raise their blood alcohol levels to approximately 0.07% during each of four daily sessions. All of the sessions were conducted in the same distinctive environment. In the fifth session, however, beer was consumed by some subjects in the same environment and by others in a distinctly different setting after which all subjects were assessed on several perceptual motor and cognitive tasks. When alcohol consumption and assessment occurred in the usual drinking environment, performance on most of the tasks was disrupted by alcohol to a lesser extent than when consumption and assessment occurred in the novel environment. Presumably, subjects who were administered alcohol and assessed in the usual drinking environment had acquired conditioned compensatory responses that attenuated the effects of alcohol.

To the extent that conditioned compensatory responses are acquired by drinkers outside the laboratory setting, they would account in part for the development of tolerance and the necessity experienced by heavy drinkers to increase their alcohol consumption in order to attain the same effects as they experienced initially. In essence, this increased consumption represents the drinker's operant compensatory response, which is presumably reinforced to the extent that it counteracts the classically conditioned compensatory response elicited by environmental cues.

The occurrence of withdrawal symptoms following detoxification and subsequent experiences of craving alcohol reported by drinkers who have become dependent upon alcohol can also be explained in part by a classical conditioning model. In fact, these phenomena can be conceptualized as manifestations of the same conditioned compensatory responses that account for tolerance to alcohol when it is consumed, except that in the case of dependence compensatory conditioned responses occur in the *absence* of alcohol consumption. According to the model, when a dependent drinker is exposed to environmental stimuli previously associated with alcohol consumption, they act as conditioned stimuli to elicit physiological and subjective changes in the direction opposite to the effect of alcohol. In the event that the alcohol abuser does not drink, the conditioned compensatory responses are not counteracted by the effects of alcohol but are instead expressed as subjective craving, tremulousness, nausea, and so on. If the abuser were to drink in these circumstances, alcohol consumption would presumably be particularly reinforcing inasmuch as it would relieve withdrawal symptoms.

Empirical support for the classical conditioning model of alcohol withdrawal in humans is still limited. Ludwig and Stark (1974) and Mathew, Claghorn, and Largen (1979) have analyzed retrospective self-reports of alcohol abusers regarding the circumstances in which they have experienced the greatest withdrawal distress. Their findings, that withdrawal is greatest and relapse most likely in the presence of alcohol-associated cues, are consistent with the classical conditioning model. Similarly, the widely recognized effects of the sight, smell, and taste of beverage alcohol in eliciting craving and loss of control among alcohol abusers would also be predicted by the model. Perhaps the most compelling evidence has been obtained by Lightfoot (conditioned responses 19 ; cited in Siegel, 1983), who demonstrated alcohol-compensatory in research subjects who had been administered a placebo in an environment in which they had previously been administered alcohol.

Genetic Factors

Evidence for a genetic component in the etiology of alcoholism derives from familial, twin, adoption, cross-cultural, and selective-breeding studies. Adoption studies, however, provide the strongest evidence. Goodwin and his colleagues (Goodwin, Schulsinger, Hermansen, Guze, & Winokur, 1973) found that sons of alcoholics were four times more likely to become alcoholic than sons of nonalcoholics, regardless of whether they were raised by alcoholic parents. That is, biological parentage was shown to be more important than the drinking status of the adoptive parents. Moreover, Cloninger, Bohman, and Sigvardsson (1981) found that alcohol abuse in adoptive parents did not increase the risk of alcoholism in male adoptees, whereas abuse in biological parents did.

The risk of alcoholism increased from 14.7% when neither biological parent was alcoholic to 33.3% when both biological parents were alcoholic (Cloninger, 1983). Interestingly, however, these rates do not apply to women.

Although many physiological responses to alcohol ingestion and the metabolism of alcohol are known to be under genetic control, it is unclear which of these heritable factors are involved in the etiology of alcoholism. Presumably, genetic factors could predispose an individual to alcoholism in at least three different ways: (a) by increasing the positively reinforcing properties of alcohol consumption, (b) by increasing functional tolerance to the effects of alcohol, and (c) by increasing the rate of alcohol metabolism or dispositional tolerance to alcohol. The influence of each of these factors upon drinking behavior has been studied, mainly in animal studies, but cross-cultural and prospective human studies have also been reported.

Cappell and LeBlanc (1983) reviewed studies that examined selectively bred rat strains that differed in their preference or consumption of alcohol. They concluded that alcohol-preferring rat strains are less susceptible to the effects of alcohol upon the central nervous system than nonpreferring strains. Evidence for the reverse relationship, however, is less clear. Strains differing in neurosensitivity sometimes do not differ in preference.

Individual differences occur not only in initial sensitivity but also in the amount of acquired functional tolerance with chronic administration. Evidence suggests that rats with stronger initial sensitivity also become tolerant less rapidly than rats with weaker initial sensitivity (Erwin & McClearn, 1981). Evidence from human populations is less direct. The flushing response in Mongols has been attributed to an exaggerated sensitivity to the aversive effects of alcohol. Mongols generally exhibit stronger reactivity in heart rate, blood pressure, and facial flushing and report more subjective discomfort following alcohol consumption than do Caucasians (Pardo & Hall, 1983). They also have a lower rate of alcoholism than Caucasians. In addition, prospective studies by Schuckit (1982) have shown that males with a family history of alcoholism demonstrate more positive responses to alcohol (greater reduction in muscle tension and less intense subjective feelings of intoxication) than males without a family history of alcoholism, who are matched on drinking history.

Individual differences in metabolic or dispositional tolerlance have also been observed and appear to be genetically determined. The rate of metabolism of alcohol, for example, is more concordant in monozygotic twins than in dizygotic twins (Erwin & McClearn, 1981). Studies have shown that alcohol-preferring and nonpreferring rats sometimes differ metabolically, but the differences in metabolic rate do not appear to account adequately for differences in drinking behavior. Acetylaldehyde levels appear to be a more influential factor. Acetylaldehyde, the by-product of the metabolism of alcohol by alcohol dehydrogenase (ADH), has toxic effects upon accumulation. Alcohol-preferring rats have low levels of acetylaldehyde after consumption, whereas nonpreferring rats show exaggerated levels after consumption. Elevation of acetylaldehyde levels can also suppress drinking in rats, presumably through the mechanism of aversive control (Cappell & LeBlanc, 1983).

Some findings from the study of human racial differences parallel data from animal research. The oxidation rate of alcohol does not differ between Mongols and Caucasians, but Mongols have been found to develop higher levels of acetylaldehyde after consumption than Caucasians (Ewing, 1983). In addition, Pardo and Hall (1983) have demonstrated in Japanese subjects an atypical form of the ADH enzyme that produces acetylaldehyde unusually rapidly with the result that higher levels accumulate. This particular ADH allele is present in 6% of Europeans and in 85% of Mongols (Cloninger, 1983). There are, however, some contrary data. Schuckit (1982), for example, found that males with a positive family history for alcoholism have higher levels of acetylaldehyde after alcohol consumption than those with a negative history. Cloninger (1983) and Wallace (1983) reported similar findings. It is not yet clear how these apparently contradictory findings will be reconciled.

A study by Thurman *et al.* (1982) demonstrated that some rats were able to increase their rate of alcohol metabolism rapidly, whereas others were not. This effect has also been observed in some humans. The relationship between acquired metabolic tolerance and alcohol consumption, however, is relatively unknown (Cappell & LeBlanc, 1983).

The finding that strong versus weak withdrawal reactions can be bred selectively in rats suggests that at least some aspect of dependence is heritable. In addition, dependent rats have been found to prefer alcohol to a greater extent than nondependent rats. Not all of the evidence, however, is consistent (Cappell & LeBlanc, 1983). Nevertheless, it has been suggested that severity of dependence may relate to craving for alcohol in humans (Hodgson, 1984).

Fluid and Electrolyte Balance

Investigations of the effect of alcohol on fluid and electrolyte balance indicate the existence of another self-regulatory physiological mechanism that may contribute to alcoholism. This area of research, overlapping as it does with studies of physiological substrates of thirst and fluid intake generally, would appear to be basic to an understanding of the physiological determinants of alcohol consumption, but it has largely been overlooked.

It has been well established that acute alcohol ingestion inhibits the secretion of vasopressin in both animal and human subjects (Cicero, 1983). Shortly afterward, diuresis occurs which, together with simultaneous solute retention, produces a physiological state of dehydration in the drinker (Beard & Knott, 1971). It has been demonstrated, moreover, that the dehydration resulting from the consumption of a moderate dose of alcohol (0.8g of ethanol/kg) is sufficient to produce a significant increase of nonalcoholic fluid intake among both social drinkers and alcoholics (Lawson, 1977). Unlike social drinkers whose subjective thirst ratings were higher after the alcoholic than the nonalcoholic beverage, and whose subsequent ad-lib intake correlated with thirst ratings, the alcoholics did not discriminate subjectively between the two beverage conditions despite the fact that they drank significantly more following alcohol than following placebo.

These research findings indicate that acute alcohol consumption increases subsequent nonalcoholic drinking and that this dipsogenic effect of alcohol is mediated physiologically by the same mechanisms that regulate thirst and drinking. Whether these same mechanisms account in part for continued alcohol consumption during an acute drinking episode is not known. There is evidence, however, that chronic excessive beer drinking may cause disruptions of fluid and electrolyte metabolism which in turn sustain drinking (Beard & Sargent, 1979; Sargent, Simpson, & Beard, 1975).

Implications of Biological Factors Associated with Alcohol Consumption for the Behavioral Treatment of Alcoholism

The preceding section was a brief overview of several biological mechanisms that effect alcohol consumption. Although limited in number, the mechanisms selected for discussion are representative of a larger domain of biological factors, at least to the extent that they exert their influence at different points in the drinking history of the alcoholic. Genetic factors, for example, begin to exert their effects during the alcoholic's earliest drinking episodes, whereas the influence of changes in fluid and electrolyte metabolism may occur either during initial or later stages in the etiology of alcoholism. Tolerance and dependence are typically acquired only after prolonged excessive drinking, by which point neuropsychological deficits are becoming increasingly apparent. Despite the fact that these mechanisms occur at different points in the alcoholic's drinking history, they all have important implications for the behavioral treatment of alcoholism.

Neuropsychological Deficits

Research on the neuropsychological deficits associated with alcohol abuse have implications for the optimal timing of behavioral intervention, the specific type and duration of treatment procedures, and the very goal of treatment itself.

The extent of cognitive impairment during alcohol withdrawal has led several researchers to recommend the delay of treatment for 2 to 3 weeks until recovery is observed in some cognitive functions (Carlen & Wilkinson, 1983; Miller & Saucedo, 1983). These researchers argue that progress is severely limited by a patient's inability to retain verbal material. In contrast, Eckardt and Ryback (1981) recommend that treatment begin as soon as active withdrawal symptoms dissipate to avoid deterioration of the patient's motivation for change, especially as the value of treatment delay has not yet been empirically tested.

The value of treatment delay may, though, depend on the severity of cognitive impairment. Treatment outcome has been shown to relate to the degree of impairment at intake and to the degree of neuropsychological improvement over the course of treatment. In addition, less severely impaired patients are more likely to complete treatment than more severely impaired patients (Miller & Saucedo, 1983). However, the predictive value of neuropsychological impairment with regard to treatment outcome is not consistent (Eckardt & Ryback, 1981). In addition, research studies that have examined the role of neuropsychological deficit in treatment outcomes are frequently methodologically inadequate. Parsons (1983), for example, reported that patients rated as showing more improvement and having better prognosis demonstrated neuropsychological skills superior to the skills of those rated as less improved. However, treatment methods were not described and treatment evaluation was based solely on therapists' ratings. Further investigation is required in this area.

Cognitively oriented forms of psychotherapy, occupational rehabilitation, and educational counseling are expected to yield minimal effects in patients who have impaired memory and abstracting abilities (Eckardt & Ryback, 1981). Memory and learning deficiencies may also impede behaviorally oriented treatments. New coping responses may require more repetition than is usual in nonimpaired populations before they become established as alternative responses.

Another treatment issue concerns the data relating neuropsychological performance to continued abstinence versus moderate drinking. The evidence is not unequivocal, but some researchers have found that neuropsychological performance deteriorates with the resumption of drinking of even a moderate degree (Eckardt & Ryback, 1981; Parsons, 1983). Miller and Saucedo (1983) suggest that moderate drinking may be inadvisable for patients whose cognitive dysfunction has progressed beyond a certain point. Given a return in learning and memory deficits with the resumption of drinking, and possible state-dependent effects produced by acute intoxication, maintenance of new skills acquired from treatment may be less likely with a controlled drinking program than with an abstinence-oriented program. That is, severity of impairment may interact with treatment goal in determining long-term outcome.

Tolerance and Dependence

The available research on the classical conditioning model of drug dependence indicates that tolerance and drug compensatory conditioned responses once acquired can be retained following longer periods of abstinence. Thus, to the extent that abstinence is maintained in an environment free of alcohol-associated stimuli such as in a residential treatment facility, subsequent reexposure to such environmental stimuli would, according to the classical conditioning model, elicit alcohol-compensatory conditioned responses which would in turn increase the risk of relapse. The clinical implications of the model are clear: either the detoxified abuser should be returned to an environment distinctly different from the one in which dependence was acquired, or specific therapeutic strategies should be implemented prior to discharge to extinguish alcohol-compensatory conditioned responses.

There are, of course, practical limitations to the extent of environmental change possible for most individuals following treatment for alcohol abuse. It may, for example, be extremely difficult to arrange employment for the unemployed, or marital reconciliation for the separated. Moreover, even if substantial environmental changes were to occur, it is highly unlikely that the former abuser would succeed indefinitely in avoiding all alcohol-associated environmental stimuli. It would appear, therefore, that specific strategies should be routinely incorporated in the treatment of all dependent abusers to ensure that alcohol-compensatory conditioned responses are extinguished. The cue-exposure–response prevention techniques employed by Rankin *et al.* (1983) and Marlatt's programmed relapse procedure (1985) would theoretically elicit alcohol-compensatory conditioned responses in the absence of the usual pharmacological unconditioned responses and thereby promote extinction of conditioned responses.

As suggested by Siegel (1983), the classical conditioning model of alcohol dependence also has implications for the treatment of negative affective states such as anxiety and depression in dependent abusers. According to Siegel, these affective states may act in three different ways to increase the likelihood of relapse: (a) as conditioned stimuli which elicit physiologically based alcohol-compensatory conditioned responses; (b) as components of compensatory conditioned responses which are elicited by alcohol-associated environmental cues; and (c) as stimuli that potentiate the elicitation of alcohol-compensatory conditioned responses in the presence of alcohol-associated conditioned stimuli. In all cases, it is clear that a comprehensive treatment program would include not only procedures to extinguish associations previously established between extroceptive, alcohol-associated cues and alcohol but also procedures to extinguish conditioned associations between aversive affective states and alcohol. To minimize the possibility that aversive affective states will act to potentiate the effects of alcohol-associated conditioned stimuli, Siegel recommended further that the extinction of alcohol-compensatory conditioned responses be conducted in the context of the relevant affective state. We strongly concur with this recommendation and suggest that procedures such as stress innoculation training (Meichenbaum, 1977) be implemented for this purpose.

Consistent with Siegel's classical conditioning model of tolerance and attendance, it has been well established that tolerance and dependence are acquired more rapidly on second and subsequent occasions than they are originally. Thus, an alcoholic who has a history of tolerance and dependence separated by periods of remission should be viewed as being at risk for more rapid reacquisition of drinking habits and therefore as unsuitable for treatment programs in which the goal is moderation or controlled drinking. Interestingly, research on the predictors of successful controlled drinking outcomes in such programs yields a similar caution (Miller, 1983).

It should not be surprising, given the adequacy of a learning model in accounting for the phenomena of tolerance and dependence, that responses indicative of these conditions generalize to other drugs. To the extent that tolerance to the effects of alcohol has been acquired, it is likely that the individual has thereby also become tolerant to the effects of drugs such as benzodiazepines, sedative hypnotics, morphine, and tetrahydrocannabinol (Cappel & LeBlanc, 1983). Similarly, to the extent that alcohol dependence has been acquired, the individual will experience relief from withdrawal symptoms following the administration of drugs such as the benzodiazepines. The clinical implications of cross-tolerance and cross-dependence are clear. Assessment, both initially and throughout treatment, should include specific examination of all drug use to ensure that treatment does not merely result in the substitution of one harmful substance for another and that the use of drugs other than alcohol does not inadvertently maintain conditioned responses that are targeted for extinction during treatment.

Genetic Factors

In a preceding section, a brief overview was presented of the evidence regarding the heritability of alcoholism, and it was suggested that any of a number of genetically controlled physiological and metabolic processes might be implicated. Certainly, the possibility that the disorder is in part genetically transmitted would not deter the behaviorally oriented clinician from initiating treatment. What, then, one might ask, are the implications of these findings for the behavioral treatment of alcoholism?

Although history taking alone will not enable the clinician to distinguish alcoholics for whom the disorder is in part genetically transmitted from those in whom it is not, it is clear that assessments should include specific inquiry regarding the drinking habits of family members and that a clear distinction should be made between biological relatives and those related by marriage and adoption. In the event the alcoholic is both male and positive for a family history of alcoholism, the clinician should recognize the possibility that currently available treatment techniques may not be as effective as they are with alcoholics without the family history, that the duration of treatment may be extended, and that abstinence may be a more judicious goal than moderation.

Nathan (1986) has recently recommended that individuals with a positive family history, whether they are seeking treatment for alcoholism or for an unrelated condition, should be forewarned about their increased risk to develop alcoholism, informed that they may be different from those without a family history of alcoholism, and cautioned that they may be particularly susceptible to alcohol dependency. Although the intent of such counseling is unquestionably laudable, there is no empirical support for offering such advice. On the contrary, one could argue that merely providing such well-intended cautions might itself put the individual at risk for developing alcoholism. It is well established, for example, that beliefs and expectations regarding the effects of alcohol can have a powerful influence on a range of behaviors in alcoholics and nonalcoholics including alcohol consumption itself (Wilson, 1978). In our opinion, it remains for future research to determine whether the benefits of providing such information to our patients outweigh the potential risks. In the meantime, we advocate that clinicians inform their patients that it is at presnt impossible to determine the relative contribution of genetic and environmental factors for any individual alcoholic.

Fluid and Electrolyte Balance

Although the potential role of alcohol-induced effects on fluid and electrolyte metabolism in the etiology of alcoholism is yet to be fully explored, the available research suggests that the implementation of two procedures might enhance the effect of behavioral interventions. Since it has been demonstrated that alcohol is a dipsogenic substance, patients, especially those in controlled drinking programs, should be advised that their drinking will result in a mild state of physiological dehydration which they can easily correct by consuming nonalcoholic beverages. It is interesting to note, parenthetically, that alternating between alcoholic and nonalcoholic beverages has been recommended for those attempting to moderate their alcohol consumption because it increases the intervals between successive alcoholic beverages (Miller & Munoz, 1982). Research on the effects of alcohol on fluid and electrolyte metabolism, however, would suggest that it is advisable also because it may reduce an introceptive stimulus for further drinking.

A second procedure suggested by this body of research is cognitive relabeling. As cited previously, although both social drinkers and alcoholics increased their nonalcoholic fluid intake following acute alcohol consumption, only the social drinkers rated themselves as being thirstier after alcohol than after placebo, and only in the case of the social drinkers was ad-lib fluid intake correlated with suggestive ratings of thirst. This finding is consistent with research on blood alcohol discrimination training (Nathan, 1980) and on the effects of nonalcoholic fluid preloading (Brown & Williams, 1975) which has shown that alcoholics are relatively insensitive to interoceptive stimuli associated with the consumption of alcoholic and nonalcoholic beverages. Coversely, it has been demonstrated that alcoholics are relatively more sensitive to external cues relating to both nonalcoholic and alcoholic beverages (Brown & Williams, 1979; Ludwig, Wikler, & Stark, 1974). In attempting to integrate these findings, Lawson (1977) has suggested that alcoholics may, in the presence of alcohol-related external cues, cognitively mislabel their state of physiological dehydration as a craving for alcohol rather than merely as thirst. If subsequent research were to support this hypothesis, it would suggest that alcoholics would benefit from cognitively relabeling internal states associated with craving.

The objective of this chapter has been to examine the research on biological processes associated with alcoholism to determine what implications, if any, it has for behavioral treatment of alcoholics. Despite the limited scope of the overview, the findings of this sample of research were shown to have implications for the assessment of alcoholics prior to and during treatment, the scheduling of treatment, the components of treatment, and the very goal of treatment itself.

Interestingly, it was noted that some procedures suggested by our review of the biological research are already being implemented by behavioral clinicians, although the rationales for their use are different from those suggested by the biological literature. Perhaps nowhere is this convergence of the behavioral and biological research more evident than it is in the use of cue-exposure response prevention. This procedure was originally introduced in the treatment of alcoholics because of the evident similarity between excessive drinking and obsessive-compulsive disorders for which cue-exposure response prevention had proved so effective. Our review of the biological literature, however, suggests a very different rationale for implementing this procedure—specifically to extinguish conditioned, anticipatory compensatory drug responses.

Despite such evidence of convergence between the clinical implications of behavioral and biological research, it is essential, in our opinion, for behavioral clinicians treating alcoholics to be informed of research advances in the biology of alcoholism. Such knowledge will not only enable us to refine existing treatment procedures but will also suggest new ones. Only by integrating the findings of both these research domains can we hope to develop maximally effective interventions for our patients.

ACKNOWLEDGMENTS. The authors would like to express their sincere appreciation to Ms. Tania Deans for her patient and meticulous preparation of the manuscript and to Dr. Wolfgang Linden for his continued support and encouragement.

References

Azrin, N. H., Sisson, R. W., Meyers, R., & Godley, M. (1982). Outpatient alcoholism treatment by disulfiram and community-reinforcement therapy. *Journal of Behavior Therapy and Experimental Psychiatry, 13,* 105–112.

Beard, J. D., & Knott, D. H. (1971). The effect of alcohol on fluid and electrolyte metabolism.

In B. Kissin & H. Begleiter (Eds.), *The biology of alcoholism: Vol. 1. Biochemistry*. New York: Plenum Press.

Beard, J. D., & Sargent, W. Q. (1979). Water and electrolyte metabolism following ethanol intake and during acute withdrawal from alcohol. In Majchrowicz and Noble (Eds), *Biochemistry and Pharmacology of Alcohol* (Vol. 2). New York: Plenum Press.

Bigelow, G. E., Stitzer, M. L., Griffiths, R. R., & Liebson, I. A. (1981). Contingency management approaches to drug self-administration and drug abuse: Efficacy and limitations. *Addictive Behaviors, 6*, 241–252.

Brown, R. A., & Williams, R. J. (1979). The effects of cues of quantity visible and preferences on drinking by alcoholic and non-alcoholic subjects. *British Journal of Social Psychology, 18*, 99–104.

Brown, R. A., & Williams, R. J. (1975). Internal and external cues relating to fluid intake in obese and alcoholic persons. *Journal of Abnormal Psychology, 84*, 660–665.

Cappell, H., & LeBlanc, A. E. (1983). The relationship of tolerance and physical dependence to alcohol abuse and alcohol problems. In B. Kissin & H. Begleiter (Eds.), *The pathogenesis of alcoholism: Biological factors*. (pp. 359–414). New York: Plenum Press.

Carlen, P. L., & Wilkinson, D. A. (1983). Assessment of neurological dysfunction and recovery in alcoholics: CT scanning and other techniques. *Substance and Alcohol Actions Misuse, 4*, 191–197.

Chaney, E. F., O'Leary, M. R., & Marlatt, G. A. (1978). Skill training with alcoholics. *Journal of Consulting and Clinical Psychology, 46*, 1092–1104.

Cicero, T. J. (1983). Endocrine mechanisms in tolerance to and dependence on alcohol. In B. Kissin & H. Begleiter (Eds.), *The pathogenesis of alcoholism: Biological factors* (pp. 285–357). New York: Plenum Press.

Cloninger, C. R. (1983). Genetic and environmental factors in the development of alcoholism. *Journal of Psychiatric Treatment and Evaluation, 5*, 487–496.

Cloninger, C. R., Bohman, M., & Sigvardsson. (1981). Inheritance of alcohol abuse. *Archives of General Psychiatry, 38*, 861–868.

Eckardt, M. J., & Ryback, R. S. (1981). Neuropsychological concomitants of alcoholism. In M. Gallanter (Ed.), *Currents in alcoholism: Recent advances in research and treatment* (Vol. 8). New York: Grune & Stratton.

Elkins, R. L. (1980). Covert sensitization treatment of alcoholism: Contributions of successful conditioning to subsequent abstinence maintenance. *Addictive Behaviors, 5*, 67–89.

Erwin, V. G., & McClearn, G. E. (1981). Genetic influences on alcohol consumption and actions of alcohol. In M. Gallanter (Ed.), *Currents in alcoholism: Recent advances in research and treatment* (Vol 8). New York: Grune & Stratton.

Ewing, J. A. (1983). New trends in biomedical research on alcoholism. *Journal of Psychiatric Treatment and Evaluation, 5*, 557–563.

Foy, D.W., Miller, P. M., Eisler, R. W., & O'Toole, D. H. (1976). Social skills training to teach alcoholics to refuse drinks effectively. *Journal of Studies on Alcohol, 37*, 1340–1345.

Goldfried, M. R., & Sprafkin, J. N. (1974). *Behavioral personality assessment*. Morristown, NJ: General Learning.

Goodwin, D. W., Schulsinger, F., Hermansen, L., Guze, S. B., & Winokur, G. (1973). Alcohol problems in adoptees raised apart from alcoholic biological parents. *Archives of General Psychiatry, 28*, 238–243.

Hemmingsen, R., & Kramp, P. (1980). Haematological changes and state of hydration during delirium tremors and related clinical states. *Acta Psychiatric Scandinavica, 62*, 511–518.

Hemmingsen, R., Kramp, P., & Rafaelsen, O. J. (1983). Organic cerebral reactions in alcoholism: Psychobiological aspects of treatment. *Substance and Alcohol Actions Misuse, 4*, 225–234.

Hodgson, R. (1984). Craving and priming. In G. Edwards & J. Littleson (Eds.), *Pharmacological treatment for alcoholism*. London: Groom Helm.

Hunt, G. M., & Azrin, N. H. (1973). A community-reinforcement approach to alcoholism. *Behavior Research and Therapy, 11*, 91–104.

Kwentus, J., & Major, L. F. (1979). Disulfiram in the treatment of alcoholism. *Journal of Studies on Alcohol, 40*, 428–446.

Lawson, D. (1977). The dipsogenic effect of alcohol and the loss of control phenomenon. In M. Gross (Ed.), *Alcohol intoxication and withdrawal: Vol. 3b. Studies in alcohol dependence* (pp. 547–568) New York: Plenum Press.

Ludwig, A. M., & Stark, L. H. (1974). Alcohol craving: Subjective and situational aspects. *Quarterly Journal of Studies on Alcohol, 35*, 889–905.

Ludwig, A. M., Wikler, A., & Stark, L. H. (1974). The first drink: psychobiological aspects of craving. *Archives of General Psychiatry, 30*, 539–547.

Marlatt, G. A. (1985). Cognitive assessment and intervention procedures for relapse prevention. In G. A. Marlatt & J. R. Gordon (Eds.), *Relapse prevention: Maintenance strategies in the treatment of addictive behaviors* (pp. 201–279). New York: Guilford Press.

Mathew, R. J., Claghorn, J. L., & Largen, J. (1979). Craving for alcohol in sober alcoholics. *American Journal of Psychiatry, 136*, 603–606.

Meichenbaum, D. (1977). *Cognitive-behavior modification: An integrative approach*. New York: Plenum Press.

Mello, N. (1983). A behavioral analysis of the reinforcing properties of alcohol and other drugs in man. In B. Kissin & H. Begleiter (Eds.), *The biology of alcoholism: The pathogenesis of alcoholism* (Vol.7, pp. 133–198). New York: Plenum Press.

Miller, P. M. (1972). The use of behavioral contracting in the treatment of alcoholism: A case report. *Behavior Therapy, 3*, 593–596.

Miller, W. R. (1982). Treating problem drinkers: What works? *Behavior Therapist, 5*, 15–18.

Miller, W. R. (1983). Controlled drinking: A history and a critical review. *Journal of Studies on Alcohol, 44*, 58–83.

Miller, W. R., & Hester, R. K. (1980). Treating the problem drinker: Modern approaches. In W. R. Miller (Ed.), *The addictive behaviors: Treatment of alcoholism, drug abuse, smoking, and obesity*. Oxford: Pergamon Press.

Miller, W. R., & Munoz, R. F. (1982). *How to control your drinking*. Albuquerque, NM: University of New Mexico Press.

Miller, W. R., & Saucedo, C. F. (1983). Assessment of neuropsychological impairment and brain damage in problem drinkers: A critical review. In C. J. Golden (Ed.), *Diagnosis and rehabilitation in clinical neuropsychology* (pp. 141–195). Springfield, IL: Charles C Thomas.

Nathan, P. (1980). Etiology and process in the addictive behaviors. In Miller (Ed.), *The Addictive behaviors: Treatment of alcoholism, drug abuse, smoking and obesity*. Oxford: Pergamon Press.

Nathan, P. E. (1986). Some implications of recent biological findings for the behavioral treatment of alcoholism. *Behavior Therapist, 8*, 159–161.

Page, R. D. (1983). Cerebral dysfunction associated with alcohol consumption. *Substance and Alcohol Actions Misuse, 4*, 405–421.

Pardo, M. P., & Hall, T. B. (1983). Genetic implications of the alcohol-induced flushing response phenomenon in orientals. In M. Gallanter (Ed.), *Currents in alcoholism: Recent advances in research and treatment* (Vol. 8). New York: Grune and Stratton.

Parsons, O. A. (1983). Cognitive dysfunctions and recovery in alcoholics. *Substance and Alcohol Actions Misuse, 4*, 175–190.

Pattison, E. M., Sobell, M. B., & Sobell, L. C. (1977). *Emerging concepts of alcohol dependence*. New York: Springer.

Rankin, H., Hodgson, R., & Stockwell, T. (1983). Cue exposure and response prevention with alcoholics: A controlled trial. *Behavior Research and Therapy, 21,* 435–446.

Sargent, W. Q., Simpson, J. R., & Beard, J. D. (1975). Renal hemodynamics and electrolyte excretions after reserpine and ethanol. *Journal of Pharmacology and Experimental Therapeutics, 193,* 356–362.

Schuckit, M. A. (1982). A study of young men with alcoholic close relatives. *American Journal of Psychiatry, 139,* 791–794.

Siegel, S. (1983). Classical conditioning, drug tolerance, and drug dependence. In R. G. Smart, F. B. Glaser, Y. Israel, H. Kalant, R. E. Popham, & W. Schmidt (Eds.), *Research advances in alcohol and drug problems* (Vol. 7). New York: Plenum Press.

Tarter, R. E., & Alterman, A. J. (1984). Neuropsychological deficits in alcoholics: Etiological considerations. *Journal of Studies on Alcohol, 45,* 1–9.

Tarter, R., Alterman, A. J., & Edwards, K. (1984). Alcoholic denial: A biopsychological interpretation. *Journal of Studies on Alcohol, 45,* 214–218.

Thurman, R. G., Paschal, D., Abu-Murad, C., Pekkanen, L., Bradford, B. V., Bullock, K., & Glassman, E. (1982). Swift increase in alcohol metabolism (SIAM) in the mouse. *Journal of Pharmacology and Experimental Therapeutics, 223,* 45–49.

Wallace, J. (1983). Alcoholism: Is a shift in paradigm necessary? *Journal of Psychiatric Treatment and Evaluation, 5,* 479–485.

Wilson, G. T. (1978). Booze, beliefs and behavior: Cognitive factors in alcohol use and abuse. In P. E. Nathan, G. A. Marlatt, & T. Lobert (Eds.), *Alcoholism: New directions in behavioral research and treatment.* New York: Plenum Press.

CHAPTER 3

Causes and Effects of Obesity

Implications for Behavioral Treatment

Donna Romano White and Norman M. White

It is often said, "You are what you eat." One interpretation of this aphorism is that weight is determined by the amount eaten. If this were true, then the cause, and, by implication, the treatment, of obesity would be quite simple: eat less. In fact, many individuals treat themselves for obesity quite successfully using this method (Schacter, 1982). In other cases, however, obesity proves more difficult to deal with and many therapists are confronted with clients who have found it impossible to lose weight on their own.

As with any other condition requiring treatment, successful intervention with obesity depends on a knowledge of etiology. In this chapter, we take the approach that many factors, both biological and learned, which may act in various combinations, contribute to obesity. We review a number of these factors, from both animal and human literature, for which reasonable evidence suggests a role in causing obesity. Although there is certainly no shortage of data and theories on this topic, present knowledge is inadequate for identification of which factors among a large number of possibilities cause obesity in individual cases. It would be unreasonable to expect any single treatment to be successful for all obese clients regardless of cause, and it is in this context that we review the efficacy of behavior therapy approaches to obesity. We will argue that our inability to identify those clients for whom behavior therapy is the

Donna Romano White • Centre for Research in Human Development, Concordia University, Montreal, Québec, Canada H3G 1M8. *Norman M. White* • Department of Psychology, McGill University, Montreal, Québec, Canada H3A 1A1.

treatment of choice partially accounts for the disappointing outcomes achieved by behavioral interventions. These limitations do not mean that we must abandon behavioral treatment. However, it may be that our expectations of these interventions, on both group and individual levels, must be modified.

Another problem for the clinician treating obesity is that overweight itself has been shown to produce metabolic and behavioral changes which may make weight reduction and the maintenance of weight loss difficult. We review animal and human literature on a series of factors that are affected by the condition of obesity and examine behavior therapy in the light of these consequences of overweight. Our review leads to the conclusion that behavioral programs have, in general, failed to consider these factors and their effects. We propose modifications in current behavioral treatments that take account of this information.

Causes of Obesity

Because no weight gain at all is possible without food intake, factors that control eating are one group of potential causes of obesity, and we examine first how aberrations in the control of these *ingestional* variables can cause obesity. After food has been eaten, its energy content can be disposed of in any of three ways: by work (exercise), by thermogenesis (heat production), or by storage (deposition of adipose tissue). Constitutional or pathological individual differences in the control of any or all of these three proceses could lead to obesity; therefore these *postingestional* factors are also discussed.

Ingestional Factors

Because ingested food is the source of deposited fat, it stands to reason that any condition leading to overconsumption could be a cause of obesity. A variety of potential causes associated with both the initiation and the termination of eating have been identified.

Properties of Available Food

There is ample evidence from both human and animal studies that the availability and palatability of food have a powerful influence on amount consumed and consequently on body weight. When the available food is made more accessible (that is, when the amount of effort required to obtain it is low) rats voluntarily increase their intake and consequently their body weights (Collier, Hirsch, & Hamlin, 1972; Kaufman & Collier, 1982; Logan, 1964). Similarly, increases in the fat content (Corbit & Stellar, 1964; Schlemmel, Mickelson, & Gill, 1970), palatability (Hirsch & Walsh, 1982; Ingle, 1949; Muto & Miyahara, 1972) or the variety (Rothwell & Stock, 1979; Sclafani & Springer, 1976) of food offered rats cause increases in consumption and long-term weight gains. In humans, dietary changes also cause increases in consumption and body weight (Miller, Mumford, & Stock, 1967; Simms *et al.*, 1968).

It has often been observed that Western industrialized society is replete with abundant, easily available, highly palatable, heavily advertised food. These environmental conditions are, of course, similar to the experimental conditions that cause obesity in both animals and humans, so perhaps the relevant question is why everyone is not obese. There are two probable answers to this question. One could be individual differences in innate or learned responses to food. A second possibility is that there are differences in individuals' cognitive and ideational processes with respect to the food environment and to eating itself.

Learned and Innate Responses to Food Stimuli

All living organisms from the lowest amoebae up to and including humans have innate behavioral mechanisms for obtaining food (Maier & Schnierla, 1964). The observable behavior includes a sequence involving approach and consumpton and is initiated in the presence of an adequate external stimulus and an internal state. In mammals, these behavior sequences are modified and strengthened by experience, through a process of stimulus–response learning reinforced by the consumption of food. With sufficient repetition, these response tendencies become independent of both the internal state and the reinforcement that produced them: The external stimulus alone is sufficient to elicit approach and consumption. This phenomenon has been explicitly demonstrated in rats (Weingarten, 1983). The occurrence of such a learning process is adventitious and therefore impossible to observe directly in humans; however, at least one series of experiments illustrated the existence of such learned responses by showing differences in subjects' salivary responses to seeing and thinking about foods of varying palatability (Wooley & Wooley, 1973; Wooley, Wooley, & Woods, 1975). Additional evidence for this kind of phenomenon has been reviewed by Booth (1977) and by Bellisle (1979). Individual differences in the nature and strength of these appetitive responses to food could be a cause of overeating and obesity.

Social and Cognitive Influences on Consumption

Although individuals who are obese are known to differ from those who are not on a number of cognitive variables, the present concern is whether such variables can be a cause of obesity. A cognitive variable could cause obesity if it resulted in a set of behaviors toward food or eating that led to overconsumption. A psychoanalytic model of this type suggesting that obesity can originate in the nature of the infant–mother interaction during the early feeding has been proposed by Bruch (1973). Studies of somewhat older children have shown that the tendency to obesity exists among children adopted by obese parents (Garn, 1976), suggesting that such tendencies can in fact be acquired. Rodin (1982) has reported data suggesting that a high level of responsiveness to external stimuli ("externality": Schacter, 1971) including food may predict obesity. However, Woody and Constanzo (1981) report data that they interpret as refuting the notion that externality is a cause of obesity. These authors suggest that a combination of biological predisposition and parental attitudes (which differ for male and female children) are major causes and that externality is a result of obesity. The notion that parental attitudes and other socializing forces can be major causes of obesity is supported by the data on adopted children as well as by the results of studies on the effects of socioeconomic status (Garn, Clark, & Guire, 1975; Goldblatt, Moore, & Stunkard, 1965) and cultural factors (Dwyer, Feldman, & Mayer, 1967; Goldblatt *et al.* 1965) on the incidence of obesity. Although it is possible to comprehend in a general way how such factors could be causes of obesity, there has been relatively little work (Woody and Costanzo, 1981, is a notable exception) on specifying exactly how they can lead to overeating.

Postingestional Factors

Feedback Errors

Virtually every conception of the control of eating includes provision for some form of feedback. In its simplest terms, this means that some consequence of food intake acts to inhibit further consumption. In some theories the consequences of eating that act in this way are known as "satiety factors." An obvious potential cause of obesity is a change in or failure of the action of one or more feedback factors. If the feedback inhibition of eating is reduced or eliminated, consumption increases, leading to weight gain.

The three "classic" satiety factors were originally proposed as components of theories of the regulation of eating: the glucostatic (Mayer, 1953), thermostatic (Brobeck, 1948) and lipostatic (Kennedy, 1953) theories of feeding. As implied by their names, these theories proposed that eating is controlled by inhibitory feedback in the form of changes in blood glucose, temperature, or circulating lipid levels. More recently, a class of substances thought to be specific satiety factors has been proposed. Cholecystokinin (CCK), a hormone released in the gut, is the best studied of these.

It should be noted that, with the exception of conditioned satiety, evidence for these feedback mechanisms as causes of obesity in humans is lacking and might be very difficult to obtain. Studies on individuals who are already obese do not provide the type of evidence required because it is impossible to distinguish the causes of obesity from its effects in such individuals. Therefore, the data reviewed here are almost entirely from the animal literature. Nevertheless, as research provides more information about these factors and their substrates of action, it may be possible to devise specific tests for feedback failures in humans.

Blood Glucose. Ingestion of a meal is accompanied by increases in blood glucose which begin within a few minutes after eating starts (Strubbe, Steffens, & de Ruiter, 1975). Injections of exogenous glucose decrease consumption in starved animals (Booth, 1972; Mayer & Bates, 1952; Ramirez & Friedman, 1982). There are two substrates on which glucose could act to inhibit consumption. First, there is evidence that dopaminergic nigrostriatal neurons (which course through the lateral hypothalamus) mediate normal food intake (Stricker & Zigmond, 1976) and body weight levels (Glick, Greenstein, & Waters, 1974; Glick & Stanley, 1975). Several lines of evidence suggest that blood glucose acts to inhibit the function of these neurons. Release of dopamine from the terminals of these neurons is inhibited when they are perfused with glucose (McCaleb & Myers, 1979); elevated blood glucose inhibits the firing rate of nigrostriatal neurons (Saller & Chiodo, 1980); and diabetic rats, which have chronically elevated blood-glucose levels, also have increasd numbers of dopamine receptors (Lozovsky, Saller, & Kopin, 1981), evidence for chronically reduced dopamine function. The increase in blood glucose that accompanies ingestion of certain foods may therefore act directly on dopamine neurons to inhibit the further intake of food. Second, there is evidence that glucose acts directly on the liver and that the liver influences intake through the autonomic nervous system. Injections of glucose into the blood supply of the liver inhibit eating in starved animals (Russek, 1970; Russek, Lora-Vilchis, & Islas-Chaires, 1979). Similar injections influence the firing rate of single cells in the hypothalamus and cutting the sympathetic innervation of the liver blocks this effect (Schmitt, 1973). Increased blood glucose may therefore act through the liver to control intake, thereby controlling body weight.

Temperature. Although there has been little recent work on this factor in terms of the control of consumption, it remains a possible cause of obesity. Ingestion of a meal increases body temperature (Brody, 1945) and it is well known that such temperature increases or simply maintaining animals in a hot environment (Brobeck, 1948) decreases consumption of food. There is little evidence for the specific substrate of action of this factor, but the demonstration that directly warming the hypothalamus inhibits eating (Andersson & Larsson, 1961) suggests that this part of the brain may normally respond to the changes in body temperature that accompanying eating. In this way, temperature could act as a satiety factor in the control of intake and therefore of body weight.

Lipids. In its original form (Kennedy, 1953), the lipostatic theory postulated that some circulating factor related to fat deposition might act as a satiety factor that controls eating on a long-term basis. Circulating triglycerides, the concentration of which is correlated with deposition of body fat (Albrink & Meigs, 1965; Gordon, 1960), could act in this way, because injection of exogenous triglycerides inhibits eating in starved animals (Maggio & Koopmans, 1982). The mechanism of action of this suppressive effect is not presently understood, but if the elevated triglyceride levels that accompany increased deposition of fat can control consumption in normal individuals then abnormalities in this mechanism are an avenue for the occurrence of obesity.

Satiety Hormones. Each of the satiety factors discussed so far has a physiological function and acts to inhibit consumption as a secondary role. Recently, research has focused on the possible existence of a class of factors for which the sole function may be signaling satiety. CCK is a peptide hormone which is thought to be released in the gut when the lumen is contacted by food (Smith, 1984; Smith, Jerome, Cushin, Eterno, & Simansky, 1981). It appears to act locally, possibly on the exposed parasympathetic nerve endings in the lining of the stomach, or on the smooth muscle of that organ (Smith, 1984). Injection of exogenous CCK specifically inhibits consumpiton of food in starved rats and humans (Smith, Gibbs, Jerome, Pi-Sunyer, Kissileff, & Thornton, 1981). It is of interest that CCK is also present in the brain wherein it may act as a neurotransmitter in a neural system that mediates satiety centrally (McCaleb & Meyers, 1981). Other substances also inhibit eating when injected peripherally or centrally, and these too have often been proposed as satiety hormones. Neurotensin (Nemeraff & Prange, 1982; Stanley, Eppel, & Hobel, 1982) is an example: however, evidence that this substance acts specifically to signal satiety is lacking at present.

The feedback factors described in this brief review present a very large number of possibilities for errors in the control of consumption. In any one of the cases a failure of release, transport, action on the substrate, or action of the substrate itself could cause a failure of satiety and consequent overeating. Potential causes of such failures include individual genetic differences, genetic errors, disease processes, and aging.

Conditioned Satiety

The original argument in favor of conditioned satiety as a factor controlling consumption (LeMagnen, 1955) was based on the assumption that absorption and feedback during a meal could not occur quickly enough to influence the same meal. Although there is now some question about whether this assumption was correct, there is good evidence for a genuine process of classical conditioning in rats (Booth, 1972; Davis & Campell, 1973) and humans (Booth, Lee, & McAlvey, 1976) leading to satiety. Although Booth (1977) argued that the conditioned stimulus for satiety was some postabsorptive factor, Stunkard (1975) suggested that the sensory properties of the ingested food are the stimuli that become associated with the satiety response. This notion receives strong support from a series of experiments with humans (Wooley, 1972; Wooley, Wooley, & Dunham, 1972) which show that the visual appearance and taste of milkshake preloads exerted almost total control over both verbal reports of satiety and subsequent consumption of food, even when these sensory properties were manipulated orthogonally to the actual caloric content of the preloads. Individual differences in the acquisition of these conditioned satiety responses could result in a sufficiently weak response to permit overconsumption and consequent obesity.

Metabolic Mechanisms

Ingested food can be disposed of in any of three ways: by storage, as heat, or by exercise. Individual differences in any of these processes could shift the normal distribution of ingested calories to fat deposition.

Several metabolic mechanisms related to fat deposition and heat production were recently described by McMinn (1984). Two of these are described here as an illustration of these mechanisms.

Lipoprotein lipase is an enzyme in the membranes of fat cells (adipocytes) that breaks down circulating triglycerides for storage in the cells. Genetically obese rats have elevated lipoprotein lipase activities at two weeks of age, before they become obese (Gruen, Hietanen, & Greenwood, 1978), suggesting that this enzyme activity may be the cause of obesity in these animals. Obese humans have elevated lipoprotein lipase activity compared to normal weight controls (Schwartz & Brunzell, 1981). When obese individuals lose weight, lipoprotein lipase activity increases (Schwartz & Brunzell, 1981), suggesting that obesity is not the cause of the elevated enzyme activity but that the reverse is the case. Therefore, it is possible that idividual differences in lipoprotein lipase activity are a cause of individual differences in body weight.

Brown adipose tissue is a specialized form of fat that appears to be involved in thermogenesis in rats (James, Trayhurn, & Garlick, 1981). McMinn (1984) suggests three ways in which this thermogenic mechanism might be defective: there may be decreased blood flow in the brown adipose tissue of obese rats (Thurlby & Trayhurn, 1980); the normal innervation of brown adipose tissue which may stimulate the tissue to thermogenesis (Perkins, Rothwell, Stock, & Stone 1981) may be ineffective; or the tissue itself may simply be less than normally efficient at thermogenesis (Himms-Hagen & Desautels, 1978). A failure of thermogenesis in any one of these ways would, in the absence of any change in work performed, leave more energy to be stored as fat, leading to obesity.

Activity Level

The final possible postingestive cause of obesity concerns the amount of ingested food energy consumed by work or exercise. Two studies (Bullen, Reed, & Mayer, 1964; Durnin, Lonergan, Good, & Ewan, 1974) suggest that there are preexisting differences in the activity levels of individuals. Chronically low levels of activity could lead to obesity in the presence of constant levels of food intake and thermogenesis. Although this is clearly a logical possibility, more research is required before conluding that this factor actually operates in some cases.

Treatment Considerations

Any particular case of obesity might be attributable to any or all of the possible causes reviewed here. The ultimate challenge for treatment is to make a differential diagnosis in the individual case and to apply the treatment that is appropriate to removal of the specific cause or causes. Obviously, it would be surprising if errors in feedback or metabolic postingestional factors were responsive to behavioral treatment; as potential biological causes, these problems would require medically oriented treatments. On the other hand, behavioral methods might be appropriate for cases in which the problem is related to responsiveness to food stimuli, attitudes toward food and eating, deficiencies in conditioned satiety, or insufficient activity level. One purpose of this section is to summarize briefly the status of behavioral interventions aimed at conditioning such responses.

More recent behavioral approaches have tended to combined a number of techniques into a treatment "package." Studies of such behavioral approaches to weight loss are not lacking in the literature. Comprehensive reviews of results (e.g., Abramson, 1977, 1983; LeBow, 1981; Stunkard & Mahoney, 1976) and methodology (Jeffrey, 1976; Wilson, 1978) are available elsewhere. Our purpose is to summarize and evaluate these interventions, with special emphasis on their efficacy. We argue that, in view of the multiple causes of obesity and our inability to distinguish causes in individual clients, present conclusions about the efficacy of behavioral treatments require reinterpretation. Finally, we discuss the implications of individual causal variation for the use of treatment packages in behavior therapy.

Early Conditioning Studies

Early behavioral interventions focused on helping clients learn to eat less rather than on attempts to increase activity (LeBow, 1977). These studies were directed at simple stimulus–response (including covert stimulus–response) changes and attempted to demonstrate efficacy of interventions such as aversive conditioning (e.g., Foreyt & Kennedy, 1971; Morganstern, 1974), covert sensitization (e.g., Cautela, 1967; Diament & Wilson, 1975), "coverant" conditioning (e.g., Horan & Johnson, 1971; Tyler & Straughan, 1970), and therapist reinforcement techniques (e.g., Foxx, 1972; Jeffrey, Thompson, & Wing, 1978). With the exception of therapist reinforcement techniques, such interventions produced some behavior change but did not have significant impact on body weight. Furthermore, clients did not use such techniques outside the laboratory situation. Therapist reinforcement studies resulted in substantial weight loss, but only as long as the therapist controlled both the environment and the reinforcement contingencies (e.g., reviews by Abramson, 1973; Leon, 1976). Such simple conditioning techniques were quickly abandoned and replaced with package treatments that aimed at helping clients improve self-control strategies for managing their eating environments.

Self-Control Packages

Short-Term Efficacy. More recent work has focused on treatment packages which involve a number of behavioral techniques such as self-monitoring, slowing eating, stimulus-control techniques, and attitude restructuring taught over 10–12 weeks to all clients. Several reviews of behavioral therapy have been based upon studies of such short-term package programs. In a survey of 21 behavioral studies from 1969 to 1974, Jeffrey, Wing, and Stunkard (1978) found a mean weight loss of 11.5 pounds. Foreyt, Goodrick, and Gotto (1981) reviewed 16 group studies wherein average treatment length was 12 weekly sessions; the majority of the patients were female and mean pretreatment weight was 86 kg, 52% above "ideal" weight. During treatment the rate of group or mean weight loss was about one half kilogram per week.

Brightwell and Sloan (1977) concluded that behavioral treatments can lead to short-term weight loss in most individuals who use them. Stunkard and Mahoney (1976) characterized short-term behavioral interventions as "superior to all other treatment modalities for managing mild to moderate obesity" (p. 54).

In spite of these positive evaluations, several difficulties with short-term treatment programs were acknowledged. First, the short-term weight losses achieved in behavioral programs are often described as disappointing: most clients are still overweight at the end of treatment. The conclusion is that behavioral programs produce statistically significant, but not clinically significant, weight loss. Secondly, not all individuals in these programs lose weight. Behavioral programs have been criticized because outcome is characterized by marked individual variability. According to Wilson (1980), some clients lose substantial amounts of weight; others lose little or none. Wilson does point out that few individuals gain weight over the course of treatment. However, behaviorists have been critical of their programs in the light of marked individual variability in outcome.

Long-Term Efficacy. The goal of self-control packages is to provide clients with management techniques that allow them to continue to lose weight after therapist–group contacts are terminated. Most early behavioral programs did not include long-term follow-up evaluations. However, more recent studies have provided such data. Brightwell and Sloan (1977) reviewed 15 studies, which met fairly stringent criteria for length of follow-up and provision of data on pretreatment and posttreatment weights. These reviewers conclude that there is little evidence that weight loss continues after all contact with the therapist has ceased.

More recently, Foreyt *et al.* (1981) reviewed 16 group studies that reported data at least 1 year after treatment. They found that not only are initial weight changes small, but further weight losses do not occur and variability during follow-up is large. In the studies reviewed, the average rate of weight loss was zero during the 1st year following treatment. They conclude that "self-management for continued weight loss over the long term has not been demonstrated" (p. 164).

Attempts to obtain continued weight loss following the treatment period have taken the form of booster sessions rather than extended treatment periods. Abramson (1983) reviewed four studies that utilized booster sessions and concluded that attempts to promote continued weight loss by the addition of booster sessions were generally unsuccessful.

It must be noted that booster sessions, when used, have generally been infrequent, consisting of only three or four contacts over several months. Only one study in the literature actually utilized an extended treatment period. Craighead, Stunkard, and O'Brien (1981) conducted a large-scale pharmacological study in which one of the conditions was behavioral treatment for 6 months, the longest active treatment period reported to date, and full 1-year follow-up was done. Average weight loss for clients in the behavioral treatment condition was 11.4 kg. Furthermore, patients in the behavioral condition regained only 1.8 kg during the course of 1 year following treatment and were superior in maintaining weight losses to a medication group and a medication plus behavior therapy group.

Reinterpretation of Efficacy

The criteria by which behavioral treatments have been judged have been summarized by Foreyt *et al.* (1981):

> In order to be judged a success, any treatment for obesity should produce, for most of those treated, a loss of body fat that has a significant effect on health and psychological well-being, and which is maintained for at least several years at a reasonable cost of time, effort, and money. (p. 160)

Although behavioral techniques produce short-term weight loss in most clients, weight losses achieved are regarded as clinically insignificant and group weight loss has not been found to continue during the maintenance period. Furthermore, there is marked individual variability in weight loss and weight loss maintenance. Given the potential multiple possibilities in causation of obesity, questions should be asked about whether these results constitute treatment failure.

Group versus Individual Efficacy. It is unreasonable to expect any one treatment or any treatment that focuses on one set of learned causes to be successful for all obese clients. Behavioral interventions will be most helpful to clients with learned eating patterns that lead to obesity rather than to those with physiologically caused obesity. The marked individual variability in treatment outcome is at least partially a function of our inability to diagnose those clients whose obesity is biologically based.

In view of these facts, the group or mean data presented on efficacy of behavioral treatments in both the short- and long-term studies must be reevaluated in terms of individual success. It should be noted that both reviews (Brightwell & Sloan, 1977; Foreyt *et al.*, 1981) of long-term follow-up indicate that at least a subgroup of patients can maintain their weight loss. For example, Foreyt *et al.* (1981) note that the mean posttreatment weight loss for clients in the 16 studies reviewed was 5.9 kg (range 3.2 to 10.1 kg) and mean weight loss at 1 year after treatment was 6.1 kg (range .5 to 12.6 kg). Apparently, therefore, behavior therapy was successful with a subgroup of the clients who account for these data.

A study of Levitz, Jordan, LeBow, and Coopersmith (1980) attempted to investigate weight loss maintenance only in clients who were successful in the initial 20 weeks of a behavioral program. Levitz *et al.* attempted to follow 190 people who had lost at least 6.8 kg in a 20-week behavioral program. Of this sample, 154 persons (116 women and 51 men) were called again and agreed to participate. Results indicated that 54% of the sample retained a significant weight loss 1 to 5 years later. These results indicate that weight loss can be maintained for a substantial proportion of clients who participate successfully in behavioral interventions.

Individualizing Programs

In view of the individual variation in response to behavioral programs, it becomes necessary to reconsider the use of treatment packages. As indicated, the package treatment is a series of behavioral techniques that are to be implemented by all clients regardless of whether they are consistent with individual needs. Treatment packages tend to average about 10–12 weeks and to end at this time whether or not behavior has changed or weight loss has occurred. Therapists tend to meet clients on a weekly basis rather than to arrange for an individualized schedule of meetings. The treatment is often carried out in groups. As Wilson (1980) has noted, "Most behavioral programs have become prematurely standardized and unimaginative in both form and content" (p. 329).

This standard package approach is unacceptable from both a behavioral and biological standpoint. From a behavioral perspective, treatment should include a detailed individual investigation of the client's eating behaviors including events prior to, during, and subsequent to eating. The client is taught to record and eventually to self-monitor these behaviors. Analysis of recorded behaviors with the therapist leads to specification of problematic eating sequences and procedures designed to change the behavior are instituted. Changes can be applied to antecedent events (stimulus-control procedures), consequent events (contingency management or changes in reinforcement), or directly to eating behaviors. The selection of procedures should be tailored to individual needs and based upon observations of the individual. Such individualized treatments need to be reinstituted in behavior therapy in view of the multiple possible causes of obesity and the variability of causal factors among clients.

This individualization of behavior therapy programs in terms of both evaluation and treatment is important for several reasons. First, it gives impetus to the continued use of behavioral techniques in the treatment of obesity. Until we can relate treatment to cause, it seems important to continue to offer behavior therapy because it does help many clients. We must be aware of the fact that behavioral programs can be improved. We must also keep in mind the fact that behavioral techniques will be ineffective for some clients no matter how carefully individualized and improved the programs are. For these clients, as noted by Wooley, Wooley, and Dryenforth (1979), it may be "advantageous to define more broadly the goals of treatment so as to deal with the severe problems in self-esteem stemming from social prejudice and repeated failure" (p. 21) in dieting, possibly because of biological factors.

Effects of Obesity

As is the case with the factors that cause obesity, some factors associated with the condition of overweight itself affect ingestion of food. Other factors are postingestive in that they involve changes in the disposition of food energy after it has been consumed. Both types of changes can be considered as *adaptations to obesity* that may, in some cases, act to impede attempts to reduce consumption and increase activity. However, there is also reason to think that in many cases these factors are subject to readaptation as weight is lost.

Ingestional Adaptations

Responsiveness to Food Stimuli

Cabanac and Duclaux (1970) had human subjects rate the taste of a glucose solution before and after they drank a pint of glucose. Normal weight subjects rated the taste "pleasant" before drinking, but "unpleasant" afterwards. Obese subjects rated the glucose solution pleasant both before and after drinking. The authors concluded that obese individuals' responses to taste stimuli are unaffected by their internal states. Similar data exist for rats made hyperphagic (and consequently obese) with ventromedial hypothalamic lesions. These animals consume more of palatable foods than normal animals (Graff & Stellar, 1962; Miller, Bailey, & Stevenson, 1950) and it has been shown (Franklin & Herberg, 1974) that this syndrome is caused by the fact that the animals are obese, not directly by the lesions. A sensory change of this type in humans would obviously make it difficult to reduce intake, but evidence that lesioned rats fail to exhibit this syndrome after they have been starved down to their normal weights suggests that it follows body weight closely and is therefore clearly reversible.

Arousability

The increased responsiveness to palatable foods observed in humans and rats has its obverse in the fact that such individuals also eat less of unpalatable foods than normals. This fact, together with other more direct observations, has led to the suggestion that obese individuals are "external"; that is, they are more responsive than normal individuals to external stimuli of all kinds (Schacter, 1971).

This notion has been elaborated by Rodin (1982) and her co-workers. They have shown that, compared to normal controls, obese individuals respond with shorter latencies in reaction-time tests with complex stimuli and are more distracted by irrelevant stimuli. The fact that they are more responsive to all kinds of stimuli including food may be related to the maintenance of obesity because it causes them to eat more. They have also demonstrated that compared to normal individuals obese individuals are more emotionally aroused by electric shock or by aversive auditory material and that emotional arousal leads to overeating in both obese and normal people. Taken together, these findings suggest that a pattern of response associated with obesity contributes to the maintenance of this condition. The extent to which this pattern might reverse when an obese individual loses weight is unclear at present.

Cognitive Changes

Although there may be as many cognitive patterns associated with obesity as there are obese individuals, at least two common patterns have been described. One is a general unhappiness with the condition of obesity (presumably this has its origin in the value society places on thinness), which is exacerbated by repeated futile attempts at weight loss (Rodin, 1982). This state of mind makes it difficult for an individual to undertake the difficult project of dieting yet another time.

Another demonstration of a cognitive barrier to weight loss in the obese has been called the "what-the-hell" effect by Herman and Polivy (1975). These workers had human subjects drink several milk shakes as a preload and then participate in what was stated to be a taste test of ice cream, the real object being to see how much would be eaten after the preload. The surprising result was that individuals who were supposed to be dieting ate more ice cream than nondieting controls. The authors suggest that this occurred because the dieters decided that because the milkshakes had vitiated their diets for that day, they were no longer constrained in how much they could eat!

Postingestional Adaptations

A variety of hormonal changes accompany obesity. Overweight individuals exhibit elevated levels of fasting plasma glucose, decreased glucose tolerance, increased free fatty acid levels, and reduced levels of stimulated growth hormone release, among others. Although some of these abnormalities may make weight loss more difficult, there is at present no direct evidence for this and several studies suggest that all of these abnormalities reverse themselves after weight loss (Kalkoff, Kim, Cerletty, & Ferrou, 1971; Knittle & Ginsburgh-Fellner, 1972). In the case of other postingestive adaptations, the implications for weight loss are clear, and some of these are considered here.

Hyperinsulinemia

Obese individuals have higher basal levels of circulating insulin than normal individuals (Simms *et al.*, 1968). The consequence of this condition is that, compared to normal individuals, in the obese a greater proportion of ingested nutrients is converted to fat leading to more rapid return to a state of energy depletion, reinitiation of eating, and further weight gain. At least some data (Salans, Knittle, & Hirsch, 1968) suggest that insulin falls to normal levels after weight loss.

Thermogenesis

Metabolic rate, measured by resting oxygen consumption and equivalent to thermogenesis in the absence of changes in activity, adapts to increases in body weight by increasing when rats consume large quantities of a palatable diet (Rothwell & Stock, 1979). In an experiment described by Keesey and Corbett (1984), thermogenesis increased during a period when rats gained weight by overeating a high fat diet but returned to normal after weight gain ceased. When the obese rats were restricted to eating 50% of their *ad lib* intake, they began to lose weight. This loss was accompanied by a decrease in thermogenesis, suggesting a decrease in metabolic rate. Such a decrease would have the effect of retarding weight loss because more ingested energy would be left for disposition as fat. However, some data (Shetty, Jung, James, Barrand, & Callingham, 1981, Figure 1) suggest that metabolic rate readapts to lower weight levels within months after weight is lost. McMinn (1984) reviews evidence suggesting that these changes in thermogenesis may be caused by changes in the amount and function of brown fat tissue.

Fat Cell Number

Fat is stored in cells. When an individual gains weight, the size of each cell in the adipose tissue depots increases. If weight gain continues, the existing fat cells stop growing and new fat cells begin to appear (Faust, 1984). This adaptive neoplastic process has been observed to continue until the number of fat cells was at least doubled in rats (Hirsch & Knittle, 1970), and in humans the amount of deposited fat is positively correlated with number of fat cells (Gurr, Jung, Robinson, & James, 1982; Hirsch, Knittle, & Salans, 1966). When an individual loses weight the size of each fat cell decreases (Salans *et al.*, 1968). However, the number of fat cells remains at its elevated level and, for the present at least, it appears that there is no way to reverse the increase in number. Moreover, there is some evidence that in the presence of palatable food the hypercellular (recovered obese) rat eats more than the normocellular rat of equivalent body weight (Faust, 1984). If these data are confirmed and extended to humans, one implication is that increases in cell number, to the extent that they may occur in highly obese individuals, may make reduction of intake and weight loss difficult. Another implication is that it would be difficult for a formerly obese hypercellular individual to maintain normal levels of consumption. However, the importance of fat cell number as a barrier to weight loss and its maintenance in formerly obese individuals has been questioned in a recent review (Kirtland & Gurr, 1979).

Lipoprotein Lipase

An increase in lipoprotin lipase, the enzyme that converts triglycerides into fat for storage in fat cells, is evident in formerly obese individuals several months after weight loss (Schwartz & Brunzell, 1978). This metabolic reaction to weight loss would certainly impede further loss and maintenance. On the other hand, a decrease in lipoprotein lipase activity was observed when food intake was restricted (Taskinen & Mikkila, 1979), a change that would promote weight loss. Although it appears that this enzyme has an important influence on weight, its precise role in the treatment of obesity remains to be elucidated.

Activity Level

As already discussed, there is some evidence for the notion that a propensity to low activity levels may be a cause of obesity, but regardless of whether or not this is the case, the negative relationship between body weight and activity level in humans is very well established (Stern, 1984). Because work is one of the ways in which ingested food energy can be disposed of, increase in activity level is an obvious complement to decrease in food intake in the treatment of obesity. A recent review of the role of exercise in obesity (Thompson, Jarvie, Lahey, & Cureton, 1982) points out that physical activity increased metabolic rates during and for some time after exercise, making this an effetive method for disposing of ingested and stored-food energy supplies. Presumably, psychological methods can be used to encourage obese individuals to increase their activity levels.

Implications for Treatment

The set of factors discussed in this section are caused by obesity and tend to act to maintain this state. Unlike the factors that cause obesity, however, it appears likely that these factors exist for all moderately to severely obese individuals, because they are the results of the obesity itself. Any therapeutic measures that are attempted must, therefore, take these factors into account and attempt to deal with them. We have divided our discussion of the treatment implications of these factors into irreversible and reversible effects. Although the evidence is often tenuous and more research is undoubtedly needed, our review indicates that most of the metabolic adaptations to obesity may be reversible.

Irreversible Effects

Of the metabolic factors discussed, only one, hypercellularity, appears to be irreversible, although the evidence is not conclusive on this point (Kirtland & Gurr, 1979). However, if the current animal research is confirmed for humans and it proves impossible to reduce fat cell number and to maintain reduced food intake in hypercellular individuals, then behavior therapy will not produce lasting weight reduction in these cases. Furthermore, repeated attempts to intervene using behavioral methods or even drastic dieting such as fasting or protein sparing will fail for such clients and produce depression and a sense of failure. For these reasons, it seems important to identify hypercellular clients and to consider alternative treatments or treatment goals for them.

Laboratory tests for hypercellularity are not part of current routine medical practice. Stunkard (1984) has suggested a classification system based upon severity of obesity. It is possible that his definition of excessive obesity, greater than 100% overweight, together with early age of onset of obesity, might be used as a rough diagnostic indication of hypercellularity.

Hypercellular clients should be made aware that they will not be able to reduce to some "ideal" level and that weight losses they do achieve will probably be difficult to maintian. Weight loss that involves reducing the size of fat cells should be possible, but further weight decrease is probably not possible.

Therefore, the goal weight for hypercellular clients would be far above the ideal or average weights indicated in tables such as the Metropolitan Life Insurance norms (1959). Once these biological limitations are understood by the client and the practitioner, behavioral techniques might be used to help such individuals reach and maintain a more realistic goal weight.

Stunkard (1984) suggests that radical medical treatments, known as gastric restriction procedures, are currently the treatment of choice for excessive obesity. He notes that all techniques relying on reduction of food intake have failed with such clients. He reviews evidence to support the effectiveness of gastric restriction procedures in producing large weight losses with relatively few untoward consequences. Further evaluation of these surgical interventions is needed to confirm the lack of negative side effects and to provide data on long-term maintenance of weight loss. Although promising, they should be regarded as experimental.

Reversible Effects

Many of the effects of obesity may be reversible. In this section, we discuss the treatment implications of several potentially reversible effects: metabolic adaptations, arousal and cognitive structure, and activity patterns.

Metabolic Adaptations. It has been argued that physiological adaptations to obesity other than hyperplasia may act to inhibit and limit weight loss (Brownell, 1982; Wooley *et al.*, 1979). These researchers have suggested that both hyperinsulinemia and thermogenesis may act to make weight loss difficult. In fact, it has become fashionable to refer to the biological adaptations associated with obesity as evidence of a "set point" for body weight. Proponents of "set point theory" have argued that ideal body weight is set or predetermined and that the biological tendencies to maintain this preset body weight are so strong that reduction of weight below its set point is virtually impossible to achieve and maintain.

There are many problems with the set point notion. First, the existence of a body-weight set point is not supported by the empirical evidence. Evidence that overeating leads to weight gain in both animals and humans has already been reviewed. It is important to note that in the case of the animal studies at least, the increased intake was completely voluntary, apparently motivated solely by an increase in the palatability of the available food. Conversely, there is clear evidence that when the effort required to obtain food is increased (Collier *et al.*, 1972), or its palatability decreased (Ferguson & Keesey, 1975; Kratz, Levitsky, & Lustick, 1978) animals voluntarily reduce their intake and lose weight. It has been observed (e.g., Keesey & Corbett, 1984) that the amounts of weight gained and lost by the subjects in these experiments are less than would be predicted by calculations of the energy equivalents of the increase or decreases in consumption. These discrepancies undoubtedly occur because of the physiological adaptations to changes in consumption and body weight that have already been discussed. But they in no way refute the clear finding that, as a matter of fact, body weight is simply not maintained at a constant level, or set point, in a variety of different conditions of type and availability of food.

A second problem with the notion of set point is that the evidence reviewed suggests that (with the exception of hypercellularity) the factors that adapt to increased weight can readapt to decreased weight. Such changes in the operation of factors influencing body weight suggest that there is no biologically or homeostatically preset value for this parameter. The concept of altered set point, which has been used to explain adaptation and readaptation, is a complete contradiction in terms which does little to improve our understanding of the mechanisms of weight control. It is an example of how, in spite of its undeniable theoretical elegance and parsimony, the body-weight set-point concept acts to impede progress in understanding the causes of obesity. The concept has assumed a status similar to that once held by the concept of instinct in psychology. As was pointed out by Beach (1955), rather than providing testable hypotheses, such theoretical concepts are accepted as explanations and thus act to prevent the kinds of detailed analyses that lead to the identification of specific factors that contribute to behavior.

A final reason for eschewing the body-weight set-point concept is that it is counterproductive in the therapeutic environment. It provides obese individuals with a cognitive framework for concluding that weight loss is impossible. However, in most cases this would be an erroneous conclusion because most adaptations to obesity are reversible.

There is a primary difference, however, in the way in which weight is typically gained and lost in our society. Weight gain leading to obesity usually occurs over a period of years with several long-term plateaus. Logically, it would seem that given such a pattern of weight gain in humans, the body has time to adapt slowly to increasing weight levels. The pattern of weight reduction is usually quite different. The usual expectation is that weight be lost steadily and consistently until an ideal goal is reached. Some programs aim to make the weight reduction period as short as possible and to achieve goal weight as rapidly as possible. Lay-led groups such as Weight Watchers support slower losses of 2 pounds per week; however, clients are still urged to stay on a low-calorie regime and to continue weight loss until all their "overweight" is lost. This mentality also underlies behavioral programs: lose weight steadily until an ideal goal weight is reached; maintain the weight loss.

It appears reasonable to question such an approach in light of the biological adaptations to obesity described. If current evidence regarding the reversibility of biological adaptations to obesity can be supported, it would seem reasonable to allow the body periods of readaptation after moderate amounts of weight loss and before attempting further weight loss. Such an approach might be more conducive to achieving permanent weight loss.

Many dieters are familiar with weight plateaus and frequently describe such phenomena—as well as their frustration—to clinicians. Instead of responding with skepticism about whether the individual is really sticking to the program or attributing the problem to a predetermined set point, our hypothesis is that a maintenance period is required when these plateaus are reached because time may be required for adaptation of the various metabolic and behavioral factors associated with overweight. Rather than further reducing food intake and urging continued weight loss, the usual responses to such plateaus, a slightly increased food-intake regime, consistent with keeping off weight already lost (true maintenance), is suggested. Weight reduction could be reinstituted after a substantial period of successful maintenance when metabolic functions have adapted to the lower weight and when the client is psychologically prepared for undergoing another period of deprivation.

There are, of course, difficulties with such an approach. In our impatient, give-me-a-miracle-to-make-me-thin-immediately world, it is difficult to take such a long-term view of weight management. The possible payoff, permanent weight reduction without having to fight your own body, may well be worth the time.

Arousal and Cognitive Adaptations. There are few data on how well behavioral techniques deal with these factors. Cognitive restructuring or attitude change is a component of many behavioral packages, although it is rarely discussed in detail when programs are described. Stimulus control methods have played a major role in behavioral packages since their inception (Stuart, 1967).

One problem with evaluating whether attitudes toward food or eating and arousal change following behavioral interventions is that measures of such variables have not been included as part of the evaluation of behavioral treatment: weight loss is often the sole criterion for success. Brownell and Stunkard (1978) note that even a general relationship between behavioral change and weight loss has not been demonstrated. Foreyt *et al.* (1981) have advanced the notion that weight loss in the behavioral treatment program could be due to social pressure associated with therapist contact and peer pressure from group members in a clinical setting. As noted by Leon (1976), group support in and of itself is not associated with successful weight reduction, but group support might act in combination with behavioral techniques to produce weight loss. Clinicians should investigate the importance of group support and possibly utilize this variable directly in behavioral programs.

There is even greater need to increase our understanding of variables that might help sustain weight loss. Even the definition of the maintenance period seems contradictory in the behavioral literature: the posttreatment period is called maintenance, but continued weight loss is to be achieved. Clients are expected to use the same methods learned during the treatment period, yet maintenance conditions differ from treatment conditions in that therapist and peer contact are withdrawn. No strategies specific to the maintenance period have been developed, although Wilson (1980) has suggested that improved booster sessions, induction of self-efficacy to counter anticipated negative cognitive reactions, and the use of social support in the client's natural environment are possibilities. More understanding of these factors is needed before their role in maintenance can be specified, but they provide some initial direction to developing better maintenance strategies.

The need to understand whether behavioral techniques actually act to alter cognitive effects of obesity and to develop differential treatment and maintenance interventions aimed at helping clients make habit and life-style changes rather than focusing all of our intervention efforts on weight loss is consistent with our proposal that a series of weight loss and weight loss maintenance periods may be required for permanent weight reduction. Such an approach would also require behaviorists to approach clients as individuals and to help them identify optimal periods for weight reduction versus maintenance. It would require clients and therapists to take a broad, long-term view of weight control.

Exercise Effects. Exercise has recently received attention in the literature from both a behavioral and biological standpoint. Abramson (1983) noted that one of the most promising behavioral innovations in recent years is the increasing focus of energy expenditure in obesity treatment. Previous work on weight reduction had not included systematic study of exercise. LeBow (1977) reported that only 20% of approximately 100 reports he reviewed included increasing activity as one of the treatment goals for obese clients.

Recently, Thompson *et al.* (1982) reviewed controlled group studies that used exercise along with other intervention procedures. They found five such studies, four of which indicated that exercise in combination with diet or a behavioral management procedure produced greater weight loss than did single exercise, dietary, or behavioral interventions. Thompson *et al.* also note that in three of these studies which provided follow-up data exercise enhanced maintenance effects. Methodological problems with these studies force Thompson *et al.* to interpret them cautiously. Nonetheless, the efficacy research does appear to provide support for the continued investigation of exercise as part of treatment for obesity within the behavioral framework.

Increased activity is also consistent with a biological framework. Thompson *et al.* (1982) note that metabolic effects of exercise may make a significant contribution to energy expenditure and may counter some of the metabolic effects of obesity that serve to maintain overweight. These reviewers conclude that exercise produces energy output through a direct effect on metabolic rate during the activity and an indirect effect subsequent to the activity. Also, exercise may elevate dietary-reduced basal metabolic rate, thus countering the negative metabolic effects of calorie restriction. Finally, exercise decreases storage fat rather than lean body mass, whereas dietary interventions tend to reduce both variables. Attempts to increase lean body mass may counter the lowering of basal metabolic rate that is associated with dieting.

A Biobehavioral Treatment Model

Any treatment model for obesity must consider biological and behavioral causes of the condition. Given that our present kowledge of cause is inadequate for identification of which factors among many cause obesity in individual cases, it cannot be expected that behavioral interventions will succeed with all clients. However, in view of the relative success of these methods, they must suffice until differential diagnosis is possible. To maximize success, the behavioral interventions offered must be individualized. It is necessary to help patients who fail to maintain weight losses reconsider their weight reduction goals and come to understand the possible role of causal biological factors that may impede maintenance at what are presumed to be ideal levels.

Any treatment model for obesity must also consider biological and behavioral effects of the condition. Research has indicated a large number of adaptations to obesity which would operate in moderate to severe cases. At least one of these effects, hypercellularity, may not be reversible with weight loss. However, current evidence indicates that most of the adaptations to obesity may be reversible following weight loss.

A treatment model that considers these adaptations to obesity would take a broad, long-term view of weight managment, linked to changes in life-style. As well as individualization of treatment, efforts would have to be directed toward understanding the mechanisms of weight loss and weight maintenance and developing specific strategies particularly for the maintenance period. From a biobehavioral perspective, efforts to increase activity as well as to change eating behavior would be necessary. Finally, the proposed model would involve, especially for moderately obese individuals, periods of weight reduction followed by maintenance periods in which the body can adjust to changes in biological functioning.

References

Abramson, E. E. (1973). Behavioral approaches to weight control. *Behavior Research and Therapy, 11*, 547–556.

Abramson, E. E. (1977). Behavioral approaches to weight control: An updated review. *Behavior Research and Therapy, 15*, 355–363.

Abramson, E. E. (1983). Behavioral treatment of obesity: Some good news, some bad news, and a few suggestions. *Behavior Therapist, 6*, 103–106.

Albrink, M. J., & Meigs, J. W. (1965). The relationship between serum triglycerides and skinfold thickness in obese subjects. *Annals of the New York Academy of Science, 131*, 673–683.

Andersson, B., & Larsson, B. (1961). Influences of local temperature changes in the preoptic area and rostral hypothalamus on the regulation of food and water intake. *Acta Physiologica Scandinavica, 52*, 75–89.

Beach, F. A. (1955). The descent of instinct. *Psychological Bulletin, 62*, 401–410.

Bellisle, F. (1979). Human feeding behavior. *Neuroscience and Biobehavioral Reviews, 3*, 163–169.

Booth, D. A. (1972). Feeding inhibition by glucose loads compared between normal and diabetic rats. *Physiology and Behavior, 8*, 801–805.

Booth, D. A. (1977). Satiety and appetite are conditioned reactions. *Psychosomatic Medicine, 39,* 76–81.

Booth, D. A., Lee, M., & McAlvey, C. (1976). Acquired sensory control of satiation in man. *British Journal of Psychology, 67,* 137–147.

Brightwell, D. R., & Sloan, C. L. (1977). Long term results of behavior therapy for obesity. *Behavior Therapy, 8,* 898–905.

Brobeck, J. R. (1948). Food intake as a mechanism of temperature regulation. *Yale Journal of Biology and Medicine, 20,* 545–552.

Brody, B. (1945). *Bioenergetics and growth.* New York: Hafner.

Brownell, K. D. (1982). Obesity: Understanding and treating a serious prevalent and refractory disorder. *Journal of Consulting and Clinical Psychology, 6,* 820–840.

Brownell, K. D., & Stunkard, A. J. (1978). Behavior therapy and behavioral change: Uncertainties in programs for weight control. *Behavior Research and Therapy, 16,* 301.

Bruch, H. (1973). *Eating disorders.* New York: Basic Books.

Bullen, B. A., Reed, R. R., & Mayer, J. (1964). Physical activity of obese and nonobese adolescent girls appraised by motion picture sampling. *American Journal of Clinical Nutrition, 14,* 211–223.

Cabanac, M., & Duclaux, R. (1970). Obesity: Absence of satiety aversion to sucrose. *Science, 168,* 496–497.

Cautela, J. R. (1967). Covert sensitization. *Psychological Reports, 20,* 459–468.

Collier, G., Hirsh, E., & Hamlin, P. H. (1972). The ecological determinants of reinforcement in the rat. *Physiology and Behavior, 9,* 705–716.

Corbit, J. D., & Stellar, E. (1964). Palatability, food intake, and obesity in normal and hyperphagic rats. *Journal of Comparative and Physiological Psychology, 58,* 63–67.

Craighead, L. W., Stunkard, A. J., & O'Brien, R. M. (1981). Behavior therapy and pharmacotherapy for obesity. *Archives of General Psychiatry, 38,* 763–768.

Davis, J. D., & Campbell, C. S. (1973). Peripheral control of meal size in the rat: Effect of sham feeding on meal size and drinking rate. *Journal of Comparative and Physiological Psychology, 83,* 379–387.

Diament, C., & Wilson, G. T. (1975). An experimental investigation of the effects of covert sensitization in an analogue eating situation. *Behavior Therapy, 6,* 499–509.

Durnin, J. V., Lonergan, M. E., Good, J., & Ewan, A. (1974). Cross-sectional nutritional and anthropometric study with an interval of 7 years on 611 young adolescent school children. *British Journal of Nutrition, 32,* 169–179.

Dwyer, J., Feldman, J. J., & Mayer, J. (1967). Adolescent dieters: Who are they? Physical characteristics, attitudes, and practices of adolescent girls. *American Journal of Clinical Nutrition, 20,* 1045.

Faust, I. (1984). Role of the fat cell in energy balance physiology. In A. J. Stunkard & E. Stellar (Eds.), *Eating and its disorders.* New York: Raven.

Ferguson, N. B. L., & Keesey, R. E. (1975). Effect of a quinine-adulterated diet upon body weight maintenance in male rats with ventromedial hypothalamic lesions. *Journal of Comparative and Physiological Psychology, 89,* 478–488.

Foreyt, J. P., & Kennedy, W. A. (1971). Treatment of overweight by aversion therapy. *Behavior Research and Therapy, 9,* 29–34.

Foreyt, J. P., Goodrick, G. K., & Gotto, A. M. (1981). Limitations of behavioral treatment of obesity: Review and analysis. *Journal of Behavioral Medicine, 4,* 159–174.

Foxx, R. M. (1972). Social reinforcement of weight reductions: A case report on an obese retarded adolescent. *Mental Retardation, 10,* 21–23.

Franklin, K. B. J., & Herberg, L. J. (1974). Ventromedial syndrome: The rat's "finikiness" results from the obesity, not from the lesions. *Journal of Comparative and Physiological Psychology, 87,* 410–414.

Garn, S. (1976). The origins of obesity. *American Journal of Diseases of Children, 130*, 465–467.

Garn, S., Clark, D. C., & Guire, K. E. (1975). Growth, body composition, and development of obese and lean children. In M. Winick (Ed.), *Childhood obesity*. New York: Wiley.

Glick, S. D., & Stanley, M. E. (1975). Neurochemical correlate of body weight in rats. *Brain Research, 96*, 153–155.

Glick, S. D., Greenstein, S., & Waters, D. H. (1974). Lateral hypothalamic lesions and striatal dopamine levels. *Life Sciences, 14*, 747–750.

Goldblatt, P. B., Moore, M. E., & Stunkard, A. J. (1965). Social factors in obesity. *Journal of the American Medical Association, 192*, 1039–1044.

Gordon, E. S. (1960). Non-esterified fatty acids in the blood of obese and lean subjects. *American Journal of Clinical Nutrition, 8*, 740–743.

Graff, H., & Stellar, E. (1962). Hyperphagia, obesity and finikiness. *Journal of Comparative and Physiological Psychology, 55*, 418–424.

Gruen, R., Hietanen, F., & Greenwood, M. R. C. (1978). Increased adipose tissue lipoprotein lipase activity during the development of the genetically obese rat (fa/fa). *Metabolism, 27*, 1955–1966.

Gurr, M. I., Jung, R. T., Robinson, M. P., & James, W. P. T. (1982). Adipose tissue cellularity in man: The relationship between fat cell size and number, the mass and distribution of body fat and the history of weight gain and loss. *International Journal of Obesity, 6*, 419–436.

Herman, C. P., & Polivy, J. (1975). Anxiety, restraint, and eating behavior. *Journal of Abnormal Psychology, 84*, 666–672.

Himms-Hagen, J., & Desautels, M. A. (1978). Mitochondrial defects in binding of purine nucleotides and a failure to respond to cold by an increase in binding. *Biochemical and Biophysical Research Communications, 83*, 628–634.

Hirsch, J., & Knittle, J. L. (1970). Cellularity of obese and nonobese human adipose tissue. *Federation Proceedings, 29*, 1516–1521.

Hirsch, E., & Walsh, M. (1982). Effect of limited access to sucrose on overeating and patterns of feeding. *Physiology and Behavior, 25*, 129–134.

Hirsch, J., Knittle, J. L., & Salans, L. B. (1966). Cell lipid content and cell number in obese and nonobese human adipose tissue. *Journal of Clinical Investigation, 45*, 1023.

Horan, J. J., & Johnson, R. G. (1971). Coverant conditioning through a self-management application of the Premack principle: It effects on weight reduction. *Journal of Behavior Therapy and Experimental Psychiatry, 2*, 243–249.

Ingle, D. J. (1949). A simple means of producing obesity in the rat. *Proceedings of the Society for Experimental Biology and Medicine, 72*, 604–605.

James, W. P. T., Trayhurn, P., & Garlick, P. (1981). The metabolic basis of subnormal thermogenesis in obesity. In P. Bjorntorp, A. Cairella, & A. Howard (Eds.), *Recent advances in obesity research* (Vol. 3, pp. 220–227). London: Wiley.

Jeffrey, D. E. (1976). Treatment outcomes: Issues in obesity research. In B. J. Williams, S. Martin, & J. P. Foreyt (Eds.), *Obesity: Behavioral approaches in dietary management*. New York: Brunner/Mazel.

Jeffrey, R. W., Thompson, P. D., & Wing, R. R. (1978). Effects on weight reduction of strong monetary contracts for calorie restriction or weight loss. *Behavior Research and Therapy, 16*, 363–369.

Jeffrey, R. W., Wing, R. R., & Stunkard, A. J. (1978). Behavioral treatment of obesity: The state of the art, 1976. *Behavior Therapy, 9*, 189–199.

Kalkoff, R. K., Kim, H. J., Cerletty, J., & Ferrou, C. A. (1971). Metabolic effects of weight loss in obese subjects. *Diabetes, 20*, 83–91.

Kaufman, L. W., & Collier, G. (1982). Cost and meal patterns in wild-caught rats. *Physiology and Behavior, 30*, 445–449.

Keesey, R. E., & Corbett, S. W. (1984). Metabolic defense of the body weight set point. In A. J. Stunkard & E. Stellar (Eds.), *Eating and its disorders*. New York: Raven.

Kennedy, G. C. (1953). The role of depot fat in the hypothalamic control of food intake in the rat. *Proceedings of the Royal Society, 140*, 578–592.

Kirtland, J., & Gurr, M. I. (1979). Adipose tissue cellularity: A review, 2. The relationship between cellularity and obesity. *International Journal of Obesity, 3*, 15–56.

Knittle, J. L., & Ginsburg-Fellner, F. (1972). Effect of weight reduction on *in vitro* adipose tissue lipolysis and cellularity in obese adolescents and adults. *Diabetes, 21*, 754–761.

Kratz, C. M., Levitsky, P. A., & Lustick, S. L. (1978). Long-term effects of quinine on food intake and body weight in the rat. *Physiology and Behavior, 21*, 321–324.

LeBow, M. D. (1977). Can lighter become thinner? *Addictive Behaviors, 2*, 87–93.

LeBow, M. D. (1981). *Weight control: The behavioral strategies*. Chichester, England: Wiley.

LeMagnen, J. (1955). Sur le mécanisme d'établissment des appétits caloriques. *Compes Rendus de l'Académie des Sciences, 240*, 2436–2438.

Leon, G. R. (1976). Current directions in the treatment of obesity. *Psychological Bulletin, 83*, 557–578.

Levitz, L. S., Jordan, H. A., LeBow, M. D., & Coopersmith, M. L. (September, 1980). *Weight loss five years after behavioral treatment*. Unpublished report based upon data presented at a meeting of the American Psychological Association, University of Manitoba, Winnipeg, Manitoba.

Logan, F. A. (1964). The free behavior situation. *Nebraska Symposium on Motivation 12*, 99–128.

Lozovsky, D., Saller, C. F., & Kopin, I. J. (1981). Dopamine receptor binding is increased in diabetic rats. *Science, 214*, 1031–1033.

Maggio, C. A. & Koopmans, H. S. (1982). Food intake after intragastric meals of short, medium, or long triglyceride. *Physiology and Behavior, 28*, 921–926.

Maier, M. R. F., & Schnierla, T. C. (1964). *Principles of animal psychology*. New York: Dover.

Mayer, J. (1953). Glucostatic mechanisms of regulation of food intake. *New England Journal of Medicine, 249*, 13–16.

Mayer, J., & Bates, M. F. W. (1952). Blood glucose and food intake in normal and hypophysectomized, alloxan-treated rats. *American Journal of Physiology, 168*, 812–819.

McCaleb, M. L., & Myers, R. D. (1979). Striatal dopamine release is altered by glucose and insulin during push–pull perfusion of the rat's caudate nucleus. *Brain Research Bulletin, 4*, 651–656.

McCaleb, M. L., & Myers, R. D. (1981). Cholecystokinin acts on the hypothalamic "noradrenergic system" involved in feeding. *Peptides, 1*, 47–49.

McMinn, M. R. (1984). Mechanisms of energy balance in obesity. *Behavioral Neuroscience, 98*, 375–393.

Metropolitan Life Insurance Company (1959). New weight standards for men and women. *Statistical Bulletin, 40*, 1–4.

Miller, N. E., Bailey, C. J., & Stevenson, J. A. F. (1950). Decreased "hunger" but increased food intake resulting from hypothalamic lesions. *Science, 112*, 256–259.

Miller, D. S., Mumford, P., & Stock, M. J. (1967). Gluttony: 2. Thermogenesis in overeating man. *American Journal of Clinical Nutrition, 20*, 1223–1229.

Morganstern, K. P. (1974). Cigarette smoke as a noxious stimulus in self-managed aversion therapy for compulsive eating. *Behavior Therapy, 5*, 255–260.

Muto, S., & Miyahara, C. (1972). Eating behavior of young rats: Experiments on selective feeding on diet and sugar solution. *British Journal of Nutrition, 28*, 327–337.

Nemeraff, C. B., & Prange, A. J. (Eds.) (1982). Neurotensin, a brain and gastrointestinal peptide. *Annals of the New York Academy of Science, 400*.

Perkins, M. N., Rothwell, N. J., Stock, T. W., & Stone, T. W. (1981). Activation of brown adipose tissue thermogenesis by the ventromedial hypothalamus. *Nature, 189*, 401–402.

Ramirez, I., & Friedman, M. I. (1982). Suppression of food intake by intragastric glucose in rats with impaired glucose tolerance. *Physiology and Behavior, 31*, 39–43.

Rodin, J. (1982). Obesity: Why the losing battle? In B. B. Wohlman (Ed.), *Physiological aspects of obesity: A handbook*. New York: Van Nostrand Reingold.

Rothwell, N. J., & Stock, M. J. (1979). Regulation of energy balance in two models of reversible obesity in the rat. *Journal of Comparative and Physiological Psychology, 93*, 1024–1034.

Russek, M. (1970). Demonstration of the influence of an hepatic glucosensitive mechanism on food intake. *Physiology and Behavior, 5*, 1207–1209.

Russek, M., Lora-Vilchis, M. C., & Islas-Chaires, M. (1979). Food intake inhibition elicited by intraportal glucose and adrenaline in dogs on a 22-hour fasting/2-hour feeding schedule. *Physiology and Behavior, 24*, 157–161.

Salans, L. B., Knittle, J. L., & Hirsch, J. (1968). The role of adipose cell size and adipose tissue insulin sensitivity in the carbohydrate intolerance of human obesity. *Journal of Clinical Investigation, 47*, 153–165.

Saller, C. F., & Chiodo, L. A. (1980). Glucose supresses basal firing and haloperidol-induced increases in the firing rate of central dopaminergic neurons. *Science, 210*, 1269–1271.

Schacter, S. (1971). *Emotion, obesity, and crime*. New York: Academic.

Schacter, S. (1982). Recidivism and self-cure of smoking and obesity. *American Psychologist, 37*, 436–444.

Schlemmel, R., Mickelsen, O., & Gill, J. L. (1970). Dietary obesity in rats: Body weight and body fat accretation in seven strains of rats. *Journal of Nutrition, 100*, 1041–1048.

Schmitt, M. (1973). Influences of hepatic portal receptors on hypothalamic feeding and satiety centers. *American Journal of Physiology, 225*, 1089–1095.

Schwartz, R. S., & Brunzell, J. D. (1978). Increased adipose tissue lipoprotein lipase in moderately obese men after weight reduction. *Lancet, 1*, 1230–1231.

Schwartz, R. S., & Brunzell, J. D. (1981). Increase of adipose tissue lipoprotein lipase activity with weight loss. *Journal of Clinical Investigation, 67*, 1425–1430.

Sclafani, A., & Springer, D. (1976). Dietary obesity in adult rats: Similarities to hypothalamic and human obesity syndromes. *Physiology and Behavior, 17*, 461–471.

Shetty, P. S., Jung, R. T., James, P. T., Barrand, M. A., & Callingham, B. A. (1981). Postprandial thermogenesis in obesity. *Clinical Science, 60*. 519–525.

Simms, E. A. H., Goldman, R. F., Gluck, C. M., Horton, E. S., Kelleher, P. C., & Row, D. W. (1968). Experimental obesity in man. *Transactions of the Association of American Physicians, 81*, 153–169.

Smith, G. P. (1984). Gut hormone hypothesis of postprandial satiety. In A. J. Stunkard & E. Stellar (Eds.), *Eating and its disorders*. New York: Raven.

Smith, G. P., Gibbs, J., Jerome, C., Pi-Sunyer, F. X., Kissileff, H. R., & Thorton, J. (1981). The satiety effect of cholecytokinin: A progress report. *Peptides* (Suppl. 2), *2*, 57–59.

Smith, G. P., Jerome, C., Cushin, B. J., Eterno, R., & Simansky, K. J. (1981). Abdominal vagotomy blocks the satiety effect of cholecystokin in the rat. *Science, 213*, 1036–1037.

Stanley, B. G., Eppel, M., & Hobel, B. G. (1982). Neurotensin injected into the paraventricular hypothalamus suppresses feeding in rats. *Annals of the New York Academy of Science, 400*, 425–427.

Stern, J. S. (1984). Is obesity a disease of inactivity? In A. J. Stunkard & E. Stellar (Eds.), *Eating and its disorders*. New York: Raven.

Stricker, E. M., & Zigmond, M. J. (1976). Recovery of function after damage to central catecholamine-containing neurons: A neuro-chemical model for the lateral hypothalamic syndrome. In A. N. Epstein & J. M. Sprague (Eds.), *Progress in psychobiology and physiological psychology* (Vol 6.) New York: Academic.

Strubbe, J. H., Steffens, A. B., & de Ruiter, L. (1975). Plasma insulin and the time pattern of feeding in the rat. *Physiology and Behavior, 18*, 81–86.

Stuart, R. B. (1967). Behavioral control of overeating. *Behavior Research and Therapy, 5*, 357–365.

Stunkard, A. J. (1975). Satiety is a conditioned reflex. *Psychosomatic Medicine, 37*, 383–387.

Stunkard, A. J. (1984). The current status of treatment for obesity in adults. In A. J. Stunkard & E. Stellar (Eds.), *Eating and its disorders*. New York: Raven.

Stunkard, A. J., & Mahoney, M. J. (1976). Behavioral treatment of the eating disorders. In H. Lutenberg (Ed.), *Handbook of behavior modification and behavioral therapy*. Englewood Cliffs, NJ: Prentice-Hall.

Taskinen, M. R., & Nikkila, E. A. (1979). Effects of caloric restriction on lipid metabolism in man. *Atherosclerosis, 32*, 289–299.

Thompson, J. K., Jarvie, G. J., Lahey, B. B., & Cureton, K. J. (1982). Exercise and obesity: Etiology, physiology and intervention. *Psychological Bulletin, 91*, 55–78.

Thurlby, P. L., & Trayhurn, P. (1980). Regional blood flow in genetically obese (ob/ob) mice. *Pfluegers Archiv. European Journal of Physiology, 385*, 193–201.

Tyler, V. O., & Straughan, J. H. (1970). Coverant control and breath holding as techniques for the treatment of obesity. *Psychological Record, 20*, 473–478.

Weingarten, H. P. (1983). Conditioned cues elicit feeding in sated rats: A role for learning in meal initiation. *Science, 220*, 431–432.

Wilson, G. T. (1978). Methodological considerations in treatment outcome research. *Journal of Consulting and Clinical Psychology, 46*, 687–702.

Wilson, G. T. (1980). Behavior modification and the treatment of obesity. In A. J. Stunkard (Ed.), *Obesity*. Philadelphia: Saunders.

Woody, E. Z. & Constanzo, P. R. (1981). The socialization of obesity-prone behavior. In S. Brehm, S. Kassin, & F. Gibbons (Eds.), *Developmental social psychology*. New York: Oxford University Press.

Wooley, O. W., Wooley, S. C., & Dunham, R. B. (1972). Can calories be perceived and do they affect hunger in obese and nonobese humans? *Journal of Comparative and Physiological Psychology, 80*, 250–258.

Wooley, O. W., Wooley, S. C., & Woods, W. W. (1975). Effect of calories on appetite for palatable food in obese and nonobese humans. *Journal of Comparative and Physiological Psychology, 89*, 619–625.

Wooley, S. C. (1972). Physiologic versus cognitive factors in short-term food regulation in the obese and nonobese. *Psychosomatic Medicine, 34*, 62–68.

Wooley, S. C., & Wooley, O. W. (1973). Salivation to the sight and thought of food: A new measure of appetite. *Psychosomatic Medicine, 35*, 136–142.

Wooley, S. C., Wooley, O. W., & Dyrenforth, S. R. (1979). Theoretical, practical, and social issues in behavioral treatments of obesity. *Journal of Applied Behavioral Analysis, 12*, 3–25.

CHAPTER 4

Biobehavioral Approaches to Smoking Control

J. Allan Best, Patricia E. Wainwright, David E. Mills, and Susan A. Kirkland

> Smoking-related diseases are such important causes of disability and premature death in developed countries that the control of cigarette smoking could do more to improve health and prolong life in these countries than any other single action in the whole field of preventive medicine. (WHO Expert Committee, 1979)

Researchers involved in smoking control face the perplexing question of why, given a reasonable understanding of the adverse effects of smoking, people still start and continue to smoke. Furthermore, although the majority of smokers express a desire to quit, those that attempt to do so are generally unsuccessful (Pechacek, 1979). Numerous programs have been developed that aim not only to aid smokers in their attempts to break the habit but also to prevent the onset of smoking in individuals who represent a population at risk. Unfortunately, these efforts—both smoking prevention and smoking cessation—have been notoriously ineffective (Bernstein & McAlister, 1976; Best & Bloch, 1979; Evans, Henderson, Hill, & Raines, 1979; Flay, d'Avernas, Best, Kersell, & Ryan, 1983; Leventhal & Cleary, 1980; Lichtenstein & Danaher, 1976; Pechacek, 1979; Thompson, 1978). At best, recent interventions such as social-influences prevention programs and nicotine-replacement-therapy cessation strategies appear promising but have not been fully evaluated.

J. Allan Best, Patricia E. Wainwright, David E. Mills, and Susan A. Kirkland. • Department of Health Studies, University of Waterloo, Waterloo, Ontario, Canada N2L 3G1.

Reviewers argue persuasively that our failure to develop effective intervention methods stems from inadequate analyses of the behavior (Best & Hakstian, 1978; Lichtenstein, 1982; Pechacek & Danaher, 1979; Pomerleau, 1980, 1981). Indeed, our understanding of smoking behavior lags far behind our knowledge of its physiological effects. Clearly, cigarette smoking involves more than a physiological addiction to the pharmacological components of tobacco. Motivational and situational factors have been implicated, but there is a paucity of empirical data addressing the interplay of these and other social, psychological, and pharmacological factors. There exist even fewer data characterizing the dynamic processes of behavior change involved in smoking prevention and cessation. Factors influencing cigarette smoking appear to vary as the individual moves from initiation to maintenance, to cessation, and resumption or relapse (Best & Hakstian, 1978; Best, Owen, & Trentadue, 1978; Leventhal & Cleary, 1980; Ontario Council of Health, 1982; Pechacek & McAlister, 1979). Thus, if we are to develop effective interventions for smoking control we must address the following issues:

1. *Smoking initiation:* What factors influence experimentation and initiation of smoking, and how might the relative contributions of these factors change over the course of the initiation process? Simply, the question is, Why do individuals begin smoking?
2. *Smoking maintenance*: Once a pattern of regular or chronic smoking has developed, what are the factors that maintain this behavior? That is, why do people continue to smoke, often even in the presence of compelling reasons for change?
3. *Smoking reductions*: Given a stabilized rate of smoking, what are the acute effects of smoking reduction? In essence, the question is, What is smoking withdrawal?
4. *Maintenance of smoking reduction and/or recidivism*: If significant smoking reduction is achieved, what are the factors that might precipitate relapse in the long term? In other words, why do people often fail in their efforts to maintain a reduced (or zero) rate of smoking?

Note that we speak of smoking reduction to include two perhaps quite different phenomena: cutting down on smoking and quitting entirely. Available research on smoking reduction processes refers almost exclusively to cessation, despite the fact that many smokers try to cut down rather than quit. Intervention programs can be designed to eliminate the behavior entirely or to change the behavior to reduce potential risk. Less hazardous smoking might be achieved through substance changes (switching to lower tar and nicotine cigarettes), through other behavior changes (reducing the number of cigarettes smoked per day or reducing the yield of each cigarette by taking fewer puffs, inhaling less deeply), or a combination of the two. However, conclusive evidence of the relative feasibility and health consequences of these two modes of change is not currently available (Ontario Council of Health, 1982). Understandably, then, health professionals might argue that cessation is a better program objective than reduced exposure. For the purposes of this discussion, however, we will use the general term *smoking reduction* to refer to either condition.

The purpose of this chapter is to discuss the possible interplay between behavioral and biological factors that influence smoking and thereby contribute to our understanding of why interventions succeed or fail. First, a brief description of three relevant models of learning will be presented. Second, two central biobehavioral issues will be discussed: the pharmacological aspects of nicotine in smoking, and self-regulatory and compensatory mechanisms controlling smoking behavior. Third, we will propose preliminary models of the processes smokers encounter. Current behavioral approaches to smoking prevention and reduction will be discussed in light of these accounts. Finally, implications for both intervention and research will be outlined.

Smoking Behavior and Learning

Three distinct models of learning, well known to psychologists, have been related to smoking behavior. *Social learning theory* (Bandura, 1977) builds on operant conditioning (Skinner, 1953) to describe social influences and reinforcement mechanisms. *Associative learning theory* (Hunt, Matarazzo, Weiss, & Gentry, 1979) attempts to explain the habit aspects of chronic smoking. *Classical conditioning theory* (Siegel, 1982; Stewart, deWit, & Eikelboom, 1984) provides a way of integrating pharmacological and physiological factors in a comprehensive learning-theory analysis of smoking behavior. Interested readers are referred to thoughtful discussions by others of the different ways in which diverse biobehavioral theories and data can be integrated around smoking (cf. Ashton & Stepney, 1982; Best & Hakstian, 1978; Glad, Tyre, & Adesso, 1976; Leventhal & Cleary, 1980; Mausner & Platt, 1971; Pechacek & Danaher, 1979; Pomerleau, 1980, 1981; Raw, 1978; Russell, 1974).

Different kinds of learning may occur and operate simultaneously. Indeed, the learning principles described above do not constitute pure examples of one form of learning, and the three theories outlined share some common features. For example, all are concerned with discrete environmental situations and a scientific analysis of environment–behavior relationships. All focus attention on the antecedents and consequences of smoking. In addition, however, each theory has distinguishing features, and each has a relatively distinct focus.

Operant and Social Learning Theories

Behavior that produces positive results tends to be repeated. Thus, smoking is an operant to the extent that it acts to produce effects people desire—feeling accepted by peers, relief from boredom, relaxation—positive reinforcers that contribute to the development and maintenance of smoking behavior. A primary reinforcer is one that is unlearned. For example, the act of smoking may produce biological effects that are naturally reinforcing to the organism (see the following section on the role of nicotine). Smoking also may be maintained by secondary reinforcers. For example, if an individual finds some social situations stressful and repeatedly smokes to relieve that stress, the cigarette itself may come to serve as a secondary reinforcer with the ability to reduce stress in subsequent social situations. Stimuli preparatory to the act of smoking (e.g., the sight of a cigarette) function as secondary reinforcers for behavior preceding them (e.g., picking up a pack of cigarettes) as well as discriminative stimuli that set the occasion for behavior to follow them (e.g., lighting a cigarette and inhaling). These chains of smoking behavior develop such that smoking is controlled by both cues (events signaling potential reinforcement for smoking) and consequences (the process of reinforcement itself). From this perspective, an understanding of smoking requires both an analysis of the cues triggering smoking (e.g., sight of other smoking, physiological reactions associated with stress) and the consequences of smoking (e.g., relief from boredom, feelings of social belonging) (Best & Hakstian, 1978). Note that a range of social, psychological, and biological events can serve as both cues and consequences.

Negative reinforcement refers to situations in which a behavior is strengthened, not because it produces positive consequences, but because it prevents or relieves negative consequences. As smoking becomes established, various states of discomfort become associated with nonsmoking, providing an escape–avoidance contingency for smoking behavior. Once smoking comes to relieve withdrawal, it may, through the process of stimulus generalization, come to relieve other disphoric states as well, for example, anger, tension, and boredom (Best & Hakstian, 1978; Tomkins, 1966). Thus, smoking may serve as a generalized primary and secondary reinforcer providing both positive and negative reinforcement over a remarkably wide range of life situations (Pomerleau, 1980).

Principles of operant learning suggest that the chains of behavior involved in smoking are strengthened in several ways. Because the act of smoking over the years is performed tens of thousands of times, in a wide variety of situations, the conditioned links between smoking cues and behavior will become very strong indeed. Repeated, consistent reinforcement will serve to strengthen links; the complexity of cue and consequence relationships will make the behavior highly resistant to change.

Two more concepts are central to initiation and reduction processes. First, social learning theory emphasizes modeling as an important mechanism (Bandura, 1977). Thus, children "learn" smoking behavior by watching parents and peers doing it, in addition to the learning that may occur through reinforcement as they begin to experiment with smoking (Flay *et al.*, 1983). Second, smoking reduction involves self-control. If smoking reliably produces immediate, powerful reinforcers, then not smoking in a smoking situation requires an act of self-control—postponing immediate satisfaction, or reinforcement, for long-term benefit. Behavioral self-management theory and procedures can be brought to bear in developing "nonsmoking behaviors"—behavioral responses to smoking situations that serve as operants and thus, as strengthened with time, come to produce reinforcement without smoking (Best, 1980).

Associative Learning Theory

Hunt and his colleagues (Hunt *et al.*, 1979) discuss the concepts of associative learning and habit as they relate to health behavior. The theory begins by assuming operant learning principles and then extends these in several significant ways. A habit is defined as "a stable pattern of behavior marked by automaticity and unawareness and influenced by associative learning as well as reinforcement" (Hunt *et al.*, 1979, p. 112). A two-process theory of learning is thus proposed. Smoking behavior originally develops through operant learning. However, as it becomes overlearned and habitual, associative learning gradually takes over. The behavior becomes increasingly automatic, occurring without much awareness, and is performed so quickly that there is little opportunity for motivational arousal and reinforcement. Smoking becomes progressively independent from reinforcement, to the point of being "functionally autonomous," characterized by continued maintenance of behavior patterns long after the apparent disappearance of original reinforcing consequences. As a result, habitual smoking displays a strong resistance to extinction.

Classical Conditioning Theory

In recent years, classical conditioning theory has enjoyed growing popularity as a model for understanding addiction and its development (Pomerleau, 1980, 1981; Siegel, 1982; Solomon, 1977; Solomon & Corbit, 1973, 1974; Stewart *et al.*, 1984; Ternes, 1977). Again, the model takes nothing away from operant and associative learning accounts of smoking; rather, it extends the models to account for additional aspects of smoking behavior.

Classical conditioning accounts of smoking are distinguished by a concern with stimulus–stimulus relationships, that is, an understanding of how antecedents or cues come to trigger a seemingly reflexive action. The theory has particular value in explaining drug tolerance and withdrawal phenomena. Solomon's (Solomon, 1977; Solomon & Corbit, 1973, 1974) opponent process theory of acquired motivation builds on classical conditioning to explain addictive phenomena. The model assumes central nervous system mechanisms which operate homeostatically to regulate affect. A stimulus, such as nicotine, may elicit an unconditioned alpha-process. The alpha-process will in turn trigger an opposite beta-process to return the organism to homeostasis. The key postulate of opponent process theory is that the beta-process will become conditioned to stimulus aspects of the drug-taking (smoking) situation. Thus, cues associated with smoking (e.g., the sight of a cigarette, a stressful situation) come to trigger the opponent beta-process. Environmental events, particularly those that affect mood or signal performance demand, modulate the reinforcement value of nicotine self-administration. As a consequence, more of the drug, in this case nicotine, will be required to produce an alpha-process sufficiently strong to offset the beta-process and produce central nervous system (CNS) gratification. In other words, tolerance will develop. If an individual does not smoke in the presence of conditioned smoking cues, there will be no alpha-process to balance the conditioned beta-response, homeostasis will be disrupted, and aversive physiological reactions (withdrawal) will ensue. Smoking as an operant thus is positively reinforced by producing pleasure and negatively reinforced by terminating withdrawal, setting up an addictive cycle whereby the individual smokes as much as to avoid withdrawal as to produce pleasure.

Most opponent process research has been done with addictive drugs other than nicotine, notably opiates, and primarily using animal models (see Siegel, 1982, for a review). Though the data seem to fit classical conditioning principles and the opponent process theory rather well, it may be the case that this is not the complete story. Recent data from animal experiments indicate that in many cases, rather than opposing the effects of the drug, many conditioned drug effects directly mimic the positive affective aspects of drug use (reviewed by Stewart, *et al.*, 1984). These authors propose that the self-administration of opiates and stimulants is maintained by the effect of conditioned stimuli in producing a state similar to that produced by the drug and thereby "priming" the organism to respond to drug-related stimuli and to increase drug-seeking behavior. This mechanism may be more useful in explaining the development of dependence in situations in which the pattern of use would not support the development of physiological withdrawal symptoms. An important aspect of the model of conditioned drug effects is that it suggests how environmental stimuli can precipitate craving for a drug even after an extended period of abstinence has ended physical dependence.

Biobehavioral Processes in Smoking

Many of the processes discussed above assume that there is an altered physiological state induced by smoking. In this section we will consider these pharmacological effects, followed with a discussion of how such effects might influence self-regulatory behavior.

Pharmacology of Nicotine

The products of combustion of tobacco include various "tars" and carbon monoxide in addition to the alkaloid nicotine. Although the other components do have physiological actions and contribute to the long-term health hazards associated with smoking, the acute effects of inhaling cigarette smoke have been mainly attributed to nicotine. The free base, which is present under alkaline conditions, is lipid-soluble and therefore is readily absorbed through the cell membranes of the lungs, skin, buccal and nasal mucosa, gastrointestinal tract, bladder, and renal tubules. This has important clinical implications in that nicotine levels in the body can be altered by manipulating the pH at sites of absorption or excretion. For example, nicotine chewing gum is buffered at an alkaline pH to enhance absorption (Russell, Raw, & Jarvis, 1980) and the urine can be acidified to enhance excretion (Beckett, Rowland, & Triggs, 1965; Schachter, Kozlowski, & Silverstein, 1977).

The liver microsomal enzyme system is the major site of metabolism, with 80–90% of the compound being modified prior to excretion by the kidneys. The major metabolites are cotinine and nicotine-*N*-oxide, which are pharmacologically inactive (Russell & Feyerabend, 1978). A considerable proportion of nicotine taken orally is metabolized during its first passage through the liver before ever becoming available for distribution by the systemic circulation, accounting for the low activity of nicotine administered in the form of oral tablets. There is some evidence that chronic cigarette smoking may increase the activity of the hepatic metabolic system, leading to an increase in the deactivation of nicotine as well as of other drugs (Beckett & Triggs, 1967). This will lead to an increase in dosage requirements to compensate for an increase in the breakdown of the drug and constitutes the basis for the phenomenon known as metabolic tolerance (Goodman Gilman, Goodman & Gilman, 1980).

The plasma half-life ($t_{1/2}$) of nicotine is close to 2 hours (Benowitz, Jacob, Jones, & Rosenberg, 1982). Accordingly, observations have been made that blood nicotine concentrations accumulate for 4–6 hours with regular smoking, and elevated concentration persist in the blood overnight (Benowitz, Kuyt, & Jacob, 1981). The actual concentration attained will be a function of the dosage size and interval as well as the plasma half-life. It is appropriate to note here that there will be differences among individuals with respect to the rate of nicotine metabolism. These differences arise as a function of various factors such as genetic variation (including sex, age, and health status), as well as prior exposure to drugs or chemicals. There is some evidence that aging and declining metabolic rates may be reflected in declining rates of smoking (Garvey, Bosse, & Seltzer, 1974).

If the motivation of smoking behavior is that of maintaining the plasma nicotine concentration within certain limits, this can be achieved most efficiently by a dosage regimen that provides an initial high "loading" dose, followed by smaller maintenance doses at appropriate intervals. It is possible that individual variability in metabolic processes as well as differences in tissue sensitivity with respect to the effects of nicotine are factors contributing to the individual differences in smoking schedules.

The preferred method of nicotine self-administration is through inhalation. Because of the large surface area of the lungs accompanied by the slightly alkaline pH of the surface fluids, absorption of nicotine is both rapid and efficient. It has been shown that the increase in plasma nicotine concentration as a result of repeated inhalations of cigarette smoke is similar to that following a "bolus" intravenous injection of a similar dose (Russell & Feyerabend, 1978). This means that with successive inhalations the tissues will be intermittently exposed to peak concentrations of nicotine that are much higher than those that would be attained were the same dose to be administered continuously. It has been shown that the response of cells to the same dose of nicotine differs as the mode of administration is varied (Armitage, Hall, & Sellers, 1969). Other methods of nicotine administration, such as nicotine chewing gum, are unable to simulate this pattern of exposure, and this may explain why cigarette smoking is more popular than chewing tobacco or taking snuff.

The nicotine in the blood travels from the lungs to the heart and thence to the entire body. It is estimated that it takes 7–8 seconds for the nicotine from a single puff to reach the brain (cited in Russell & Feyerabend, 1978). Nicotine is not distributed evenly throughout all the body tissues and is actively sequestered by the nervous system, leading to concentrations in the brain much greater than those in the blood. However, because of its high lipid solubility, nicotine can diffuse freely out of cells; thus, it also leaves the brain quickly and so the maintenance of these high concentrations will depend on replenishment from the concentrated "boli" obtained through repeated inhalations.

Many of the physiological actions of nicotine can be attributed to its structural similarity to the neurotransmitter acetylcholine and its consequent ability to act on certain of the cholinergic receptors (reviewed in Goodman Gilman *et al.*. 1980). Acetylcholine is the neurotransmitter released by preganglionic fibres to all ganglia in the autonomic nervous system and the adrenal medulla. In addition, it is released by postganglionic parasympathetic fibres to effector organs as well as being the neurotransmitter of motor fibers to skeletal muscle. Receptors are regions on the presynaptic or postsynaptic cell membrane that recognize the structure of a drug in a specific way. An agonistic drug binds the receptor and activates the receptor complex which then mediates the biological effect. Conversely, an antagonist drug will block this effect. In some cases a drug will initially act as an agonist when it binds to the receptor, but if it is not readily displaced it will prevent the receptor from being further stimulated and thereby act as an antagonist. The cholinergic receptors can be divided into two populations on the basis of their sensitivity to either nicotine or another naturally occurring alkaloid, muscarine. All the receptors responsive to acetylcholine in both the autonomic ganglia and in skeletal muscle are also responsive to nicotine and are termed nicotine receptors. Although both acetylcholine and nicotine stimulate the receptors, nicotine, unlike acetylcholine, is not rapidly inactivated, so the combination with the receptor is of relatively longer duration. In fact, as the dosage increases, nicotine will eventually block the receptors so that at toxic doses no further transmission is possible. This accounts for the biphasic action of the drug wherein the initial effect is stimulatory but later on inhibition predominates.

The peripheral effect of small doses of nicotine is that of activation of the sympathetic division of the autonomic nervous system. As the dose increases, stimulation of the sympathetic ganglia is followed by a similar effect on the parasympathetic ganglia, then later blockade of the parasympathetic and then the sympathetic ganglia. Consequently, the physiological effects of nicotine are dose-dependent; however, those seen after cigarette smoking are generally those of sympathetic stimulation. Epinephrine is released from the adrenal medulla and norepinephrine from sympathetic nerve endings (Cryer, Haymond, Santiago, & Shah, 1976). This increase in catecholamine release has several biological effects, including vasoconstriction and an increase in heart rate, blood pressure, and blood sugar. As a result of the lowered peripheral blood flow, skin temperature decreases (Stephens, 1977). The influence of nicotine on the chemoreceptors in the carotid and aortic bodies leads to a modest increase in respiratory rate. It can also cause nausea and vomiting by stimulating the chemoreceptor trigger zone of the medulla oblongata and by activating the vagal reflexes involved in emesis. An interesting observation is that, like acetylcholine, nicotine stimulates sensory receptors. This may contribute to the experimental finding that cigarette smoking is accompanied by a decreased consumption of sweet-tasting, highly caloric foods (Grunberg, 1982). It is possible that this could explain, in part, the lower body weight commonly found in cigarette smokers and the fact that weight gain is often an unwanted consequence of smoking reduction.

Nicotine as an Addictive Substance

The effects of nicotine on the central nervous system are crucial to an understanding of smoking behavior. Smoking has been described as an addictive or dependent behavior in that an individual will go to great lengths to continue smoking and will show difficulty in ceasing voluntarily. The question is whether the pharmacological effects of nicotine act as reinforcers which serve to maintain the behavior. In this context there are two types of reward to consider: either the positive reinforcing effect of nicotine through its effect on the central nervous system, or the negative reinforcing effect of nicotine through its ability to prevent the aversive physical symptoms associated with withdrawal of the drug. There is evidence that nicotine enhances the activity of the central catecholamine "reward" system (Crow & Deakin, 1978) and can act as a positive reinforcer of operant behavior in rats (Balfour, 1982). Pomerleau, Fertig, Seyler, and Jaffe (1983) have shown that smoking releases the peptide beta-endorphin in humans, which suggests that the effects of smoking may be mediated through the opioid peptides that play an important role in homeostasis (Kostrelitz & Hughes, 1978). These peptides have been shown to be endogenous ligands for the receptors which are normally occupied by morphine and other structurally related drugs. At high doses their activity resembles that of these drugs, including a capacity to engender dependence. The large molecule, beta-endorphin, is produced by the pituitary, whereas two smaller pentapeptides, methionin-enkephalin and leucine-enkephalin, which are fragments of beta-endorphine, are also found in the CNS. They act by modulating ongoing neural activity in the brain and thereby altering neurotransmission (Van Ree & De Wied, 1981). Physiological changes such as these may provide the basis for the positively reinforcing effects of nicotine.

There are two phenomena that must be considered in a discussion of how the negative reinforcing effects of nicotine might be maintaining its self-administration; these are tolerance and physical dependence (Cappell & LeBlanc, 1981). Tolerance has been described as the condition in which there is a reduction in the effect of a standard dose of a drug as a result of continued use, and the ability to reinstate this effect by a concomitant increase in dose. In human subjects, measures such as change in heart rate and skin temperature have been used to assess tolerance to the effects of nicotine; greater tolerance is evident as decreased physiological reactivity (Pomerleau, Fertig & Shanahan, 1983). It is important to note that tolerance may develop at different rates to the various effects of a drug; data from animal studies using morphine suggest that tolerance develops more rapidly to the aversive than to the positive effects (Stewart *et al.*, 1984).

Physical dependence is described as an altered state of CNS activity engendered by chronic exposure to a drug, and it is common for this to compensate for the effects produced by the drug; this may in fact account for some of the observed effects described as tolerance. Usually the symptoms of physical dependence do not become apparent until the drug is removed, when they are perceived as withdrawal symptoms. When smokers stop smoking they do experience a wide variety of physiological and psychological symptoms (Shiffman, 1979). These include nausea, headache, gastrointestinal disturbances, and increased appetite, as well as disturbances of arousal such as drowsiness, fatigue, and insomnia. Psychological complaints are reflected in an inability to concentrate and increased irritability and hostility, as well as increased anxiety. The reported severity of these symptoms in subjects deprived of nicotine can be attenuated through smoking high- or low-nicotine research cigarettes (Pomerleau, Fertig, & Shanahan, 1983) or with nicotine chewing gum (Schneider, Jarvik, & Forsythe, 1984). Recent research (Pomerleau, Fertig, Seyler, & Jaffe, 1983a) has indicated that heavy smokers, as determined by plasma cotinine level, are more nicotine-dependent than light smokers. It would also appear that this population may be better able to regulate nicotine levels than the light smokers. Abrupt smoking cessation as well as smoking reduction precipitate withdrawal effects; these improve more rapidly following "cold turkey" cessation than following gradual withdrawal (Shiffman, 1979). It has been suggested that subjects in the latter group are in a state of permanent withdrawal; an alternative explanation might be that the nicotine is acting as a "primer" which stimulates further drug-seeking behavior. A recent study (Glassman, Jackson, Walsh, Roose, & Rosenfeld, 1984) has indicated that clonidine, an alpha-2-adrenergic agonist, is as effective as the tranquilizer Alprazolam in reducing most withdrawal symptoms with a specific effect on cigarette craving. This suggests a relationship between central noradrenergic activity and the effects of withdrawal from nicotine.

Self-Regulatory Aspects of Smoking

A great deal of anecdotal information has accumulated in the form of self-reports from smokers, that subjective distress leads to increases in smoking behavior. This concept has largely been supported by experimental evidence indicating that stress is one of the most frequently cited cues for smoking (Emery, Hilgendorf, & Irvin, 1968; Frith, 1971; Ikard, Green, & Horn, 1969) and that exposure to experimental stress leads to an increase in smoking activity (Golding & Mangan, 1982; Rose, Ananda, & Jarvik, 1983; Schachter, Silverstein, Kozlowski, Herman, & Liebling, 1977). However, not all researchers have been able to confirm this relationship; in fact, several studies have reported that smoking activity decreases during performance of stressful tasks (Ashton & Watson, 1970; Fuller & Forrest, 1973). This apparent contradiction in results may be attributed to individual differences in the tendency to increase or decrease habitual substance consumption in response to varying levels of stress (Conway, Vickers, Ward, & Rahe, 1981), as well as interference with performance of habitual behaviors by certain stressors (Ashton & Watson, 1970). Stress has also been implicated in precipitating relapses following attempts at smoking cessation (Pomerleau, Adkins, & Pertschuk, 1978; Shiffman, 1979), and it has been reported that less anxious smokers are more likely to be successful in quitting the habit (Pomerleau *et al.*, 1978; Schwartz & Dubitzky, 1968).

One theory explaining the relationship between stress and smoking is based on the nicotine-addiction theory of smoking and the idea that smoking behavior is modulated by the "tracking" or monitoring of blood nicotine levels and the drive to regulate these levels within a certain range. Proponents of this theory suggest that stress induces physiological changes that increase the turnover rate of nicotine in the body, lowering blood-nicotine levels. Increases in smoking activity during stress serve to restore blood nicotine to prestress values in order to prevent physical withdrawal symptoms.

Support for this theory is based on a series of studies examining urine acidity and smoking behavior. As mentioned above, nicotine excretion by the kidney is directly related to urine acidity; for example, for a given nicotine intake, the more acidic the urine, the greater the nicotine excretion rate (Beckett *et al.*, 1965; Haag & Larson, 1942). In a series of studies, Schachter and co-workers attempted to demonstrate that stress-induced increases in urine acidity caused stress-related increases in smoking. First, it was demonstrated that a wide variety of stressors, ranging from electric shock to public speaking, elicited increases in urine acidity in both smokers and nonsmokers (Schachter, Silverstein, Kozlowski, Herman, & Wiebling, 1977). Following this, in order to demonstrate the dependence of smoking behavior on urine acidity, the smoking behavior of seven individuals whose urine acidity was manipulated by administration of vitamin C (acid), placebo, and bicarbonate (alkaline), was followed over 2 days. Results of this study suggested that an increase in the acidity of the urine was accompanied by increased nicotine consumption. The final study in this series examined the effects of altering urine acidity on smoking activity during low- and high-stress conditions (Schachter, Silverstein, & Perlick, 1977), demonstrating that prevention of acidic urine during high-stress situations attenuated the smoking increase in comparison to control subjects.

The results of these studies, along with others suggesting that smokers track and regulate circulating nicotine levels (Ashton & Watson, 1970; Frith, 1971; Schachter, 1977) led Schachter *et al.* (1977) to speculate that urinary acidity, regulated by the kidney, is the crucial mediator of the smoking stress relationship in heavy smokers. If these theories are correct, switching smokers to low nicotine cigarettes may create a greater health hazard by leading these individuals to smoke more, exposing them to higher levels of the harmful constituents of tobacco smoke in their drive for nicotine. In addition, it suggests that the physical drive for nicotine during stress will be difficult, if not impossible, to attenuate by behavioral manipulations.

However, there is much controversy over the theory that a nicotine drive is completely responsible for the smoking–stress relationship, as Schachter himself points out. One problem with the theory is that the urinary changes in response to stress are relatively slow, whereas the smoking response is relatively rapid. If urine acidity were the sole mediator of the behavior, one would expect a well-defined latent period between the initiation of stress and the smoking increase. Another major point of contention is that not all smokers can be demonstrated to track nicotine (Finnegan, Larson, & Haag, 1945; Goldfarb, Jarvik, & Glick, 1970), and classification of smokers into heavy and light categories to explain this reality is largely arbitrary, with no physiological basis. In light of these limitations, it would appear that renal control of smoking behavior during stress is only a partial answer to the question.

The second major theory as to why smoking increases during stress considers smoking behavior as a homeostatic mechanism, an activity that assists the body in restoring itself to equilibrium in the face of stress. There are many ways in which smoking might perform this function. Perhaps the most obvious is through alteration of the neuroendocrine response to stress. Smoking has been shown to increase circulating levels of the stress-responding hormones epinephrine (Hill & Wynder, 1947), and cortisol (Seyler, Fertig, Pomerleau, Hunt, & Parker, 1984), and nicotine inhalation increases antiviral protein (AVP) in humans (Rowe, Kilgore, & Robertson, 1980). Similarly, nicotine administration to animals results in increases in ACTH, beta-endorphin, and corticosterone release (deVolx, *et al.*, 1981). All of these hormones are believed to play adaptive roles during stress in humans.

It has also been suggested that the neuroendocrine responses to nicotine may enhance learning and memory during stress in both animals and humans. Effects attributed to nicotine include improved memory consolidation (Andersson, 1975; Flood, Bennett, Orme, Rosenzweig, & Jarvik, 1978) and increased rate of learning of reward or avoidance tasks (Morrison & Armitage, 1967). The mechanism of action in these situations is not known; it is possible that nicotine acts directly on learning and memory centers of the hippocampus through its activity as an acetylcholine agonist (Andersson, 1975), or it may act indirectly on such centers through stimulation of AVP and ACTH release (VanRee & DeWied, 1981).

Another manner in which smoking may enhance psychological reaction and performance during stress is through alteration of arousal and mood. The relationship between performance and arousal is explained by the Yerkes-Dodson Law which states that the quality of performance relates to arousal level as an inverted U-shaped function. Performance is poor when subjects are underaroused, as well as when overaroused, peaking at an intermediate arousal level. Thus, an individual who is overaroused in a stressful situation may actually increase performance with administration of a depressant drug, whereas an underaroused animal may increase performance by administration of a stimulant (Corcoran, 1965).

In light of the biphasic effects of nicotine, a smoker may experience either stimulation or depression, depending on the dose administered. Several investigators have observed that smoking is followed by EEG changes indicative of arousal (Knott & Venables, 1977), whereas smoking abstinence leads to EEG changes indicative of decreased arousal (Ulett & Itil, 1969). Studies on humans have also shown that smoking in a relaxing environment leads to increased central nervous system arousal (as determined by EEG), whereas smoking in a stressful environment (white noise) decreases arousal (Mangan & Golding, 1978).

One would expect that changes in arousal levels would serve to increase performance during stressful tasks. Although smoking may either increase or decrease performance in short-term reaction time tasks (Ashton, Savage, Telford, Thompson, & Watson, 1972; Myrsten, Post, Frankenhauser, & Johansson, 1972), it has been observed to increase performance in comparison to both deprived smokers and nonsmokers in vigilance tasks (Tarriere & Hartenmann, 1964; Wesnes & Warburton, 1978).

Despite the evidence cited describing the relationship between nicotine and arousal, one troubling paradox remains. This is that although nicotine and smoking cause significant increases in physiological arousal, especially of autonomically innervated organs, they frequently reduce behavioral and self-report measures of emotion and elicit feelings of relaxation and tranquility (Gilbert, 1979). A number of investigators have examined various behaviors and moods relating to this paradox. Several studies report decreases in muscle tension in the face of autonomic arousal from nicotine administration, suggesting that this is responsible for the relaxing effect smokers describe (Gilbert, 1979; Gilbert & Hagan, 1980). Others report lowered pain (Pomerleau, Turk, & Fertig, 1984) and anxiety levels in subjects following nicotine administration (Hutchinson & Emley, 1973; Gilbert, 1979). Conversely, increased anxiety and irritability have been demonstrated in deprived smokers (Perlick, 1977; Silverstein, 1977), and resumption of smoking has consistently led to subjective well-being, improved mood states, and decreased levels of aggression in these individuals (Auge, 1973; Cherek, 1981; Frankenhauser, Myrsten, & Post, 1970). Although nicotine has been found to affect these processes (Nesbitt, 1973), it is not known whether the observed suppression of emotion and improved mood result entirely from nicotine or from a combination of other factors such as oral and manipulative activities, or conditioned reactions. However, several theories have been proposed to explain the reduced affective response following smoking in the face of autonomic arousal, all centering on nicotine as the mediating agent. One theory is that of cortical desynchronization, that is, a divergence of the activities of cortical and subcortical centers in the brain so that arousal occurs in subcortical areas, leading to autonomic activation, whereas a simultaneous sedation occurs in cortical areas (Eysenck, 1973). This model also predicts differences in the arousal effects of nicotine in different personality types. According to the theory, when arousal of the cortex is initially high (introvert personality) nicotine will act as a depressant and when cortical arousal is low (extrovert personality) nicotine will act as a stimulant. Some support for this theory has come indirectly from studies demonstrating either cortical arousal or depression by nicotine (Brown, 1967; Philips, 1971), but direct evidence is lacking.

Models of Smoking Processes

The task now is to relate these basic biobehavioral principls to smoking initiation, maintenance, and change processes. Social learning theory and data serve as a starting point of discussion; other theories are introduced as the stages progress. Biological factors are added to the model at each phase in the process, albeit somewhat tentatively, given the absence of empirical literature to document the interplay. When these factors are considered together, as in the schema presented in Figure 1, important gaps in our knowledge and directions for future research become readily apparent.

Smoking Initiation

The primary determinants of smoking onset have been described as social influences (Evans *et al.*, 1979; Flay *et al.*, 1983; Kozlowski, 1979). There is a significant correlation between peer smoking and the likelihood that youth will experiment with cigarettes (Alexander *et al.*, 1983; Bewley, Bland, & Harris, 1974; Levitt & Edwards, 1970), and children are twice as likely to smoke if one parent is a smoker, four times as likely if

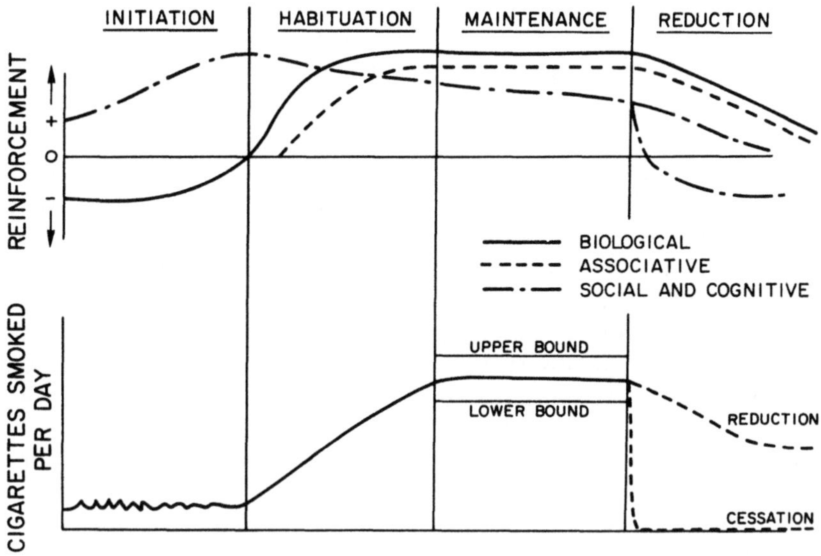

Figure 1. Biobehavioral processes in smoking initiation, maintenance, continuation, and reduction.

both parents smoke (U.S. Public Health Service, 1976). Sibling smoking and the prevalence of smoking in the school have both been shown to be independent risk factors over and above family and peer smoking (Alexander *et al.*, 1983; Best *et al.*, 1984; Flay *et al.*, 1983). Although data are less compelling, the media are also widely believed to exert a significant social influence.

Although there are few multivariate studies comparing the relative importance of social influence and other factors, the data that are available suggest that social influences do explain more variance than other factors during initiation (Bewley *et al.*, 1974; Palmer, 1970; Pederson, Baskerville, & Lefcoe, 1981). How these social influences operate is less clear. Modeling is likely to be involved; peer reward and punishment of smoking behavior probably operate as well. Smoking has also been related to problem behavior such as the taking of other drugs, early sexual activity, and poor academic performance (Bewley & Bland, 1977; Jessor & Jessor, 1977). In these instances, smoking may serve as a secondary reinforcer associated with risk-taking and rebellion. Personality characteristics, primarily extroversion and neuroticism, have been associated with smoking (Cherry & Kiernan, 1976; Mangan & Golding, 1978); cognitive and social rewards may further explain the observed relationship between smoking and factors of self-esteem and autonomy (Ahlgren, Norem, Hochhauser, & Garvin, 1982; Chassin, Presson, Sherman, & Olshausky, 1981).

Are there biological factors that affect the onset process? The first to come into play are probably the punishing, aversive consequences expected with initial acts of smoking, such as dizziness, nausea, and harsh taste. With repeated exposure, however, simple biological adaptation can account for decreasing aversiveness. Repetitive acts of smoking and the rate at which the behavior develops may be a function of how rapidly biological tolerance develops. Individual differences in metabolism and cortical arousal have been cited as possible biological influences that mediate the process of smoking initiation. For example, Silverstein, Kelly, Swan, and Kozlowsi (1982) point out that urinary pH may influence early smoking experience by altering the effective dose of nicotine. Nonsmokers with acidic urine should excrete nicotine faster than those with alkaline urine, making them less likely to experience an aversive reaction and more likely to continue attempts at smoking. Although a relationship between urinary pH and the adoption of smoking behavior has been found only in females (Silverstein *et al.*, 1982), further studies of this nature may enhance our understanding of the role that biological risk and/or protective factors play in initiation and adaptation to smoking.

Maintenance of Smoking Behavior

Initial smoking rate will be quite low, primarily dependent on cues and consequences of social and environmental events, but counterbalanced by aversive biological effects such as nausea. As tolerance increases and conditioning to positive reinforcement develops, smoking rate will increase. Smoking has been implicated in the management of (a) affect, (b) arousal, (c) analgesia, (d) anxiety and tension, and (e) aggression. These primary reinforcing effects, thought to result from the pharmacological action of nicotine, may in turn lead to secondary reinforcement through mechanisms of learning and conditioning. The habit can become increasingly tied to psychological needs, becoming an intrinsic part of the individual's life and serving many functions. According to the theory of nicotine regulation, smokers become accustomed to situation-specific levels of nicotine and titrate its intake to maintain these levels (Schachter, 1979). Furthermore, the negative reinforcement cycle of smoking to avoid withdrawal, as suggested by the classical conditioning model, may develop with repeated exposure. This multiplicity of effects, based on both biological and learning factors, may account for the apparent complexity and variation in individual reasons for smoking. Best and Hakstian (1978) investigated reasons for why people smoke using self-report data. A least squares common-factor analysis extracted 12 factors for males, 11 for females. Items comprising the factors and the biobehavioral issues discussed thus far were strikingly similar. For example, perceptions of "nervous," "worried," and "tense" loaded on one factor, labeled Nervous Tension, and reports of "finishing a meal," "drinking coffee," and "writing a letter" fell together as another factor, titled Habit.

Figure 1 depicts the hypothetical interplay of factors across the smoking processes. Social and cognitive factors are present initially and indeed must be sufficiently powerful to offset the punishing effects of smoking. However, over time the primary reinforcing properties of nicotine, in conjunction with associative learning and classical conditioning effects, can increase in relative importance as the individual becomes a habitual smoker. Thus, daily rate of smoking becomes a function of (a) reinforcement and conditioning parameters, (b) sensitivity to drug effects, and (c) development of tolerance. Each of these factors in turn will be a function of individual and environmental differences.

At what point will smoking rate asymptote? Contrary to the nicostat model, Kozlowski and Herman (1984) argue that rate will be homeostatically controlled within a range defined by relatively independent upper and lower bounds, the upper bound being a function of toxicity and the lower bound a function of reinforcement needs. Environmental influences (e.g., restrictions on smoking, prevalance of smoking models and smoking cues) and behavioral factors (e.g., duration of smoking, depth of inhalation) will affect rate of smoking within these bounds. Once the smoking habit is fully developed, smoking rate will fluctuate between these bounds in response to a variety of biobehavioral influences. The graph in Figure 1 represents an aggregate curve. What we do not know is how these bounds are determined for a particular individual. For instance, is the lower bound an absolute level, or does it operate on a relative basis, such that if a smoker gradually reduces his cigarette consumption his lower bound may lower in response?

Such an account of smoking initiation and maintenance not only is speculative but is still too general to be very useful. The purpose it does serve is that of formulating future research questions. How quickly do the various social-cognitive, biological, and associative learning processes develop and how do their relative contributions change over time? What is the role of individual differences—why do some people remain social smokers, and others very quickly become dependent smokers? How can one distinguish operationally between the strictly pharmacological effects of nicotine and those effects attributed to learning? Although their roles in maintaining smoking behavior are probably intertwined, implications for smoking reduction may differ. Answers to such questions may be needed before more effective treatment programs can be designed.

Smoking Reduction

As indicated in Figure 1, rate most commonly will decrease in response to cognitive and environmental factors, for example, pressures not to smoke, concerns about health effects, and cost. According to Bandura (1977), two types of expectations mediate behavior change: (a) the probability that a given course of action will lead to a particular outcome and (b) one's perception of personal ability to reach that outcome. Thus, the degree to which a smoker believes he or she can change habits and coping responses necessary to quit smoking can influence whether an attempt will be made.

Although the decision to quit is primarily of psychosocial significance, success in rate reduction is further affected by the physiological and behavioral aspects of nicotine dependence. Physiological withdrawal effects, if present, will be dominant in the early stages of reduction. Withdrawal symptoms appear to reflect an overshoot of homeostatic compensatory mechanisms that produce tolerance, as in the opponent process model. Since nicotine has both stimulant and depressant actions, withdrawal symptoms typically include both types of effects.

Thus, the process of smoking reduction can be considered initially to entail a reduction in rate of smoking and the achievement of reliable control. An individual's success will be a function of (a) the magnitude, duration, and direction of physiological reinforcement effects and (b) availability of alternative behaviors to obtain primary and secondary reinforcers. Nicotine gum has been used to attenuate physiological withdrawal symptoms; the concurrent use of counterconditioning, and self-management and/or stress management techniques provides behavioral alternatives to smoking. Once control is firmly establishd, the focus shifts to long-term maintenance of behavioral change wherein the use of learning principles predominates. Existing conditions at any particular point, such as psychosocial stress and social pressures, are thought to be important factors in precipitating relapse. Social support, coping skills, and cognitive restructuring may be implemented to enhance maintenance at this stage. To the extent that nicotine supplementation was used in the initial phase, the need for dealing with physiological withdrawal must eventually be faced, usually by "weaning" the ex-smoker from the nicotine-bearing substitute.

In sum, there are three major tasks involved in smoking reduction:

1. To develop and maintain motivation and incentives for change
2. To counter or successfully manage withdrawal effects
3. To extinguish smoking responses and develop or strengthen alternative behaviors

Current Approaches to Smoking Prevention and Reduction

Our aim in this section is to comment briefly on the literature dealing with smoking control from a biobehavioral perspective. Excellent reviews of both smoking prevention and smoking reduction can be found elsewhere (Best & Bloch, 1979; Evans *et al.*, 1979; Flay, 1985; Lichtenstein & Brown, 1982; Pechacek, 1979; Snow, Gilchrist, & Schenke, 1985; Thompson, 1978). In addition, the 1982 *Annual Review of Public Health* provides useful reviews of smoking control from several different perspectives.

Smoking Prevention

Traditional approaches to smoking prevention, emphasizing knowledge of the long-term health consequences of smoking, have proved to be ineffective (Evans *et al.*, 1979; Thompson, 1978). However, recent work focusing on social influences on smoking is very promising (Flay, 1985). These programs typically aim (a) to teach youth about social influences on smoking, (b) to train skills necessary to resist these influences, (c) to correct perceptions of social norms, and (d) to develop public commitment to nonsmoking. Experimental results are quite consistent, showing that rates of experimentation on a 3-year follow-up are half of those for comparison groups. From these studies, several generalizations and suggestions for future research can be made:

1. The use of social learning theory has much to offer. Despite a relatively superficial understanding of smoking initiation processes, the theory has led to the development of efficacious interventions.
2. Current smoking prevention methods are better suited to prevent smoking experimentation rather than the development of regular smoking, because they ignore biological factors and learning other than social learning. Nevertheless, these programs can lead to significant and sustained smoking cessation (Best *et al.*, 1984;

Flay *et al.*, 1985), presumably because smoking behavior initially is largely socially and cognitively controlled. Development of complementary cessation strategies for youth is indicated. We will require "needs assessment" data to determine the extent and manner to which these cessation strategies may need to attend to biological, classical conditioning, and associative learning factors.

3. Consideration of biological factors at the early initiation stage of smoking suggests additional issues and strategies. For example, the home remedy of having young experimenters smoke an entire pack in a short period of time may prove effective in that initial trials will result in strong biological punishment rather than positive social reinforcement. As another example, the increased availability in recent years of low tar and low nicotine cigarettes may have reduced the naturally aversive nature of early trials and made it easier for youth to experiment.
4. There is a need for longitudinal data on the natural history of smoking. Many studies to date have been cross-sectional in nature, and the few that are prospective have generally collected little or no process data. Such studies are needed to provide information about how smoking develops over time in individuals and in groups.

Smoking Reduction

Early reviews of smoking reduction research suggested very limited program effectiveness (cf. Bernstein, 1969; Hunt & Bespalec, 1974; Keutzer, Lichtenstein & Mees, 1968) but more recent reviews suggest slow improvements and grounds for cautious optimism (e.g., Bernstein & McAlister, 1976; Lichtenstein & Danaher, 1976; Pechacek, 1979). Nevertheless, even the most effective change programs currently achieve no greater than 50% long-term cessation rates.

A variety of techniques have been used to enhance smoking reduction. Although it is not our intention to present a comprehensive review of all such strategies, a brief description of common procedures is provided prior to a discussion of their effectiveness in treatment interventions.

Physiological strategies are employed to help an individual cope with the pharmacological aspects of nicotine addiction. Nicotine fading (Beaver, Brown, & Lichtenstein, 1981; Foxx & Brown, 1979; Prue, Krapfl, & Martin, 1981) provides for progressive reductions in nicotine intake and associated nicotine dependence, concurrent with behavioral changes.

The most promising pharmacological aid to date, nicotine-bearing chewing gum, provides partial nicotine replacement. In this manner, users can maintain a stable blood nicotine level and thus prevent the onset of severe craving and withdrawal symptoms, allowing behavioral aspects of change to be addressed separately. Randomized clinical trials report promising outcomes for abstinence rates at 6 months (Fagerstom, 1982, 1984; Schneider, Jarvik, & Forsythe, 1984), though a role for nicotine replacement in long-term maintenance has yet to be substantiated.

Counterconditioning and extinction techniques are designed first to suppress the smoking response and then to extinguish associations between environmental cues and smoking. Aversive strategies using electric shock, imaginal stimuli, and cigarette smoke itself have been developed. The most common form of the latter—rapid smoking—has proved most successful (Lichtenstein & Brown, 1982). Smokers typically are required to smoke two or three cigarettes without pause, taking puffs every 6 to 8 seconds until tolerance is reached, repeating the procedure daily at first following cessation and then less frequently. Effective suppression of smoking behavior allows extinction to occur as the quitter is exposed to smoking cues.

Alternative responses are of two kinds (Best *et al.*, 1978). *Functional responses* produce the reinforcers conditioned to smoking (e.g., tension reduction, stimulation). *Self-management behaviors* operate to control and reduce the probability of smoking behavior. To the extent that smoking is an operant behavior, alternative means of producing reinforcement must be developed in a nonsmoking life-style. Self-management behaviors are similar to counterconditioning techniques in that they suppress smoking behavior allowing for extinction and the strengthening of functional alternative responses.

Stress management techniques are designed to avoid or reduce arousal during smoking reduction. Withdrawal will produce stress, and a variety of techniques may be used to compensate. The use of tranquilizers during reduction is one example; perhaps more appropriately, environmental changes can be effected so that the prevalence and intensity of other stressors are minimized. Stress management techniques, for example the development of coping skills, provide functional alternative responses to smoking.

Social support and reinforcement strategies mobilize and organize the social environment to facilitate reduction. The strategies cut across those mentioned above, serving two functions. Significant others can help reduce environmental stressors. They can assist in the development and use of functional and self-management alternatives, and provide a source of social reinforcement for alternative behaviors.

There is limited and mixed support for a few single treatment methods, including rapid smoking (Danaher, 1977; Lichtenstein, 1982; Pechacek, 1979) and nicotine-bearing chewing gum (Fagerstrom, 1982; Hughes & Miller, 1984; Raw, Jarvis, Feyerabend, & Russell, 1980; Schneider & Jarvik, 1984). There is general consensus that multifaceted intervention programs tend to be the most effective, but little consensus on what specific techniques to include in a comprehensive program. In this respect, the literature has two major limitations.

First, with a few exceptions (e.g., Fagerstrom, 1982; Killen, Maccoby, & Taylor, 1984; Schlegel, Manske, & Shannon, 1983), the programs are inadequate from a biobehavioral perspective in that the attention given to the diverse determinants of smoking and problems of reduction is not balanced.

Second, research designs often aim to isolate the contribution of single components to program efficacy. This reductionist approach pays no attention to the fact that component strategies may be designed to address very different aspects of the problem. The biobehavioral model of smoking suggests that an integrated set of methods of change is most likely to be effective, each method logically related to others and performing a specific therapeutic role. This "curriculum" view of multifaceted programs suggests that research designs that compare one kind of curriculum to another are more useful than dismantling designs. Of course, efficiency as well as effectiveness must be considered and evaluated. The biobehavioral model also highlights the desirability of tailoring treatments to take into account individual differences in smoking determinants and change program needs. Again, the literature includes very few studies that examine the interaction between subject and treatment factors.

Maintenance of Smoking Reduction

According to Bandura (1977), factors governing cessation differ from those governing maintenance. Indeed, it has been clear to smoking researchers for many years that the more difficult task in reduction is maintenance rather than the initiation of change (cf. Bernstein, 1969; Hunt & Bespalec, 1974), though there remains a lack of research on the problems of maintenance. However, three distinct approaches appear promising.

The first focuses on the development of alternative functional responses. The aim is to "diagnose" the smoker's diverse reasons for smoking and then, for each major smoking situation, to develop a set of alternative behaviors. Several programs emphasizing this approach have been successful (Best, 1978; Brengelmann & Sedlmayr, 1977; Lando, 1977; Pomerleau *et al.*, 1978) although negative results are reported as well

(Danaher, 1977; Glasgow, 1978; Goeckner, 1979). The superiority of these programs with respect to maintenance *per se* (that is, the proportion of initially successfully quitters who remain abstinent) is consistent with but does not establish the effectiveness of training alternative behaviors (Best, 1980).

The second approach adds cognitive elements to the coping skills model. Marlatt and his colleagues (Marlatt, 1978, 1985; Marlatt & Gordon, 1980) have proposed a model of relapse focusing on the "abstinence violation effect"—the quitter's cognitive and emotional reactions to smoking incidents. Results for the few treatment studies based on this approach have been mixed thus far but are generally encouraging (Lichtenstein & Brown, 1980). One attractive feature of the model is that it could easily be expanded to include physiological sequelae to smoking incidents.

The third approach in fact focuses on physiological sequelae (Pomerleau, 1980; Siegel, 1982; Stewart *et al.*, 1984), with classical conditioning and the opponent process model as control features. The approach emphasizes the need to extinguish smoking urges by exposing the quitter to a previous smoking environment while successfully suppressing the behavior. As suggested above, a priming phenomenon could elicit increased physiological activity and craving if a smoking incident did occur (Stewart *et al.*, 1984). The model accounts for the common observation that smoking urges can occur months or even years after the behavior has been eliminated, especially when former smoking situations are reencountered, and that when these urges occur they are experienced as very "physical."

Implications and Conclusions

Can a concise biobehavioral view of smoking be stated? Clearly, both biological and psychosocial processes are centrally involved in smoking behavior, and their influences are both highly complex and variable. Furthermore, the relative contributions of biobehavioral factors change over the course of initiation, maintenance, and reduction.

In the simplest analysis, humans can be seen to use smoking and nicotine for modulating biological and psychological states in order to promote behavioral adaptation and homeostasis. Smoking is thought to serve basic functions in the areas of (a) arousal and performance and (b) affect and drive. If an individual smokes in some sense to coordinate and "optimize" these states, then smoking may serve important and legitimate biological and psychological functions. Thus, the obvious question is, What can an individual do to replace the functions smoking served?

Can these needs be met in other ways such that they do not constitute biological barriers to behavior change and smoking control? This really is an empirical question, an extremely complex and challenging one for which we have almost no data. Nevertheless, from existing data, and the models of smoking processes we have proposed thus far, we can speculate.

Arousal and Performance Functions

The Yerkes–Dodson theory of arousal and performance, combined with experimental data reviewed, suggests that people may smoke to stimulate themselves when underaroused, and smoke to sedate themselves when overaroused. What are alternate ways of increasing and decreasing arousal?

Arousal can be decreased in several ways. Various behavioral strategies for stress management make sense in this context, and there is a growing literature suggesting that exercise training can serve stress management functions (reviewed by Mobily, 1982). Methods of increasing cortical and sympathetic arousal are less obvious. Short of the use of other stimulants and drug taking (see Istvan & Matarazzo, 1984 for a relevant review of caffeine, alcohol, and tobacco use), there may be few alternative behaviors that can be performed in former smoking situations so that arousal is neatly titrated almost moment to moment, as is the case with smoking (Ashton & Stepney, 1982). A possible exception to this may be the use of biofeedback to manipulate EEG activity such that it acts as a substitute for smoking (Griffith & Crossman, 1983). Though still very exploratory at this stage, such a method of increasing arousal may hold promise for use in smoking reduction.

An intriguing notion is the therapeutic use of meditation or exercise training programs to manipulate arousal. As already noted, exercise has modulatory effects on arousal. However, exercise and meditation can serve both to increase and to decrease arousal, suggesting that either may provide comprehensive systems for modulating biological state. Few trained athletes or regular meditators are smokers, and the research of physiological effects of exercise training and meditation suggest effects similar to those produced by smoking. Unfortunately, a conclusion that meditation or exercise causes smoking reduction is precluded by the fact that meditators and athletes are self-selected. Although minimal experimental data do exist to substantiate such an argument, it would seem reasonable to hypothesize that meditation or exercise training could facilitate smoking reduction, and possibly prevent smoking initiation, by providing alternative arousal-modulating behaviors.

One aspect of arousal and performance not addressed thus far relates to the findings that nicotine may enhance learning and memory through actions on the hippocampal learning and memory centers. A critical question is whether smokers have a constitutional or acquired deficit in this respect, and in effect need such pharmacological facilitation or, alternatively, whether adaptation will occur over time with smoking reduction. One troubling possibility is that humans are not biologically well-suited to the sustained levels of alertness we find demanded by our environments and culture. Alternation of waking and sleeping as seen in animals, where high levels of arousal and alertness are reserved for few situations such as threat, may be more natural.

Affect and Drive

Smoking is associated with both positive and negative affect. Management of negative affect might be achieved with behavioral programs for anger (Davidson, 1976; Novaco, 1975), depression (McLean & Hakstian, 1979; Rehm & Kornblith, 1979), or anxiety and fear (Meichenbaum & Cameron, 1983). It is not clear that these programs produce comparable biological effects, and an important research question concerns the extent to which smoking and these alternative behaviors in fact share common pathways. *Affect* is largely a subjective experience, and quite different physiological processes may be labeled similarly, suggesting an illusion of potential substitution. Furthermore, comparability of physiological effects does not ensure therapeutic effectiveness.

Specific methods to produce positive affect are not as readily available. Psychotherapeutic change generally increases positive affect (cf. Prochaska, 1979). Yet, again, there is a growing literature on the utility of managing negative and positive affect with exercise (Folkins, 1976) and meditation (Bahrke & Morgan, 1977; Schwartz, Davidson, & Goleman, 1978).

In the larger context, smoking serves symbolic and cultural functions related to affect which vary across and within societies. As the social meaning of smoking changes, alternative rituals and symbols can produce comparable affective states. Finally, and frankly speculatively, pleasure-producing activities such as listening to music might provide biobehavioral alternatives to smoking.

Research Implications

It is abundantly clear by now that a biobehavioral view of smoking demands sophisticated, programmatic, interdisciplinary research. Biological and behavioral work is required, jointly as well as separately, with a view of basic and applied objectives and methodologies. There are three kinds of research that we feel to be necessary to further our understanding of smoking and smoking control.

First, we must establish more firmly the various functions actually served by smoking, day to day, from one person to another. We require both basic mechanisms research, with animal and human experiments, and observational and field research with smokers at the various stages of initiation, maintenance, and reduction. Objective and perceived reasons for smoking must be related to one another and to potential intervention and strategies for change.

Second, we must develop models and methods for specifying an individual's reasons for smoking. Process research to elucidate smoking behavior change is essential. We must understand why an individual does (or does not) currently smoke and be able to predict what will happen if he or she begins to change.

In relation to this is the need to consider diverse epistemological frameworks. Research and implementation thus far have been limited by a failure to integrate biological and behavioral perspectives. In a similar way, we may be limited if we are unwilling to look beyond the "cultures of science" (cf. Elkana, 1981) and the epistemology of biomedicine. An epistemology that emerges from personalistic, cultural, and symbolic studies may contribute much to our understanding. For example, an ethnographic (anthropological) methodology for studying smoking behavior may develop quite different but complementary understandings and intervention strategies, built on the clear reality that smoking is very much culturally constituted.

Third, we need ways of tailoring treatment alternatives to individual biobehavioral needs (Best, 1978; Best *et al.*, 1978). Specific therapeutic alternatives may have to be developed or refined to address the specific biobehavioral functions of smoking. For example, current products for nicotine supplementation (nicotine-bearing chewing gum) do not fully match the pharmacological effects of smoking, and other products (nicotine aerosols) might be more effective. As another example, stress management techniques such as relaxation, meditation, or biofeedback might be selected and refined to produce biobehavioral effects as much like those of smoking as possible. We recommend integrated research programs in which basic and applied research complement, and contribute to, each other.

Despite the need for ongoing research, we believe that there is sufficient understanding of smoking behavior at this point to design more effective interventions. A combination of self-report and experimental challenges could be used to profile individual reasons for smoking. (For example, the effects of nicotine deprivation or preloading in varying experimental situations may suggest specific functions served by smoking). Monitoring alternative behaviors in various naturally occurring arousal and affect management situations might be of use to predict change processes. A comprehensive treatment package with provisions for selecting components and tailoring them to individual smoking functions and change problems could be designed. A multifaceted process and outcome evaluation strategy could be developed to provide both preliminary indications of treatment efficacy and valuable formative information to guide future basic and applied research and the development of second-generation, more effective interventions.

In conclusion, we find that there is a wide-ranging body of biobehavioral knowledge that can be brought to bear on our understanding of smoking behavior and change. Researchers have neglected basic questions of determinants, but an integration of existing knowledge creates optimism and excitement about future research and intervention possibilities.

ACKNOWLEDGMENTS. The authors wish to thank Heather Ashton, Kelly Brownell, Joel Killen, Lynn Kozlowski, Eugene LeBlanc, Ovide Pomerleau, Martin Raw, Shepard Siegel, and Dennis Willms for their comments on a draft of this manuscript.

References

Ahlgren, A., Norem, A. A., Hochhauser, M., & Garvin, J. (1982). Antecedents of smoking among pre-adolescents. *Journal of Drug Education, 12*(4), 325–340.

Alexander, H. M., Callcott, R., Dobson, A. J., Hardes, G. R., Lloyd, D. M., O'Connell, D. L., & Leader, S. R. (1983). Cigarette smoking and drug use in school children: IV. Factors associated with changes in smoking behavior. *International Journal of Epidemiology, 12*(1), 59–66.

Andersson, K. (1975). Effects of cigarette smoking on learning and retention. *Psychopharmacologia, 41,* 1–5.

Armitage, A. K., Hall, G. H., & Sellers, C. M. (1969). Effects of nicotine on electrocortical activity and acetylcholine release from the cat cerebral cortex. *British Journal of Pharmacology, 35,* 152–160.

Ashton, H., & Stepney, R. (1982). *Smoking: Psychology and pharmacology.* London: Tavistock Publications.

Ashton, H., & Watson, D. W. (1970). Puffing frequency and nicotine intake in cigarette smokers. *British Medical Journal, 3,* 679–681.

Ashton, H., Savage, R. D., Telford, R., Thompson, J. W., & Watson, D. W. (1972). The effects of cigarette smoking on the response to stress in a driving simulator. *British Journal of Pharmacology, 45,* 546–556.

Auge, C. (1973). Smoking patterns, nicotine intake at different times of day and changes in two cardiovascular variables while smoking cigarettes. *Psychopharmacologia, 30,* 135–144.

Bahrke, M. S., & Morgan, W. P. (1977). Anxiety reduction following exercise and meditation. *Cognitive Therapy and Research, 2,* 323.

Balfour, D. J. K. (1982). The pharmacology of nicotine dependence: A working hypothesis. *Pharmacology and Therapeutics, 15,* 239–250.

Bandura, A. (1977). *Social learning theory.* Englewood Cliffs, NJ: Prentice-Hall.

Beaver, C., Brown, R. A., & Lichtenstein, E. (1981). Effects of monitored nicotine fading and anxiety management training on smoking reduction. *Addictive Behaviors, 6,* 301–305.

Beckett, A. H., & Triggs, E. J. (1967). Enzyme induction in man caused by smoking. *Nature, 216,* 587.

Beckett, A. H., Rowland, M., & Triggs, E. J. (1965). Significance of smoking in investigations of urinary excretion rates of amines in man. *Nature, 207*(4993), 200–201.

Benowitz, N. L., Jacob, P., Jones, R. T., & Rosenberg, J. (1982). Inter-individual variability in the metabolism and cardiovascular effects of nicotine in man. *Journal of Pharmacology and Experimental Therapeutics, 221,* 368–372.

Benowitz, N. L., Kuyt, F., & Jacob, P. (1981). Circadian study of cardiovascular and hormonal responses to smoking high or low nicotine cigarettes. *Clinical Research, 29,* 269A.

Bernstein, D. A. (1969). Modification of smoking behavior: An evaluative review. *Psychological Bulletin, 71*(6), 418–440.

Bernstein, D. A., & McAlister, A. L. (1976). The modification of smoking behavior: Progress and problems. *Addictive Behaviors, 1,* 89–102.

Best, J. A. (1978). Targeting and self-selection of smoking modification methods. In J. L. Schwartz (Ed.), *Progress in smoking cessation: Proceedings of International Conference on Smoking Cessation.* New York: American Cancer Society.

Best, J. A. (1980). Mass media, self management, and smoking modification. In P. C. Davidson & S. M. Davidson (Eds.), *Behavioral medicine: Changing health life-styles.* New York: Brunner/Mazel.

Best, J. A., & Bloch, M. (1979). Compliance in the control of cigarette smoking. In R. E. Haynes, D. W. Taylor, & D. L. Sackett (Eds.), *Compliance in Health Care.* Baltimore: Johns Hopkins University Press.

Best, J. A., & Hakstian, A. R. (1978). A situation-specific model for smoking behavior. *Addictive Behaviors, 3,* 79–92.

Best, J. A., Owen, L. E., & Trentadue, B. L. (1978). Comparison of satiation and rapid smoking in self-managed smoking cessation. *Addictive Behaviors, 3,* 71–78.

Best, J. A., Flay, B. R., Towson, S. M., Ryan, K. B., Perry, C. L., Brown, K. S., Kersell, M. W., & d'Avernas, J. R. (1984). Smoking prevention and the concept of risk. *Journal of Applied Social Psychology, 14,* 257–273.

Bewley, B. R., & Bland, J. M. (1977). Academic performance and social factors related to cigarette smoking by schoolchildren. *British Journal of Preventive & Social Medicine, 31,* 18–24.

Bewley, B. R., Bland, J. M., & Harris, R. (1974). Factors associated with the starting of cigarette smoking by primary schoolchildren. *British Journal of Preventive and Social Medicine, 28,* 37–44.

Brengelmann, J. C., & Sedlmayr, E. (1977). Experiments in the reduction of smoking behavior. In J. Steinfeld, W. Griffiths, K. Ball, & R. M. Taylor (Eds.), *Proceedings of the Third World Conference On Smoking and Health: Volume 2. Health Consequences, Education, Cessation Activities and Social Action.* New York, June, 1975. U.S. Department of HEW, Public Health Service, National Institute of Health, National Cancer Institute, DHEW Pub. No. (NIH) 77-1413, 533–543.

Brown, B. B. (1967). Relationship between evoked response changes and behavior following small doses of nicotine. *Annals of the New York Academy of Science, 142,* 190–200.

Cappell, H., & LeBlanc, A. E. (1981). Tolerance and physical dependence: Do they play a role in alcohol and drug self-administration? In Y. Israel, R. B. Glaser, H. Kalant, R. E. Popham, W. Schmidt, & R. G. Smart (Eds.), *Research advances in alcohol and drug problems* (Vol. 6, pp. 159–196.) New York: Plenum Press.

Chassin, L., Presson, C. C., Sherman, S. J., & Olshausky, R. W. (1981). Self-images and cigarette smoking in adolescence. *Personality and Social Psychology Bulletin, 7*(4), 670–676.

Cherek, D. R. (1981). Effects of smoking different doses of nicotine on human aggressive behavior. *Psychopharmacology, 75*, 339–345.

Cherry, N., & Kiernan, K. (1976). Personality scores and smoking behavior: A longitudinal study. *British Journal of Preventive and Social Medicine, 30*,123–131.

Conway, T. L., Vickers, R. R., Ward, H. W., & Rahe, R. H. (1981). Occupational stress and variation in cigarettes, coffee, and alcohol consumption. *Journal of Health and Social Behavior, 22*, 155–165.

Corcoran, D. W. J. (1965). Personality and the inverted U relation. *British Journal of Psychology, 56*, 267–273.

Crow, T. J., & Deakin, J. F. W. (1978). Brain reinforcement centres and psychoactive drugs. In Y. Israel, F. B. Glaser, H. Kalant, R. E. Popham, W. Schmidt, & R. G. Smart (Eds.), *Research advances in alcohol and drug problems* (Vol. 4, pp. 25–76). New York: Plenum Press.

Cryer, P. E., Haymond, M. W., Santiago, J. V., & Shah, S. D. (1976). Norepinephrine and epinephrine release and adrenergic mediation of smoking-associated hemodynamic and metabolic events. *New England Journal of Medicine, 295*(11), 573–577.

Danaher, B. G. (1977). Rapid smoking and self-control in the modification of smoking behavior. *Journal of Consulting and Clinical Psychology, 45*(6), 1068–1107.

Davidson, P. O. (Ed.) (1976). *Behavioral Strategies in the Management of Anxiety, Anger and Pain*. New York: Brunner/Mazel.

deVolx, B. C., Oliver, C., Giraud, P., Gillioz, P. E., Castanas, E., Lissitsky, J. C., Boudouresque, F., & Millet, Y. (1981). Effect of nicotine on *in vivo* secretions of melanoconicotropic hormones in the rat. *Life Sciences, 28*, 1067–1073.

Elkana, Y. (1981). A programmatic attempt at an anthropology of knowledge. In E. Mendelsohn & Y. Elkana (Eds.), *Sciences and cultures: Anthropological and historical studies of the sciences* (pp. 1–76). Dordrecht:D. Reidel.

Emery, F. E., Hilgendorf, E. L., & Irvin, B. C. (1968). *The psychological dynamics of smoking*. London: Tobacco Research Council Paper 10.

Evans, R. I., Henderson, A. H., Hill, P. C., & Raines, B. E. (1979). Current psychological, social and educational programs in control and prevention of smoking: A critical methodological review. In A. M. Gotto & R. Paolette (Eds.), *Atherosclerosis reviews*. New York: Raven Press.

Eysenck, H. J. (1973). Personality and the maintenance of the smoking habit. In W. L. Dunn, Jr. (Ed.), *Smoking behavior: Motives and incentives*. Washington, D.C.: Winston.

Fagerstrom, K. O. (1982). A comparison of psychosocial and pharmacological treatment in smoking cessation. *Journal of Behavioral Medicine, 5*, 343–351.

Fagerstrom, K. O. (1984). Effects of nicotine chewing gum and follow-up appointments in physician-based smoking cessation. *Preventive Medicine, 13*, 517–527.

Finnegan, J. K., Larson, P. S., & Haag, H. B. (1945). The role of nicotine in the cigarette habit. *Science, 102*, 94–96.

Flay, B. R. (1985). What do we know about the social influences approach to smoking prevention? Review and recommendations. In C. Bell & R. Battjes (Eds.), *Prevention research: Deterring drug abuse among children and adolescents*. Washington, D. C.: NIDA Research Monograph. 63.

Flay, B. R., d'Avernas, J. R., Best, J. A., Kersell, M. W., & Ryan, K. B. (1983). Cigarette smoking: Why young people do it and ways of preventing it. In P. McGrath & P. Firestone (Eds.) *Pediatric and adolescent behavioral medicine*. New York: Springer-Verlag.

Flay, B. R., Ryan, K. B., Best, J. A., Brown, K. S., Kersell, M. W., d'Avernas, J. R., & Zanna,

M. P. (1985). Are social psychological smoking prevention programs effective? The Waterloo Study. *Journal of Behavioral Medicine, 8,* 37–59.

Flood, J. F., Bennett, E. L., Orme, A. E., Rosenzwieg, M. R., & Jarvik, M. E., (1978). Memory: Modification of anisomycin-induced amnesia by stimulants and depressants. *Science, 199,* 329–336.

Folkins, C. H. (1976). Effects of physical training on mood. *Journal of Clinical Psychology, 32,* 385.

Foxx, R. M., & Brown, R. A. (1979). Nicotine fading and self monitoring for cigarette abstinence or controlled smoking. *Journal of Applied Behavior Analysis, 12,* 111–125.

Frankenhauser, M., Myrsten, A. L., & Post, B. (1970). Psychophysiological reactions to cigarette smoking. *Scandinavian Journal of Psychology, 11,* 237–245.

Frith, C. D. (1971). Smoking behavior and its reaction to the smoker's immediate experience. *British Journal of Social and Clinical Psychology, 10,* 73–78.

Fuller, R. G. C., & Forrest, D. W. (1973). Behavioral aspects of cigarette smoking in relation to arousal level. *Psychological Reports, 33,* 115–121.

Garvey, A. J., Bosse, R., & Seltzer, C. C. (1974). Smoking, weight change, and age. *Archives of Environmental Health, 28,* 327–329.

Gilbert, D. G. (1979). Paradoxical tranquilizing and emotion-reducing effects of nicotine. *Psychological Bulletin, 86,* 643–661.

Gilbert, D., & Hagan, R. (1980). The effects of nicotine and extroversion on self-report, skin conductance, electromyographic and heart responses to emotional stimuli. *Addictive Behaviors, 5,* 247–258.

Glad, W. R., Tyre, T. W., & Adesso, V. J. (1976). A multidimensional model of cigarette smoking. *American Journal of Clinical Hypnosis, 19,* 82–90.

Glasgow, R. E. (1978). Effects of a self-control manual, rapid smoking, and amount of therapist contact on smoking reduction. *Journal of Consulting and Clinical Psychology, 46,* 1439–1447.

Glassman, A. H., Jackson, W. K., Walsh, B. T., Roose, S. P., & Rosenfeld, B. (1984). Cigarette craving, smoking withdrawal and clonidine. *Science, 226,* 864–866.

Goeckner, D. J. (1979). A multifaceted approach to smoking modification: Training in alternate response strategies. *Dissertation Abstracts International, 40*(1), 450. (University Microfilms No. 7915354.)

Goldfarb, T. L., Jarvik, M. E., & Glick, S. D. (1970). Cigarette nicotine content as a determinant of human smoking behavior. *Psychopharmacologia, 17,* 89–93.

Golding, J., & Mangan, G. L. (1982). Arousing and de-arousing effects of cigarette smoke under conditions of stress and mild sensory isolation. *Psychophysiology, 19,* 449–456.

Goodman Gilman, A., Goodman, L. S., & Gilman, A. (Eds.) (1980). *The pharmacological basis of therapeutics* (6th ed.). New York: Macmillan.

Griffith, E. E., & Crossman, E. (1983). Biofeedback: A possible substitute for smoking, Experiment 1. *Addictive Behaviors, 8,* 277–285.

Grunberg, N. E. (1982). The effects of nicotine and cigarette smoking on food consumption and taste preferences. *Addictive Behaviors, 7,* 317–331.

Haag, H. B., & Larson, P. S. (1942). Studies on the fate of nicotine in the body. I: The effect of pH on the urinary excretion of nicotine by tobacco smokers. *Journal of Pharmacology and Experimental Therapeutics, 76,* 235–239.

Hill, P., & Wynder, E. L., (1974). Smoking and cardiovascular disease: Effect of nicotine on serum epinephrine and corticoids. *American Heart Journal, 87,* 491–496.

Hughes, J. R., & Miller, M. S. (1984). Nicotine gum to help stop smoking. *Journal of the American Medical Association, 252*(20), 2855–2858.

Hunt, W. A., & Bespalec, D. A. (1974). An evaluation of current methods of modifying smoking behavior. *Journal of Clinical Psychology, 30,* 431–438.

Hunt, W. A., Matarazzo, J. D., Weiss, S. M., & Gentry, W. D. (1979). Associative learning, habit, and health behavior. *Journal of Behavioral Medicine, 2*(2), 111–124.

Hutchinson, R. S., & Emley, G. S. (1973). Effects of nicotine and avoidance, conditioned suppression and aggression response measures in animals and man. In W. L. Dunn (Ed.), *Smoking behavior: Motives and incentives.* Washington, DC: Winston.

Ikard, F. F., Green, D. E., & Horn, D. (1969). A scale to differentiate between types of smoking as related to the management of affect. *International Journal of Addiction, 4,* 649–659.

Istvan, J., & Matarazzo, J. D. (1984). Tobacco, alcohol and caffeine use: A review of their interrelationships. *Psychological Bulletin, 95*(2), 301–326.

Jessor, R., & Jessor, S. L. (1977). *Problem behavior and psychosocial development: A longitudinal study of youth.* New York: Academic Press.

Keutzer, C. S., Lichtenstein, E., & Mees, H. L. (1968). Modification of smoking behavior: A review. *Psychological Bulletin, 70,*520–533.

Killen, J. D., Maccoby, N., & Taylor, C. B. (1984). Nicotine gum and self-regulation training in smoking relapse prevention. *Behavior Therapy, 15* 234–238.

Knott, V., & Venables, P. (1977). EEG alpha correlates of non-smokers, smoking and smoking deprivation. *Psychophysiology, 14,* 150–156.

Kosterlitz, H. W., & Hughes, J. (1978). Biological significance of the endogenous opiod peptides and the opiate receptors. In Y. Israel, F. B. Glaser, H. Kalant, R. E. Popham, W. Schmidt, & R. G. Smart (Eds.), *Research advances in alcohol and drug problems* (Vol. 4, pp. 1–24). New York: Plenum Press.

Kozlowski, L. T. (1979). Psychosocial influences on cigarette smoking. In *Smoking and health: A report of the Surgeon General.* U.S. Department of Health, Education and Welfare Publication No. (PHS) 79-50066. Washington, DC: U.S. Government Printing Office.

Kozlowski, L. T., & Herman, C. P. (1984). The interaction of psychosocial and biological determinants of tobacco use: More on the boundary model. *Journal of Applied Social Psychology, 14,* 244–256.

Lando, H. A. (1977). Successful treatment of smokers with a broad-spectrum behavioral approach. *Journal of Consulting and Clinical Psychology, 45*(3), 361–366.

Leventhal, H., & Cleary, P. D. (1980). The smoking problem: A review of the research and theory in behavioral risk modification. *Psychological Bulletin, 88*(2), 370–405.

Levitt, E. E., & Edwards, J. A. (1970). A multivariate study of correlative factors in youthful cigarette smoking. *Developmental Psychology,* 2, 5.

Lichtenstein, E. (1982). The smoking problem: A behavioral perspective. *Journal of Consulting & Clinical Psychology, 50*(6), 804–819.

Lichtenstein, E., & Brown, R. A. (1980). Smoking cessation methods. Review and recommendations. In W. R. Miller (Ed.), *The addictive behaviors: Treatment of alcoholism, drug abuse, smoking, and obesity.* Oxford: Pergamon Press.

Lichtenstein, E., & Brown, R. A. (1982). Current trends in the modification of cigarette dependence. In A. S. Bellack, M. Hersen, A. E. Kazdin (Eds.), *International handbook of behavior modification and therapy.* New York: Plenum Press.

Lichtenstein, E., & Danaher, B. G. (1976). Modification of smoking behavior: A critical analysis of theory, research, and practice. In M. Hersen, R. M. Eisler, & P. M. Miller (Eds.), *Progress in behavior modification.* New York: Academic Press.

Mangan, G. L., & Golding, J. (1978). An "enhancement" model of smoking maintenance? In R. E. Thornton (Ed)., *Smoking behavior: Physiological and psychological influences.* Edinburgh: Churchill Livingstone.

Marlatt, G. A. (1978). Craving for alcohol, loss of control, and relapse. A cognitive-behavioral analysis. In P. E. Nathan, G. A. Marlatt, & T. Loberg (Eds.), *Alcoholism: New directions in behavioral research and treatment.* New York: Plenum Press.

Marlatt, G. A. (1985). Relapse prevention: Theoretical rationale and overview of the model. In G. A. Marlatt & J. R. Gordon (Eds.), *Relapse prevention: Maintenance strategies in the treatment of addictive behaviors*. New York: Guilford Press.

Marlatt, G. A., & Gordon, J. R. (1980). Determinants of relapse: Implications for the maintenance of behavior change. In P. O. Davidson & S. M. Davidson (Eds.), *Behavioral medicine: Changing health life-styles*, New York: Brunner/Mazel.

Mausner, B., & Platt, E. S. (1971). *Smoking: A behavioral analysis*. New York: Pergamon Press.

McLean, P. D., & Hakstian, A. R. (1979). Clinical depression: Comparative efficacy of outpatient treatments. *Journal of Consulting and Clinical Psychology, 47*(5), 818–836.

Meichenbaum, D., & Cameron, R. (1983). Stress innoculation training: Toward a general paradigm for training coping skills. In D. Meichenbaum & M. Jaremko (Eds.), *Stress reduction and prevention* (pp. 115–154). New York: Plenum Press.

Mobily, K. (1982). Using physical activity and recreation to cope with stress and anxiety: A review. *American Corrective Therapy Journal, 36*(3), 77–81.

Morrison, C. F., & Armitage, A. K. (1967). Effects of nicotine on the free operant behavior of rats and spontaneous motor activity of mice. *Annals of the New York Academy of Sciences, 142*, 268–276.

Myrsten, K. L., Post, B., Frankenhauser, M., & Johansson, G. (1972). Changes in behavioral and psychological activation induced by cigarette smoking on habitual smokers. *Psychopharmacologia, 27*, 305–312.

Nesbitt, P. D. (1973). Smoking, physiological arousal, and emotional response. *Journal of Personality and Social Psychology, 25*(1), 137–144.

Novaco, R. W. (1975). *Anger control: The development and evaluation of an experimental treatment*. Lexington, MA: Heath.

Ontario Council of Health. (1982). *Smoking and health in Ontario: A need for balance*. Report of the Task Force on Smoking. Toronto: Author.

Palmer, A. B. (1970). Some variables contributing to the onset of cigarette smoking among junior high school students. *Social Science & Medicine, 4*, 359–366.

Pechacek, T. F. (1979). Modification of smoking behavior. In *Smoking and health: A report of the Surgeon General*. DHEW Pub. No. (PHS) 79-50066. Washington, DC: U.S. Government Printing Office.

Pechacek, T. F., & Danaher, B. G. (1979). How and why people quit smoking: A cognitive-behavioral analysis. In P. C. Kendall & S. D. Hollon (Eds.), *Cognitive-behavioral interventions: Theory, research and procedures*. New York: Academic Press.

Pechacek, T. F., & McAlister, A. (1979). Strategies for the modification of smoking behavior: Treatment and prevention. In J. Ferguson & C. B. Taylor (Eds.), *A comprehensive handbook of behavioral medicine*. New York: Spectrum Publications.

Pederson, L. L., Baskerville, J. L., & Lefcoe, N. M. (1981). Multivariate prediction of cigarette smoking among children in grades six, seven and eight. *Journal of Drug Education, 11*(3), 191–203.

Perlick, D. (1977). *The withdrawal syndrome: Nicotine addiction and the effects of stopping smoking in heavy and light smokers*. Unpublished doctoral dissertation, Columbia University, New York.

Philips, C. (1971). The EEG changes associated with smoking. *Psychophysiology, 8*, 64–74.

Pomerleau, O. F. (1980). Why people smoke: Current psychobiological models. In P. O. Davidson. & S. M. Davidson (Eds.), *Behavioral medicine: Changing health life-styles*. New York: Brunner/Mazel.

Pomerleau, O. F. (1981). Underlying mechanisms in substance abuse: Examples from research on smoking. *Addictive Behaviors, 6*, 187–196.

Pomerleau, O. F., Adkins, O., & Pertschuk, M. (1978). Predictors of outcome and recidivism in smoking cessation treatment. *Addictive Behaviors, 3*, 65–70.

Pomerleau, O. F., Fertig, J. B., Seyler, E. L., & Jaffe, J. (1983). Neuroendocrine reactivity to nicotine in smokers. *Psychopharmacology, 81,* 61–67.

Pomerleau, O. F., Fertig, J. B., & Shanahan, S. O. (1983). Nicotine dependence in cigarette smoking: An empirically based, multivariate model. *Pharmacology, Biochemistry and Behavior, 19,* 291–299.

Pomerleau, O. F., Turk, D.C., & Fertig, J. B. (1984). The effects of cigarette smoking on pain and anxiety. *Addictive Behaviors, 9,* 265–271.

Prochaska, J. O. (1979). *Systems of psychotherapy: A transtheoretical analysis.* Homewood, IL: Dorsey Press.

Prue, D. M., Krapfl, J. E., & Martin, J. E. (1981). Biochemical exposure following changes to low tar and nicotine cigarettes. *Behavior Therapy, 12,* 400–416.

Raw, M. (1978). The treatment of cigarette dependence. In Y. Israel, F. B. Glaser, H. Kalant, R. E. Popham, W. Schmidt, & R. G. Smart (Eds.), *Research advances in alcohol and drug problems.* New York: Plenum Press.

Raw, M., Jarvis, M. J., Feyerbend, C., & Russell, M.A.H. (1980). Comparison of nicotine chewing gum and psychological treatments for dependent smokers. *British Medical Journal, 1,* 481–484.

Rehm, L. P., & Kornblith, S. J. (1979). Behavior therapy for depression: A review of recent developments. *Progress in Behavior Modification, 7,* 277–318.

Rose, J. E., Ananda, S., & Jarvik, M. E. (1983). Cigarette smoking during anxiety-provoking and monotonous tasks. *Addictive Behaviors, 8,* 353–359.

Rowe, J. W., Kilgore, A., & Robertson, G. L. (1980). Evidence in man that cigarette smoking induces vasopressin release via an airway-specific mechanism. *Journal of Clinical Endocrinology and Metabolism, 51,* 170–172.

Russell, M. A. H. (1974). Realistic goals for smoking and health. A case for safe smoking. *Lancet, 1*(7851), 254–258.

Russell, M. A. H., & Feyerabend, C. (1978). Cigarette smoking: A dependence on high nicotine boli. *Drug Metabolism Reviews, 8*(1), 29–57.

Russell, M. A. H., Raw, M., & Jarvis, M. J. (1980). Clinical use of nicotine chewing gum. *British Medical Journal, 280,* 972–976.

Schachter, S. (1977). Nicotine regulation in heavy and light smokers. *Journal of Experimental Psychology: General, 106,* 5–12.

Schachter, S. (1979). Regulation, withdrawal, and nicotine addiction. In N. A. Krasnegor (Ed.), *Cigarette smoking as a dependence process.* NIDA Research Monograph 23, DHEW Pub. No. (ADM) 79-800. Washington, DC: U.S. Government Printing Office.

Schachter, S., Kozlowski, L. T., & Silverstein, B. (1977). Effects of urinary pH on cigarette smoking. *Journal of Experimental Psychology: General, 106*(1), 13–19.

Schachter, S., Silverstein, B., Kozlowski, L. T., Herman, C. P., & Liebling, B. (1977). Effects of stress on cigarette smoking and urinary pH. *Journal of Experimental Psychology: General, 106,* 24–30

Schachter, S., Silverstein, B., & Perlick, D. (1977). Psychological and pharmacological explanations of smoking under stress. *Journal of Experimental Psychology: General, 106,* 31–40.

Schlegel, R. P., Manske, S. R., & Shannon, M. (1985). Butt out: Evaluation of the Canadian Armed Forces smoking cessation program. In D. Nostbakken, W. F. Forbes, & R. Frecker (Eds.), *Proceedings of the Fifth World Conference on Smoking and Health.* Ottawa: Canadian Council on Smoking and Health.

Schneider, N. G., & Jarvik, M. E. (1984). Time course of smoking withdrawal symptoms as a function of nicotine replacement. *Psychopharmacology, 82,* 143–144.

Schneider, N. G., Jarvik, M. E., & Forsythe, A. B. (1984). Nicotine vs. placebo gum in the alleviation of withdrawal during smoking cessation. *Addictive Behaviors, 9, 149–156.*

Schwartz, G. E., Davidson, R. J., & Goleman, D. J. (1978) Patterning of cognitive and somatic processes in the self-regulation of anxiety: Effects of meditation versus exercise. *Psychosomatic Medicine, 40,* 321.

Schwartz, J., & Dubitzky, M. D. (1968). Changes in anxiety, mood, and self-esteem resulting from an attempt to stop smoking. *American Journal of Psychiatry, 124,* 138–142.

Seyler, L. E., Fertig, J., Pomerleau, O. F., Hunt, D., & Parker, K. (1984). The effects of smoking on ACTH and cortisol secretion. *Life Sciences, 34,* 57–65.

Shiffman, S. M. (1979). The tobacco withdrawal syndrome. In N. A. Krasnegor (Ed.), *Cigarette smoking as a dependent process.* National Institute on Drug Abuse Research Monograph 23. DHEW Pub. No. (ADM) 79-800, Washington, DC: U.S. Government Printing Office.

Siegel, S. (1982). Classical conditioning, drug tolerance and drug dependence. In R. C. Smart, F. B. Glaser, Y. Israel, H. Kalant, R. E. Popham, & W. Schmidt (Eds.), *Research advances in alcohol and drug problems* (Vol. 7). New York: Plenum Press.

Silverstein, B. (1977). An addiction explanation of cigarette-induced relaxation. Doctoral dissertation, Columbia University, 1976, *Dissertation Abstracts International,* 37 1029B (University Microfilms No. 76-17, 863).

Silverstein, B., Kelly, E., Swan, J., & Kozlowski, L. T. (1982). Physiological predisposition toward becoming a cigarette smoker: Experimental evidence for a sex difference. *Addictive Behaviors, 7,* 83–86.

Skinner, B. F. (1953). *Science and human behavior.* New York: MacMillan.

Snow, W. H., Gilchrist, L. D., & Schenke, S. P. (1985). A critique of progress in adolescent smoking prevention. *Children and Youth Services Review, 1,* 1–19.

Solomon, R. L. (1977). An opponent-process theory of acquired motivation: The affective dynamics of addiction. In J. D. Maser & M. E. P. Seligman (Eds.), *Psychopathology: Experimental models.* San Francisco: Freeman.

Solomon, R. L. & Corbit, J. D. (1973). An opponent-process theory of motivation: II. Cigarette addiction. *Journal of Abnormal Psychology, 81,* 158–171.

Solomon, R. L., & Corbit, J. D. (1974). An opponent-process theory of motivation: The temporal diagnosis of affect. *Psychological Review, 81,* 119–145.

Stephens, R. M. (1977). Psychophysiological variables in cigarette smoking and reinforcing effects of nicotine. *Addictive Behaviors, 2,* 1–7.

Stewart, J., deWit, H., & Eikelboom, R. (1984). Role of unconditioned and conditioned drug effects in the self-administration of opiates and stimulants. *Psychological Review, 91*(2), 251–268.

Tarriere, C., & Hartenmann, F. (1964). Investigation into the effects of tobacco smoke on a visual viligance task. In *Proceedings of the Second International Congress of Ergonomics,* (pp. 525–530). London: Taylor & Francis.

Ternes, J. W. (1977). An opponent-process theory of habitual behavior with special reference to smoking. In M. E. Jarvik, J. W. Cullen, E. R. Gritz, T. N. Vogt. & L. J. West (Eds.). *Research on smoking behavior.* NIDA Research Monograph 17. Washington DC: U.S. Government Printing Office.

Thompson, E. L. (1978). Smoking education programs, 1960–1976. *American Journal of Public Health, 68*(3), 250–257.

Tomkins, S. S. (1966). Psychological model for smoking behavior. *American Journal of Public Health, 56,* 17–20.

Ulett, J., & Itil, T. (1969). Quantitative EEG in smoking and smoking deprivation. *Science, 164,* 969–970.

U.S. Public Health Service (1976). *Teenage smoking: National patterns of cigarette smoking, ages 12 through 18 in 1972 and 1974.* NIH Pub. No. 76-931. Washington, DC: U.S. Department of Health, Education, and Welfare.

Van Ree, J. M., & DeWied, D. (1981). Brain peptides and psychoactive drug effects. In Y. Israel, F. B. Glaser, H. Kalant, R. E. Popham, W. Schmidt, & R. G. Smart (Eds.), *Research advances in alcohol and drug problems* (Vol. 6, 67–105). New York: Plenum Press.

Wesnes, K., & Warburton, D. M. (1978). The effects of cigarette smoking and nicotine tablets upon human attention. In R. E. Thornton (Ed.), *Smoking behavior. Physiological and psychological influences*. Edinburgh: Churchill Livingstone.

World Health Organization Expert Committee on Smoking Control. (1979). *Controlling the smoking epidemic*. Technical Report, Series 636. Geneva: Author.

CHAPTER 5

Considerations in the Treatment of Insomnia

P. H. Van Oot and T. D. Borkovec

Insomnia is a condition that affects nearly everyone at some time, but about one third of the population suffers from the problem chronically (Bixler, Kales, Soldatos, & Healey, 1979; Kales & Kales, 1984). It is the most common sleep-related complaint and is associated with a wide variety of psychiatric and physical disorders (Bixler *et al.*, 1979; Bixler, Kales, & Soldatos, 1979; Kales & Kales, 1984). The alleviation of insomnia is a major concern for public health practitioners, but the available treatments, as they are usually prescribed and implemented, are unreliable and often ineffective. To treat the complaint of insomnia effectively, practitioners must be aware of the variety of causes and manifestations of this complaint and its psychosocial effects. Too often a unidimensional prescriptive approach is taken without adequate consideration of the causes or effects of the problem itself. This approach is marginally effective at best and can lead to more serious or counterproductive results exacerbating the original problem unnecessarily.

This chapter focuses on the biological barriers to the behavioral treatment of insomnia and places the discussion of these barriers in a more general discussion of the problems of conceptualizing and treating insomnia. The purpose of the chapter is not to show how behavioral therapies can be improved *per se*. That is implicit. The goal, rather, is to show how the behavioral therapies can be more effectively integrated into a comprehensive, efficacious treatment package.

P. H. Van Oot and T. D. Borkovec • Department of Psychology, Pennsylvania State University, University Park, Pennsylvania 16802.

The Complaint of Insomnia

In order to treat insomnia it is essential to understand that insomnia is a symptom of either one or more combination of physiological, psychosocial, and behavioral problems and not a clinical entity unto itself. The general category of insomnia includes a heterogeneous group of sleep-disturbed individuals, and progress in obtaining information about this group has been a function of the successful specification of the various potential causes of the symptomatic inability to obtain adequate sleep. In 1979, a Diagnostic Classification of Sleep and Arousal Disorders (DCSAD) was published in the journal *Sleep* (Dement & Guilleminault, 1979). The DCSAD is the first major attempt to distinguish systematically among the various manifestations of sleep disorders and offers a detailed symptomatology of a variety of sleep-related complaints.

The DCSAD has established four major categories of sleep disturbance: "Disorders of Initiating and Maintaining Sleep" (DIMS), "Disorders of Excessive Somnolence" (DOES), "Disorders of the Sleep–Wake Schedule," and "Dysfunctions Associated with Sleep, Sleep Stages, or Partial Arousals." The focus of this chapter is primarily with the DIMS, or insomnias, but examples of the other categories that are often confused and misdiagnosed as insomnia will be considered as needed. Practitioners are strongly urged to familiarize themselves with the DCSAD, particularly if sleep complaints comprise a sizable portion of their clientele. The major limitation of the DCSAD is that specific discussions of etiology of the categories are limited or absent. This may arise from the fact that many largely inconsistent theoretical conceptualizations of the various sleep disorders presently comprise the insomnia literature. Four major problems in conceptualizing and studying insomnia present current obstacles to a complete understanding of the disorder.

First, we know very little about the nature and functions of sleep *per se*. Studies disagree about the purpose or function of the various sleep stages and states, and selective deprivation of these stages or states has not conclusively or reliably demonstrated any enduring detrimental effects. Moreover, the processes that underlie these stages and states of sleep, that is, their purpose, have not been conclusively demonstrated. Consequently, the exact implications of reduced sleep are difficult to specify (Mendelson, 1980).

Second, individuals vary greatly in the amount of sleep they need to feel and function well during the day. Cases of people who average only 3 to 4 hours of sleep per night without any deleterious medical or psychosocial consequences indicate that some humans may indeed require very little sleep (Jones & Oswald, 1968). Thus, as numerous writers have suggested, a definition of insomnia in terms of objectively verified quantity of sleep is currently impossible in at least so far as our only empirical measure of quantifying sleep, the electroencephalogram (EEG) is concerned (cf. Kales & Kales, 1984). Insomnia, therefore, remains a subjectively determined phenomenon for the most part; the client must perceive that he or she is obtaining insufficient sleep that leads to impaired daytime function (Kales & Kales, 1984; Mendelson, Gillin, & Wyatt, 1977; Williams & Karacan, 1978).

Third, the existence of numerous causes of symptomatic sleep disturbance suggests that many subtypes of the disorder exist. Some subtypes of etiological significance have been identified, whereas others have merely been hypothesized. Such heterogeneity has clear implications for interpreting past and designing future research as this research relates to clinical application and treatment development. Equivocal results in comparisons of good and poor sleepers, for example, may indicate either that the groups do not differ on the selected measures or that some subtypes of insomniacs do differ from the controls on those measures, whereas others do not. As specific causes have been identified, researchers and clinicians alike have been increasingly careful to study or treat only that subtype. Until all the etiologies have been identified, if that goal is even possible, a large residual group of insomniacs will remain heterogeneous, and a unitary conceptualization based on existing diagnostic measures (e.g., polysomnographic, psychological, or physiological) will be difficult.

Fourth, a significant theoretical issue that has enormous implications for the entire conceptualization of insomnia lies in a methodological issue. Most of the research, and subsequent clinical application of the obtained information, has been conducted from a dualist and reductionist framework. This perspective focuses on a mind–body interaction by breaking the larger question of insomnia into a variety of measurable components. A problem arises when molecular data obtained in highly specific, and therefore somewhat artificial, settings and from highly circumscribed, and therefore nonrepresentative populations, is applied indiscriminately to the general population of clinical insomniacs or is considered to be a panacea for the problem of all insomniacs. Clinical insomnia reflects a complex interaction of biological, psychological, and sociological factors that simply do not lend themselves well to the reductionist-dualist perspective that has characterized insomnia research for the past few decades. This is not to say that basic, empirical research is not useful in our understanding of the problems of insomnia; such information has contributed substantially to our understanding of some processes and many of the different forms of insomnia. Rather, the application of information so obtained should be more carefully considered. What is needed in both clinical practice and research is a reconceptualization of the entire issue more along the lines of the biopsychosocial model. This model assumes that in order adequately to conceptualize and deal with an individual's problems one must understand that people are biological organisms who think and feel in a social context (Kales, Bixler, Soldatos, Vela-Bueno, Caldwell, & Cadieux, 1982; Kales, Caldwell, Soldatos, Buxler, & Kales, 1983; Tan, Kales, Kales, Soldatos, & Boxler, in press). To place any one of these factors above the others or to fail to consider any one of them in designing and implementing treatment dooms that treatment to limited success. Moreover, as well as a concern for extraindividual variables (family, job, social environment, etc.), implied in this model is a sort of mind–body fusion, not interaction, that maintains the two are functionally inseparable.

This perspective will become clearer in the following discussion.

Traditional Treatments for Insomnia

Although insomnia is often a manifestation or symptom of some more primary disorder, it is typically perceived and treated as the primary problem because of its immediately disruptive and extremely unpleasant effects. As a result, clients tend to overlook other potentially more disruptive but less immediately obvious problems, and physicians direct their treatment at symptomatic relief of sleeplessness. This perceptual set and treatment orientation is not only faulty but potentially dangerous in certain cases.

Most individuals believe that a good night's sleep is 8 hours long and that more or less than that is unhealthy and a reason to seek treatment. Many factors affect the actual amount of sleep needed, however, including age, sex, general health, socioeconomic level, and, to some extent, geographic location. Often, however, these factors are not known or are misunderstood, and clients come to feel that their statistically normal sleep is disturbed. Because insomnia is basically a perception of inadequate sleep, this faulty or uninformed belief about "normal" sleep can be the start of a real sleeping problem based on anxiety about inadequate sleep or launching a cycle of self-medication and drug-induced insomnia. Both of these outcomes will be discussed shortly.

Chronic insomniacs tend to be individuals who are highly invested in and preoccupied by their somatic complaints. Unintentionally they create a sort of self-perpetuating situation in which their insomnia is actually encouraged and attempts to reduce the complaint are resisted.

First, chronic insomniacs tend to have a personality style characterized by an internalizing and somaticizing emotional distress. These individuals, as a group, tend to feel more depressd, inferior, and dependent than noninsomniacs do. As a result, chronic, internalized emotional arousal can produce chronic physical arousal that could interfere with sleep. Numerous studies since Monroe (Monroe, 1967) imply that some chronic insomniacs may have substantially higher levels of autonomic arousal before and during sleep than noninsomniacs. Secondly, the "sick role" that many chronic insomniacs assume serves to relieve insomniacs of considerable responsibility for themselves and places them in a position of great attention and power in family and social settings (Mechanic & Volkart, 1961; Parsons, 1951).

The families of insomniacs tend to revolve around the problems of the insomniac. Expectations for the insomniac's involvement and responsibilities in the family's problems and activities are lower than for other family members, and the complaints and problems of the insomniac can become the focus of family discussions. The entire activity pattern of the family essentially revolves around the needs and wants of the "impaired" member. This provides the insomniac with considerable secondary gain that reduces the motivation to "get well." Moreover, the family's identity is one that relies on the insomniac's complaints for its stability, and any signs of improvement may represent signs of instability and be resisted by the entire family. Thus, there is both reinforcement for maintaining the problem and covert resistance to change (Kales & Kales, 1984).

Social systems become equally involved in the maintenance of an insomniac condition. The same reduced expectations that are found in the family situation may carry over to the job and social settings. Lateness, reduced productivity, and lowered responsibility are all more readily tolerated in an "ill" person than in a healthy one. Moreover, the social services, especially welfare and disability compensations, inadvertently reinforce a "sick" role by directly paying for time lost through illness (Better, Fine, Simison, Doss, Wells, & McLaughlin, 1979). Unfortunately, the networks that pay for disability provide unequal funding and often inadequate funding, for rehabilitation or psychological counseling (Cluff, 1981). Thus, there is very little external motivation for a chronic insomniac to change, but substantial motivation for maintaining the problem.

Finally, most physicians know very little about sleep disturbances in general, many sharing the same misconceptions about insomnia as the public. Most of what they do know comes from pamphlets distributed by pharmaceutical companies to accompany information on new sedative-hypnotics or tranquilizers (Mendelson, 1980). The problems with pharmacotherapy of insomnia is discussed shortly, and these can be major. What is important to consider here is the age-old commonsense prescription for someone who has trouble sleeping: go to bed earlier, try to relax more during the day, and take something to hasten sleep. This indeed is the most common prescription from the medical model and is the traditional forms of therapy for insomnia. Numerous studies have documented, however, that the life-style of the insomniac is characterized by hypoactivity, boredom, and dependency (cf. de la Pena. 1979). Prescriptions of more rest and relaxation, therefore, merely serve to aggravate the existing problems. Additionally, the public is constantly bombarded by advertisements for new and improved sleeping aids, for alcohol, and for services in all forms to take care of what ails them. This combination of underinformed physicians and overstimulating media reinforces the patterns of passive dependency already plaguing insomniacs and further reduces the possibility of effective, enduring amelioration of the problem by other means.

What is needed to alleviate this self-reinforcing system is substantially more public and physician education about the nature and causes of insomnia. Importantly, this education should take a holistic view of the problem and consider not only the biological phenomena but also the psychological and sociological factors in insomnia. It is apparent that a simple medical model explanation of insomnia is not adequate to develop a practical treatment of insomnia in general. The development of the behavioral treatments for insomnia and several psychological treatments for the problems were developed largely as a result of the poor success of strictly medical interventions. Unfortunately, the same problem that arises in the traditional treatments for insomnia seems to have occurred in the clinical applications of the behavioral treatments for this disorder: insufficient attention to the whole problem of the client. The remainder of this chapter first describes the behavioral treatments of insomnia, touching on their rationale and discussing the methodology and research support for the most widely used forms. It will then continue with a description of the most commonly encountered biological complications that reduce the efficacy of behavioral interventions in insomnia.

Behavioral Treatments

Although drug interventions and verbal psychotherapy have been applied to the treatment of insomnia for some time, research during the past 15 years has resulted in two significant developments. First, our increased knowledge of subtypes of insomnia has led to improved clinical decisions about those clients who are likely to benefit from such interventions and those who are not. For example, psychotherapy is inappropriate for those subtypes with a likely biological basis. Moreover, the customary usefulness of brief trials of benzodiazepines or narcotics is irrelevant to some of those biologically based insomnias and in fact may have detrimental or even life-threatening consequences (e.g., in the case of sleep apneas or for women who are pregnant).

The second major development has been the successful application of several behavior therapy and related techniques. Again, such success has been limited to cases of nonbiological origin (e.g., psychophysiological and subjective insomnias, and insomnia due to learning or psychiatric disorders). Although the history of controlled treatment research in this area is relatively brief, the results are rather compelling in documenting the efficacy of these treatments when they are properly carried out. On the other hand, these positive outcomes have certain limitations. The vast majority of therapy outcome studies have depended solely upon self-report measures of sleep complaints with no attempt to demonstrate physiological change. Expectations and covert demand in these studies can produce an "improvement" in the short run but do not produce long-term change. Although some electroencephalographic evaluations have been conducted and their results are in accord with the subjective outcomes, those trials remain few in number and involve only two of the four treatment techniques to be described: biofeedback and relaxation training. Moreover, the majority of outcome research with insomnia has been applied to its most common form, sleep-onset insomnia, whereas very little work has been conducted on the problem of frequent nocturnal arousals or early morning waking. Finally, the experimental evaluations of behavioral techniques began in the early 1970s and thus were coincident with the development and dissemination of information by various sleep researchers and clinics about the different subtypes of insomnia. Consequently, many of the earlier studies failed to provide sufficient information or assessment to allow differential diagnosis of the subjects used. Although it was rare for even the earliest studies not to rule out the presence of drugs or severe biological or psychiatric problems, and although several of the subtypes of insomnia are relatively uncommon in frequency, the groups of insomniacs participating in any of these studies were quite probably rather heterogeneous. For example, only a handful of studies have specifically identified psychophysiological and subjective insomniacs and have evaluated the effects of treatment on these distinct groups. In all remaining studies we have no idea about the percentage of clients representing these two major subtypes, let alone the remainder of conditions.

Keeping these criticisms in mind, we turn to a description of these behavioral interventions and review evidence for their efficacy. The largest class of techniques thus far evaluated has involved relaxation training of some kind. Several strategies have been employed, four of which are the most common. Abbreviated progressive muscular relaxation training (Bernstein & Berkovec, 1973) is the most common and involves (a) systematic and sequential tensing and releasing of various gross muscle groups throughout the body in order to produce reductions in skeletal muscle tension, and (b) learning to attend to and identify increasingly mild forms of tension as a cue for initiating a relaxation response. Autogenic training (Schultz & Luthe, 1959) involves the repetition of a series of self-suggestions (e.g., "my arms are becoming heavy... my legs are becoming warm") designd to elicit relaxation from the body. Meditational techniques depend upon focused attention, usually to one's breathing or to a repeated word, or "mantra," as in Benson's (Benson & Hahn, 1963) technique of relaxation response. Finally, biofeedback, principally of frontalis electromyography (EMG) in the context of improving the relaxation response, has been employed as a method of teaching a general relaxation skill (cf. Hauri, 1979).

The original theoretical rationale for the application of such interventions rested upon Monroe's (1967) demonstration of greater physiological (specifically autonomic) activity among poor, as compared to good, sleepers both prior to and during sleep. Although this finding has been disputed by subsequent research (cf. Berkovec, 1982), Monroe's early data quite naturally led to the conclusion that brief relaxation strategies should be an effective form of intervention. Indeed, the subsequent controlled-outcome studies unequivocally supported their efficacy, if not the theorizing upon which their application was based. Among close to a score of controlled trials (cf. Van Oot, Lane, & Berkovec, 1984), routinely positive outcomes on subjective indices of sleep complaint have been reported. Relaxation, in the majority of studies, has been shown to be superior to no treatment and to a variety of placebo conditions, and long-term follow-up reports have revealed maintained or further improvement. Average reduction in reported latency to sleep onset from before to after treatment has been 45% over all these investigations. Moreover, EEG evaluation has been included in six of these studies, and their results objectively support the therapeutic impact of relaxation and EMG biofeedback.

Because physiological hyperactivity among insomniacs has not been consistently found and because reductions in physiological activity have not been significantly correlated with either objective or subjective improvement in the therapy outcome studies, the search for the mechanisms mediating relaxation's efficacy continues. Cognitive hyperactivity has been described as an alternative mediating characteristic of insomnia, and empirical findings seem to be more in accord with this hypothesis. Insomniacs do report a greater frequency of cognitive intrusions in the presleep period, and reductions in those reports parallel improved sleep latency upon successful treatment (e.g., Berkovec, Grayson, O'Brien, & Weerts, 1979). It may be, therefore, that relaxation procedures provide a sufficiently pleasant, monotonous condition for directed attention such that the occurrence of arousing cognitions is prevented and sleep can more easily occur.

The physiological and cognitive hyperactivity hypotheses remain strong contenders, and in the final analysis it is probably the case that each may play a role, to a greater or lesser extent in an individual case. Apparently, however, the relaxation techniques are useful for reducing both physiological activity and sleep-incompatible cognitions. Future research may succeed in developing better methods of assessing these individual differences and in allowing an ideal match between the type of mediating activity and type of relaxation strategy. For example, progressive muscular relaxation, as a somatic relaxation technique, may be best suited for lowering physiological hyperactivity, whereas meditational strategies may be particularly useful for controlling intrusive cognitive activity (Davidson & Schwartz, 1976).

Another form of biofeedback training has as its goal not the elicitation of a relaxation response, but the more direct strengthening of a physiological system involved in sleep production. The sensory-motor rhythm (SMR) has been operantly reinforced successfully in awake cats and has resulted in greater sleep duration (Sterman, Howe, & MacDonald, 1970). Moreover, evidence exists to suggest that the SMR is weak in some insomniacs (Jordan, Hauri, & Phelps, 1976). Indeed, those with weak SMR displayed objectively defined insomnia in the laboratory, whereas insomniacs with normal SMR rates showed undisturbed EEG-defined sleep, a criterion for subjective insomnia. Strength of SMR may thus relate to the differential etiology of the psychophysiological and subjective insomnias. Finally, in this latter pilot study and in a subsequent outcome investigation (Hauri, 1981), rate of learning during SMR biofeedback training was positively correlated with improvment in latency to sleep onset. In the Hauri (1981) study, subjects low in anxiety (and by implication weak in SMR) benefited from SMR training but not from EMG biofeedback, whereas the opposite was true for insomniacs high in anxiety. This emphasizes the importance of understanding the etiology of the insomnia under treatment and further exemplifies a difference in the response of different subtypes of insomnia to a given treatment.

Stimulus-control therapy (Bootzin, 1972; Bootzin & Nicassio, 1978) is based on a straightforward conditioning account of insomnia. Presumably, bed-related stimuli have been repeatedly associated with sleep-incompatible behaviors (tossing and turning, worry about falling asleep, reading, and so on). Consequently, bedtime, the bed, and the bedroom become cues for nonsleep. To create a new history of association, stimulus-control treatment attempts to pair bed-related stimuli only with rapid sleep onset. The following instructions are usually given to the insomniac to produce that new history:

1. Go to bed only when you feel sleepy and intend to fall asleep (to associate sleep behaviors only with appropriate internal ones).
2. Do not take naps (to prevent a lowering of sleep requirement during the day and to preclude the pairing of sleep with inappropriate temporal cues).
3. Arise at the same time each morning (to provide a consistent sleep parameter that will facilitate entrainment of the circadian rhythm).
4. Do not engage in any behavior in bed or in the bedroom other than sleep-related behaviors (to insure that sleep-incompatible behaviors are no longer associated with bed-related stimuli).
5. After you go to bed, if you have not fallen asleep in about 10 minutes, leave the bedroom and do something else. Once you feel sleepy again, return to bed and repeat this procedure as often as necessary until you fall asleep rapidly. This instruction is designed to insure that only rapid sleep onset is paired with bed-related stimuli and that sleep-incompatible behaviors are not allowed to continue for lengthy periods of association with those stimuli.

The several controlled evaluations of stimulus control have resulted in the largest reductions in reported latency to sleep onset (70% from before to after therapy) in the behavior-therapy literature. Direct comparisons to relaxation techniques as well as placebo conditions have favored the superiority of stimulus control, and long-term follow-up data indicate maintained improvement. Moreover, effectiveness has been demonstrated across a wide range of age, chronicity, and severity characteristics. Missing from these trials, however, are any EEG evaluations. Therefore, although we can be confident that active ingredients exist in the technique for the subjective parameters of insomnia, its degree of impact on objectively defined sleep remains unknown.

In accordance with the conditioning notion of insomnia upon which the stimulus-control strategy is based, more frequent sleep-incompatible activities in the bedroom (e.g., eating, reading, watching television) have been found among untreated insomniacs' daily monitoring reports than among those of good sleepers in only one study (Kazarian, Howe, & Csapo, 1979). However, this result has not been replicated in two other attempts (Arand, Kramer, Czaza, & Roth, 1972; Haynes, Follingstad, & McGowan, 1974). Moreover, Zwart and Lisman (1979) found that instructions simply to sit up in bed and do something other than attempting to fall alseep were just as therapeutic as the usual stimulus control package. It appears that one major measure of the technique's efficacy is a reduction in effortful attempts to fall asleep, that is, a decline in performance anxiety over trying to sleep. Effort is incompatible with sleep, and its elimination by instructions that suggest that the client not try so hard to fall asleep may produce the desired therapeutic effects.

Paradoxical intention is the last strategy for which some controlled studies exist. The client is instructed to try to stay awake for as long as possible. The rationale underlying the procedure is that remaining awake builds up sleep requirement, reduces performance anxiety, and insures rapid sleep onset once the individual does go to sleep (Frankl, 1960). Four controlled trials (two-group placebo designs and two small-sample designs) have documented the technique's efficacy and together indicate a 58% reduction in latency to subjective sleep onset (Ascher & Efran, 1978; Ascher & Turner, 1979; Ascher & Turner, 1980; Relinger & Bornstein, 1979). Again, no objective measures have as yet been obtained, follow-up information exists only for the small-sample studies, and no research has been conducted to attempt to identify the mechanism accounting for its effectiveness.

Biological Considerations

Although there are many people who suffer from psychophysiological insomnia, subjective insomnia, and the like who are appropriate candidates for the behavioral treatments mentioned, there are a substantial numer of insomniacs whose sleeping difficulties are secondary to some psychiatric or physiological disturbance. For these individuals, treatment is correctly and necessarily directed at the physical or psychiatric disturbance. Incorrect diagnosis and treatment of some of these secondary insomnias not only often results in unreliable or marginal relief of the symptoms but also can lead to serious complications if the underlying pathology or disturbance is not appropriately treated.

A discussion of every form of secondary insomnia is completely impossible in a single chapter. For discussions of insomnias secondary to the various psychiatric disturbances, therefore, the reader is referred to other sources (Kales & Kales, 1984; Mendelson *et al.*, 1977; Williams & Karacan, 1978). Many of the remaining insomnias secondary to biological pathologies or dysfunctions are rare or result from such obvious biological problems that they will be only briefly mentioned here. There are a small group of biologically based insomnias, however, that are encountered frequently enough in a clinical practice to warrant detailed consideration.

It is relatively safe to say that sleep can be disrupted by just about any noticeable change in body status. Again, the degree of the sleep disruption depends on the individual; no laws govern an individual's reaction to physical injury or dysfunction. Thus, major changes in living situation, hospitalization, significant stress of literally any kind, excessive environmental conditions (heat, cold, noise, pollution), jet lag or shift work, and an enormous host of medical conditions associated with disease, trauma, or aging all produce various degrees and kinds of insomnia. The most commonly encountered of these insomnias, however, occur as a result of drug use, respiratory and cardiovascular impairments, muscle disorders, circadian rhythm disruption, and aging. It should be remembered, however, that practically any medical problem can produce sleep impairment; gastrointestinal disorders (Armstron, Burnap, Jacobson, Kales, Ward, & Golden, 1965; Orr, Hall, Stahl, Durkin, & Whitsett, 1976), chronic kidney disorders (Daly & Hasall, 1970; Karacan, Williams, Bose, Hursch, & Warson, 1972), a variety of eating disorders and obesity (Crisp, 1980; Crisp & Stonehill, 1970; Crisp, Stonehill, & Fenton, 1971; Lacy, Crisp, Kalucy, Hartmann, & Chen, 1975; Niel, Merikangas, Foster, Merikangas, Spiker, & Kupfer, 1980), endocrine disorders (Dunleavy, Oswald, Brown, & Strong, 1974; Kales, Heuser, Jacobson, Kales, Hanley, Zweizig, & Paulson, 1967; Ross, Agnew, Williams, & Webb, 1968; Schultz, Schulte, Akiyama, & Parmelee, 1968),pregnancy (Karacan & Williams, 1970; Schweiger, 1972), and a host of neurological conditions (Broughton, 1971; Dexter & Weitzman, 1970; Freemon, 1978; Markland & Dyken, 1976) can all produce insomnia or severely disrupted sleep. The diagnosis of some of these disorders is obvious (pregnancy or obesity, for example), but often the endocrine, gastrointestinal, kidney, or neurological conditions escape detection when the primary presenting complaint is poor sleep.

Medications

Significantly contributing to the occurrences of insomnia is the widespread use of various pharmaceutical products (drugs). There is little doubt that ours is a drug-oriented society. Powerful and sometimes dangerous drugs are socially acceptable (if not desirable), readily available, and often too casually used. It is not surprising, therefore, to find a considerable number of sleep disorders that can be directly traced to drug use or abuse. Moreover, many sleeping disturbances result not from drug use *per se* but from drug interactions or withdrawal. Unfortunately, the problem of drug-related sleep disturbances is not a simple one to diagnose or treat.

Derivatives of the oxybarbiturates, the nonbarbiturate sedative hypnotics (alcohol included), and the benzodiazepine tranquilizers are the most commonly used sleeping aids. Paradoxically, these agents, our main line of defense against insomnia, account for a vast number of drug-related sleep disturbances.

Dement (1972) reported that as many as 50% of all insomniacs have had recent experience with some form of hypnotic and should be treated like other people with drug problems. These drug-related problems begin when a person begins taking sleep-inducing agents for periodic, mild insomnia. Usually the first few administrations of some form of over-the-counter medication or large doses of alcohol afford some relief. Gradually, however, this relief fades with the development of tolerance, and the initial dose is increased. Again relief is obtained, but only temporarily and as the original sleeping problem returns despite continued self-medication, the insomniac usually contacts a physician for more powrful hypnotics. The story with these is no different, however; sleep eventually becomes disrupted in spite of continued drug use. The time course for this progression of medication can be as short as a few weeks, suggesting the speed with which a drug-related problem can develop.

A few people become discouraged at this point, abandon drugs, and seek some alternative treatment. They find out very quickly, however, that upon withdrawal of the drug they experience almost total insomnia, or sleep that is very badly fragmented and marked with frequent, vivid dreams and nightmares. Returning to the drug, they find only the comfort of their original problem; only now they require drugs to maintain it. It is not uncommon, for example, to find people who have been on such medications for many months, or even years, and who derive little benefit from the drugs other than the postponement of withdrawal symptoms (cf. Mendelson, 1980).

Discussions of drug effects have, until recently, focussed either on the neurochemical or pharmacological properties of these drugs or on single-dose, one-night clinical assessments of individual drugs or multidrug comparisons. Attention has now turned to what drugs do to the sleep they induce. Moreover, serious and far-reaching questions have been raised regarding the role of tolerance, dependence, and withdrawal on the drug's overall effectiveness.

Unfortunately, an uncomplicated discussion of the effects of the various drugs on sleep is nearly impossible for several reasons. First, the methodological strategies and goals vary greatly from lab to lab, and subtle differences in such strategies can produce marked differences in outcome. Second, the between-subject and within-subject variability in sleep patterns from night to night is enormous. Even severe insomniacs, for example, have a few very good nights, especially in the lab (Kales, Kales, Bixler, & Soldatos, 1980). Third, the between- and within-subject response to the various drugs is also highly individual and can be influenced by a host of internal and external factors. Finally, the various interactions among the above-mentioned factors contribute significantly to the overall variance inherent in the drug–sleep literature.

Regardless of these problems, information on specific agents and certain general drug-related processes that directly affect sleep have been well documented. These involve the drug's effects on the architecture of the sleep they induce and the problems of tolerance, dependence, and especially withdrawal on the individual's sleep.

Sedative-Hypnotics

The hypnotic actions of alcohol and the barbiturates, based on their CNS depressant actions, as well as the tranquilizing effects of the benzodiazepine compounds have been well documented and need little elaboration here (Goodman & Gilman, 1969; Mendelson, 1980). In most people, therapeutic doses of these drugs produce light sleep, reduce sleep onset latency and the number of nocturnal awakenings, and prolong sleep duration. Each agent produces slightly different effects, but no known sedative-hypnotic produces natural sleep—and the differences between natural and drug-induced sleep can be important.

Comon to most of the CNS depressants (alcohol, the oxybarbiturates, and the nonbarbiturate sedative-hypnotics) is a marked suppression of rapid eye movement (REM) sleep. In 1968, for example, Knowles, Laverty, and Kuecher (1968) demonstrated a dose-related reduction in the amount of REM when alcohol is used. Lower doses (those not producing intoxication) suppressed REM for only the first third of the night whereas progressively higher doses initially suppressed REM for longer intervals and eventually the entire night. Williams and Salamy (1972) thoroughly reviewed the effects of acute alcohol administration on sleep, and their discussion of the effects of alcohol can be applied to the other sedative-hypnotics as well. Interestingly, although at lower doses REM was suppressed for the first third of a night, the total amount of REM for the night was not changed. The reason for this is the mini-withdrawal described by Mendelson *et al.* (1977). As alcohol or the other CNS depressants are metabolized from the body, their REM-suppressing effects wane. When blood levels of the agents drop below a certain level, REM rebound occurs, and later portions of the night are characterized by greater than normal amounts of REM. Apparently the cyclicity of REM is not affected, only the duration of the earlier episodes. Thus, low doses of the depressants do not produce changes in overall REM time during sleep but may markedly affect its distribution. At least three agents do not produce marked REM suppression: benzodiazepine, chloral hydrate, and methaqualone. All the others produce this effect to some degree.

Reductions in Stage 4 sleep are also produced by several agents: flurazepam, glutethimide, chlordiazepoxide, and pentobarbital, for example (Kales & Kales, 1972; Kales, Bixler, & Kales, 1977). Reductions in Stage 4 sleep, however, produce no known or long-lasting deleterious effects. Massive REM rebound, however, like that found in drug withdrawal (see below), or the milder rebound as that with a miniwithdrawal, can produce disrupted sleep.

The benzodiazepine tranquilizers do not appear to produce REM suppression at clinical doses. These agents are not usually prescribed for inducing sleep, however, so unqualified comparisons with the depressants are not entirely appropriate.

When the sedative-hypnotics are used for prolonged periods, a marked reduction in their effectiveness is noted and is attributable to the development of tolerance. Behaviorally defined, tolerance is the gradual reduction of the behavioral or subjective response to constant doses of the same agent administered on a regular schedule. Cross-tolerance should also be discussed in this context. This occurs when tolerance to one drug develops and is expressed in reduced response to a different but pharmacologically related agent. Tolerance to most of the depressants develops within a few days to a week of consecutive administration (Kales & Kales, 1972; Kales, Bixler, & Kales, 1977). Flurazepam and triazolam, both benzodiazepine derivatives also somewhat effective as sleep inducers, can be effective for up to 2 weeks of continuous use, but this is the upper limit of effectiveness for any of the hypnotics (Kales, & Kales, 1972; Kales, Bixler, & Kales, 1977). As tranquilizers, the benzodiazepines develop tolerance very slowly; some are effective for up to 4 months of continuous use (Goodman & Gilman, 1969). Again, this is concerned with tranquilization, not sleep induction.

With chronic use, individuals often become dependent upon the depressants. Dependence accounts for the majority of drug-related sleep complaints and presents the greatest potential danger of chronic drug use. Dependence is usually defined *post hoc* as the appearance of a withdrawal syndrome with the cessation of drug use. Both psychological and physical dependence should be considered at this point for the insomnia associated with withdrawal could be a function of either form of dependence or both. The physical aspects contributing to insomnia are discussed shortly, but the psychological effects can be just as potent sleep disrupters resulting from the apprehension and anxiety of being without the familiar agent. Moreover, if the agent has been even partially successful in inducing sleep, the stimulus cues of sedation associated with sleep are absent, making the sleeping situation less pleasant.

All commercial sedative-hypnotics, including alcohol, are basically CNS depressants. They are all, therefore, capable of producing dependence and a withdrawal syndrome. The classic depressant–withdrawal syndrome is defined by the withdrawal symptoms of the barbiturates or alcohol. This withdrawal is characterized by nausea, agitation, tremors, insomnia, and nightmares. More severe withdrawal can include the development of hallucinations, delerium tremens, convulsions, and, without proper management, sometimes death.

Except for flurazepam (a benzodiazepine), methyprylon, homatropine methylbromide, and ethinamate, all the sedative-hypnotics produce similar manifestations upon withdrawal, but to a lesser extent. Moreover, the more severe forms of withdrawal, those including hallucinations and convulsions, are rare with the nonbarbiturate sedatives. The unsettling fact about the development of dependence–withdrawal, however, is that signs of it can be seen after only one exposure to many of these agents (Goodman & Gilman, 1969; Mendelson, 1980). Most of the benzodiazepine tranquilizers do not produce a marked withdrawal syndrome though some of the shorter acting agents (flurnitrazepam, nitrazepam, and triazolam, for example) produce REM rebound (Kales *et al.*, 1977). The longer acting agents (diazepam and flurazepam, for example) do not produce a rebound effect, probably because they are metabolized from the body very slowly and the body has time to adjust to their absence (Kales *et al.*, 1977).

The whole concern with the increased REM association with rebound phenomena is that increased REM is associated with numerous other sleep disturbances. Coincident with the REM increases are frequent, vivid, or intense dreams and nightmares, frequent nocturnal arousals, and early morning waking. In more severe cases, daytime hallucinations and other REM-related phenomena may appear (cf. Mendelson, 1980). The suppression of the other stages of sleep is not accompanied by phenomena similar to REM rebound. Thus, unlike the deprivation of other stages of sleep, suppression of REM can lead to marked disturbances in subsequent sleep, particularly during withdrawal from the suppressing drug.

Stimulants, Antidepressants, and Others

The antidepressants and stimulants figure prominantly in most discussions of sleep, but there are numerous other drugs that directly or indirectly affect the quality of sleep that are beyond the scope of this chapter. The reader is referred to Goodman and Gilman (1969) or the current edition of the *Physician's Desk Reference* (PDR) (Baker, 1983) for relevant information on any drug in question.

Antidepressants can be used to alleviate insomnia secondary to depression. Both the monoamine oxidase inhibitors (MAOIs) and the tricyclic antidepressants reduce sleep onset latency, reduce the number of nocturnal arousals, and delay early morning waking—the major sleep-related symptom of depression (Hartmann, 1968a; Mendels & Hawkins, 1967; Zung, Wilson, & Dodson, 1964). In nondepressed individuals, these agents can moderately reduce the need for sleep, a form of stimulation (Hartmann, 1968).

Most antidepressants block or suppress REM to some extent (Wyatt, Chase, Scott, Snyder, & Engleman, 1970; Wyatt, Fram, Buchbinder, & Snyder, 1971). Some also increase sleep duration (Cramer & Kuhlo, 1967; Neff & Yang, 1974), but these effects have not been reliably demonstrated, and considerable controversy over the effects of the antidepressants still exists (Mendelson, 1980; Mendelson *et al.*, 1977; Neff & Yang, 1974). The tricyclics, however, and cocaine have similar effects in that they both block the reuptake of norepinephrine (NEPI) at the synapse, producing a form of stimulation. Moreover, they both block REM and reduce total sleep time (Goodman & Gilman, 1979; Post, Gillan, Goodwin, Wyatt, & Snyder, 1972). Stage 2 increases to compensate for the reduced REM time and tolerance to both agents develop over the course of several months (Hartman, 1969). Withdrawal from either agent, however, can produce a form of withdrawal syndrome that lasts up to a month (Dunleavy, Brezinova, Oswald, McLean, & Tinker, 1972). The actual effects of the antidepressants is unclear at present, and individual assessment of the effects of these agents on sleep is necessary.

The amphetamines and caffeine are the two most popular stimulants available. Both promote vigilance and alertness while postponing or markedly reducing the subjective need for sleep. Both probably operate by increasing the availability of NEPI, but the actual mechanisms of caffeine's actions are not clearly understood. (Goodman & Gilman, 1969; Mendelson, 1980).

The amphetamines are the most powerful prescription stimulants. They act to increase alertness, enhance physical performance, and postpone sleep onset. They also act to suppress REM. Tolerance to the continued use of these agents eventually develops, however, and both the arousal and REM-suppressing effects of the drugs diminish with time (Oswald, 1974). Oddly, however, in some cases a form of reverse tolerance can develop. The well-known amphetamine psychosis sometimes accompanies prolonged use or unusually large doses for a shorter period (cf. Goodman & Gilman, 1969). What this seems to reflect is a sensitization to the drug instead of a tolerance. Withdrawal from the amphetamines produces hypersomnia, depression, and abundant REM rebound characterized by shorter latencies to REM periods and by greater manifestations of Stage-3 and Stage-4 sleep in the early hours of sleep (Oswald, 1969). With the increased REM, disturbed sleep and nightmares often result. Although the drugs are rapidly metabolized from the body, it may take several months before all the drug-induced effects are gone. The withdrawal process is, therefore, prolonged and often overlooked or mistaken for something else in diagnosis.

In addition to alcohol, caffeine and nicotine are undoubtedly the most widely used drugs. To give some idea of the prevalence of caffeine use, the average cup of coffee has about 100–150 mg of caffeine, but from the intake of coffee alone Americans consume approximately 15 million pounds of caffeine per year. Caffeine is also found in tea and cola products (drinks and chocolate) which add to the popularity and overall consumption of this drug (Goodman & Gilman, 1969). Caffeine is a relatively safe drug, producing its stimulation with as little as 100 mg. Only massive doses (2–5 g, or 20–50 cups of coffee) become dangerous. Three or four cups of coffee in the morning, however, can produce a mild degree of shakiness and irritability. Caffeine is also found in a large number of weight-control agents, pain medications, and other over-the-counter drugs (Mendelson, 1980).

Tolerance to caffeine is not commonly reported, and physical dependence is still a controversial issue. Psychological dependence on caffeine, however, is commonly reported. The pharmacological effects of caffeine ingestion manifest themselves in about 45 minutes to an hour. The drug is then effective for about 2 hours thereafter (Goodman & Gilman, 1969). Reports of insomnia, hyperactivity, and tremors during sleep onset are the most common complaints following a late dinner's coffee. Once caffeine is metabolized from the body, depression, fatigue, and sleepiness may result. Such symptoms could be mistaken for some form of hypersomnia or the result of inadequate nightly sleep. This depression is immediately reversed by additional caffeine intake, however.

Nicotine is probably the most powerful natural stimulant known. Taken primarily through tobacco products, nicotine exerts its stimulation through the acetylcholine systems. The stimulation is followed, however, by the depression and lethargy associated with stimulant withdrawal. Dependence is also a major factor with nicotine, and the withdrawal syndrome is associated with intense irritability, agitation, and numerous sleep complaints similar to those associated with caffeine withdrawal. (cf. Goodman & Gilman, 1969).

A wide assortment of over-the-counter drugs also significantly affect sleep. Diet aids such as fenfluramine (Oswald, Jones, & Mannerhiem, 1968), methylphenidate (ritalin), and propanolamine and ephedrine are basically stimulants that produce various degrees of stimulation depending on the consumer and variably affect sleep in a manner similar to the other stimulants. Many of the over-the-counter sleeping aids, like ephedrine and propanolamine, were once marketed as decongestants. It was determined that these agents also produce a mild degree of sedation in a certain percentage of the population and they were therefore marketed as sleeping aids (Goodman & Gilman, 1969; Mendelson, 1980). Among these, pyrilamine maleate (Sominex, Sleep-eze, and Nytol) and doxylamine succinate (Unisome) are the most commonly encountered. These agents are of extremely questionable value in producing sleep, and when they do contribute to sleep they significantly disturb its architecture. Tolerance to the effects of these agents also develops extremely rapidly; and although not likely to produce dependence *per se*, withdrawal of these agents after prolonged use produces a form of withdrawal syndrome not unlike that of the sedative-hypnotics, only much less severe (Goodman & Gilman, 1969; cf. Mendelson, 1980). Thus, insomnia, disrupted sleep, and REM rebound-associated nightmares occur with withdrawal from these agents.

A host of other drugs, too numerous to detail here, also affect sleep. It is a safe bet, in fact, to assume that almost any drug affects sleep in some way, even though it is not known directly to depress or stimulate the central nervous system. The balances of sleep are so fine that any drug that has an effect on the smooth, integrated functioning of the body is likely to have an effect on sleep as well. If clients or patients present with a history of drug use, it is probably wise to ascertain the degree of the drug's involvement in any sleep disturbances before proceeding with any other form of assessment or treatment.

Respiratory Disorders

A substantial portion of the insomniac complaints can be traced directly to some dysfunction in respiration. Importantly, these sleep disturbances can present as either a complaint of insomnia or of daytime sleepiness. In either case the cause is essentialy the same and is a result of sleep disrupted by periods of insufficient ventilation. These dysfunctions range from simple hypoventilation to prolonged and potentially dangerous apneas. Although there has been a considerable amount of research into these problems, and a resulting literature of sizable proportions, the exact mechanisms and the sleep-disrupting effects of these problems are not precisely understood. There is ample information on the characteristics, distinguishing features, and treatments of these disturbances to permit accurate diagnosis in clinical practice, however.

A particularly important feature of these disturbances, worthy of special note, is that they can be associated with more severe cardiovascular, neurological, or pulmonary problems, which, if left uncorrected, can be fatal. Therefore reports of disturbed sleep or excessive daytime sleepiness, especially when compounded by nocturnal respiratory problems, should be given serious and immediate attention.

Normal breathing entails a wide range of irregular respiratory patterns. For the majority of people, in fact, pauses of up to 15 seconds are common and present no threat to sleep or general health (Hartmann, 1973). During sleep, especially REM sleep, however, breathing becomes much more erratic, and many otherwise harmless breathing irregularities can be accentuated to a clinically significant degree (Duron, 1972). The REM state in particular is associated with the greatest degree of irregularity in respiration. Often, however, many clients are not aware of any breathing abnormality and do not associate their disrupted sleep with a respiratory dysfunction. It is essential, therefore, that the clinician eliminate these possibilities before any treatment is prescribed.

Regardless of the specific form of disorder, the irregular, periodic, or inadequate breathing characteristic of these disorders is associated with potentially toxic levels of blood carbon dioxide and with unusual stress or performance demands in various parts of the body. Although the direct cause of this association has not yet been established, the incidence of these breathing disorders with at least one or more serious physical problems is too high for chance and warrants the assumption that the two types are related (Butler, 1974; Guilleminault, Phillips, & Dement, 1975; Reidy, Husley, Bachus, Dahl, & Levine, 1979; Sacker, Landa, Forrest, & Greeneltch, 1975).

Frequently one or more heart conditions are found in persons suffering from chronic sleep disturbances. The most common of these are either asystole or premature ventricular contranctions. Equally important, however, are ventricular hypertrophy, tachycardia, atrioventricular block, or sinus arrest. Any one of these conditions in their mild or acute forms may not present a serious or life-threatening problem. When prolonged, unusually severe, or compounded with other cardiovascular or pulmonary problems, however, they can easily become life-threatening (Barlow, Bartlett, Hauri, Hellekson, Nattie, Remmers, & Schmidt, 1980).

Hypoventilation Syndromes

Primary alveolar hypoventilation, or Ondine's curse, is characterized by cardiorespiratory disturbances resulting in chronic hypoxia. The syndrome is further characterized by incomplete or inadequate respiratory efforts resulting in reduced air exchange and chronic hypoxia-hypercapnea. In some individuals there is an almost totally absent or reduced response to blood CO_2 and hypoxia even though there are no obvious physical problems associated with the respiratory musculature. Because this syndrome does not involve complete cessation of breathing and is not associated with any obvious physical abnormalities, it may be difficult to detect. It can, however, produce the same type of physical, psychological, and behavioral effects as the more obvious breathing-related disorders and should be considered as serious. A polysomnogram is indicated to determine exactly what form of hypoventilation syndrome the client has.

Apneas

There are many people with normal waking respiratory patterns who, when asleep, display pauses or complete cessation of breathing for 150 seconds or more. People with such apneas typically go through a repeating cycle of sleep, apnea, arousal, resumption of breathing, and sleep once again (Williams, Karacan, & Hursch, 1974). This cycle can be repeated up to several hundred times per night, yet still be unknown to the sufferer (Guilleminault & Dement, 1978a,b). It has been estimated that many apnea suffers spend up to 47% of their time in bed not breathing (Sackner, Lands, Forrest, & Greeneltch, 1975). This is obviously a significant sleep-related problem.

There are three types of apnea commonly encountered; central, obstructive, and mixed. Each has its own symptomatology, etiology, and treatment indications. The importance of correct diagnosis and treatment cannot be too strongly emphasized.

Central apnea involves a temporary and periodic cessation of respiratory effort. The diaphragm and intercostal muscles of the chest simply stop functioning for brief periods. It is a very common form of apnea and occurs primarily in males (30:1), the elderly (over 60 years), and premature infants (under 30 weeks' gestation) (Guilleminault, Dement, & Holland, 1974; Guilleminault, Eldridge, & Dement, 1973; Read, Williams, Hensley, Edwards, & Beal, 1979; Steinschneider, 1972).

The clinical picture of a central apnea is not behaviorally obvious. There may be snoring, but it is not loud or abrupt. Typically, there is only a sudden, brief snort or gasp at the end of an apneic period as breathing resumes. This may or may not accompany behavioral awakening, but

EEG signs of arousal are usually present. In some cases, however, the only herald of the syndrome is the cessation of breathing followed by a large satisfying sigh or yawn. Agitated sleep, frequent movements, and complaints of frequent waking and daytime sleepiness are common in this form of apnea (Guilleminault & Dement, 1978a,b).

Central apneas are often confused with the hypoventilation syndromes. Cheyne–Stokes breathing, for example, is very similar in that breathing has a cycle of small inspirations that gradually increase in depth, then diminish and culminate in a period of apnea (Hauri, 1976). Central apnea merely involves the cessation of breathing without apparent cyclicity.

Alveolar hypoventilation (already mentioned) is also often confused with central apnea. In hypoventilation breathing continues throughout the night but becomes shallow and insufficient. With apneas, breathing stops. Distinguishing among these various disorders takes either a well-trained observer or a polysomnogram.

The central apneas reportedly respond well to respiratory stimulants (Hauri, 1976). Clomipramine and doxapram hydrochloride have been successfully used. Doxapram is also useful for hypoventilation syndromes (Lugiani & Whipp, 1979). CNS depressants, needless to say, should be avoided at all costs with these syndromes.

Phrenic nerve stimulation to trigger respirations has also been effective in treating these disturbances (Glenn, Phillips, & Gersten, 1978). This involves the surgical implantation of a nerve stimulator, however, and is a rather radical approach.

The obstructive apneas are somewhat less common but are more easily detected than the central apneas. These are defined as any condition in which airflow is blocked in the presence of continued respiratory effort. Thus, any condition in which the trachea, throat, or upper airways are blocked can create an obstructive apnea.

This form of apnea is also found in the elderly, but more often in the obese, among those with neurological conditions affecting the musculature of the throat or upper airways, among those with physical structural anomalies (e.g., scoliosis), or in those with severe infections (causing inflammation and swelling). In individuals with any of these impairments, the muscles of the upper airways relax during the sleep and the various structures sag into the throat. Airflow is impeded, and adequate ventilation stops. Arousals then occurs, and breathing resumes.

People with this type of apnea are well known, loud, snorting snorers. They also change position frequently during the night (as if struggling for breath) and wake with a sudden gasp. Frequently subjective reports of sensations of choking or dying are made. Intense anxiety or terror often accompany such episodes.

The sleep of obstructive apnea is almost devoid of Stages 3 and 4. Moreover, during any REM periods the apneic episodes are prolonged. Because the period between apneic episodes, and therefore between arousals, can be as little as 1.75 minutes, sleep is badly fragmented (Guilleminault & Dement, 1978a,b). The physical characteristics of obstructive apnea sufferers are similar to the characteristics of those with central apena: short, thick necks, and jowls (Kurtz & Krieger, 1978). A substantial number of obstructive apneics, however, are also markedly obese. The treatment for individuals in this latter category is initially weight reduction, and it has been shown that even modest weight loss is associated with substantial improvement of the condition (Bruhova, Nevsimal, Ourednik, & Stepanek, 1969; Burwell, Robin, & Whaley, 1956). In more severe cases, tracheostomy, particularly the kind that can be easily closed with a valve during waking hours, is indicated (Hill, Simmons, & Guilleminault, 1978; Sackner *et al.*, 1975). Some cases also may require surgical expansion of the upper airways or nasal resection (Hauri, 1976; Simmons & Hill, 1974). Pharmacotherapy is usually not indicated, and sedative-hypnotics are specifically contraindicated.

The mixed apneas present a symptom pattern like those of both the central and the obstructive apneas. These are defined as some combination of central and obstructive apnea and are characterized by an initial cessation of respiratory effort followed by a collapse of the upper airway structures. This form of apnea is the most commonly encountered and may be the most difficult to manage (Guilleminault & Dement, 1978a,b).

Treatment consists of both pharmacotherapy or phrenic nerve stimulation for the central apnea and, when indicated, tracheostomy or surgical expansion of the upper airways for the obstructive apnea. Losing weight in those with obesity-related problems is a good idea in its own right and is particularly indicated in this instance. Some people respond favorably to treatment of only the central apnea, for the obstructive phase appears only after the cessation of respiratory effort in most cases (Guilleminault & Dement, 1978a,b).

It should be noted that the central apneas and hypoventilation syndromes are perhaps the most common causes of sudden infant death. Particularly with some premature infants (less than 30 weeks' gestation), careful monitoring of successful, effective respiration is indicated (Butler, 1974; Guilleminault *et al.*, 1973; Steinschneider, 1972). Even if a child displays no signs of apnea, inadequate respiration can be potentially dangerous.

A special consideration for the extremely obese is also indicated. The Pickwickian Syndrome (Burwell *et al.*, 1956) is a combination of sleep disturbances and respiratory problems compounded by obesity. It is characterized by marked obesity, twitching, cyanosis, right ventricular hypertrophy and heart failure, periodic respiration, and secondary polycythemia. The insomnia and hypersomnia experienced by a Pickwickian are characterized by badly fragmented sleep. On entering sleep, the Pickwickian experiences the classic obstructive apnea syndrome. Respirations and air exchange are occluded, arousals occur, and the cycle recurs throughout the night (Williams *et al.*, 1974). The apneic episodes become more prolonged and the arousals more obvious and extended as sleep becomes progressively deeper.

The sleep of a Pickwickian has been compared to the sleep of an infant with periodic sleep-onset REM episodes, a virtual absence of Stage-3 and Stage-4 sleep, and brief periods of delta activity immediately prior to the arousals (Schwartz, Seguy, & Escande, 1967). Although the primary sleep-related complaint of a Pickwickian is hypersomnia, there is some controversy about the classification of these individuals. Kuban (1978) and others consider the disorder to be one primarily of disrupted sleep–waking mechanisms. These problems then lay the foundation for the obesity and related or subsequent problems. Spiro and Scheinberg (1978) alternatively maintain that sleep disruption is common to all obese individuals and that the Pickwickians merely suffer an unusual degree of sleep disruption due to their unusual weight. Gastaut, Duron, Papy, Tassinari, and Waltregny (1967) similarly consider the sleep disruption of the Pickwickians to be secondary to their obesity and focus on the aggrevation of breathing difficulties by the fatty deposits in the throats of these individuals. The most recent evidence, however, suggests that Pickwickians are extremely obese individuals who suffer from all the abovementioned problems because of a dysfunction in their ventilatory mechanisms, these possibly related to their sleep–waking regulators (Zwillich, Sutton, Pierson, Creagh, & Weil, 1975).

The breathing-related sleep disorders present a major diagnostic challenge to practitioners in that very subtle differences in the pattern of breath disruption has substantial implications for the form of treatment. Moreover, the urgency of proper diagnosis and treatment cannot be overemphasized. These kinds of disturbances, if left untreated or treated inappropriately, usually only intensify and can create a life-threatening situation in a relatively short time.

Circadian Rhythm Disorders

In modern society, the 24-hour social and work schedules interfere significantly with the endogenous circadian rhythms. Although the consequences of this conflict are not entirely understood, it is clear from observation and often from personal experience that sleep deprivation, shift work, and jet lag are stressful and impair alertness, memory, and general well-being. Sleep disruption is only one manifestation of disrupted circadian rhythms, and with more people doing shift work and a greater number of people routinely traveling across time zones, the number of sleep disorders due to disrupted circadian cycles is increasing. The nature of the subjective disturbance is complex and highly interactive with a variety of environmental influences. These factors and an understanding of the phenomenon of circadian cycles are important to consider in a working diagnosis of any sleep disturbance.

The DCSAD (1979) defines a limited number of sleep-related disorders directly resulting from altered circadian rhythms. These are an arbitrary collection of disturbances, some due to external factors (jet lag, shift work, and frequent changes in sleep–wake schedule), and some are largely endogenous (delayed sleep phase syndrome, advanced sleep phase syndrome, and irregular or non–24-hour sleep–wake syndrome). Subjectively these disturbances share a common complaint of not being able to sleep or awaken when the person wants to do so. What this reflects is a basic desynchronization of the internal biological and the external environmental clocks. When externally induced, a change in the rhythms begins almost immediately but can take several weeks to become "realigned" or entrained (cf. Akerstedt, 1979). A number of factors contribute to the actual manifestations of the sleep disturbance.

The nature of the circadian rhythms should be briefly explained here. The source of the rhythms appears to be a combination of external factors and the internal "biological clocks." Central pacemakers of "clocks" have been located in the hypothalamus (Conroy & Mills, 1970; Mills, 1973). The endogenous rhythms these clocks regulate persist in the absence of external cues; they retain approximately the same phase relationships and periodicity despite environmental change; and they resist change but do eventually synchronize with th environment (Akerstedt, 1979; Conroy & Mills, 1970). The behavioral manifestations of these rhythms and eventually the rhythms themselves, however, are externally influenced by such factors as light–dark cycle, temperature, availability of food, and social interactions (Aschoff, Hoffman, Pohl, & Wever, 1975; Klein & Wegman, 1975a,b).

The usual 24-hour entrainment is an apparent result of a combination of the endogenous and exogenous factors that roughly corresponds to our light–dark cycle, but both the phase and the period of the rhythms can be changed when needed. Apparently it is easier to change the phase of a cycle than it is to change its periodicity (that is, change the time at which the rhythm begins rather than change the duration of a cycle) (Aschoff, Hoffman, Phol, & Wever, 1975; Klein & Wegman, 1975a,b).

The actual nature or basis of arousal or activation is not a simple thing, however. What we consider to be activation is a general process of preparing for activity that involves a unified effort of a variety of subsystems (Duffy, 1962). Lacey (1967) divided general arousal into cortical, autonomic, and behavioral activation, the concerted action of which we call general arousal. Only in special circumstances, though, do these patterns of activation occur together. The activation patterns or rhythms of these subsystems, though interdependent, are not time-looked, and desynchrony is the rule rather than the exception. When one rhythm is out of synchrony with the others, the individual experiences distress, usually in the form of disturbed sleep, gastrointestinal disturbances, increased fatigue, and reduced higher cortical functioning (cf. Akerstedt, 1979). Moreover, when the circadian rhythms are disturbed, the entrainment or re-entrainment of the subsystems does not typically occur at the same rate, resulting in internal desynchrony. Such desynchrony and distress are commonly reported by people who work irregular shifts and by those experiencing jet lag.

With regard to the disturbances produced by changes in circadian rhythms, shift work, and jet lag are by far the most common. With jet lag, the important variable appears to be the amount of sleep deprivation that occurs. This variable may explain why eastbound flights are more stressful than westbound flights; one loses time from west to east and gains time from east to west (Aschoff, 1969; McFarland, 1975; Mills, Minors, & Waterhouse, 1978). Jet lag, fortunately, is a transient disturbance, but it can be extremely distressing and requires a month or so before the rhythms are completely resynchronized (Akerstedt, 1979). It is when individuals overrespond to the entrainment period with anxiety or heavy self-medication that chronic problems can begin.

Shift work has received considerable attention and accounts for a substantial number of insomnia reports. Shift work can include a complete day–night reversal, periodic reversals with a return to normal day–night schedules in between (rotating shift work), or irregular hours typical of emergency personnel or performers. Of these factors, the latter is the most detrimental in that no entrainment of rhythmicity is ever allowed to occur, and the body is continually stressed by desynchronicity (Akerstedt, 1979; Froberg, Karisson, Levi, & Lidberg, 1975a,b; Patkai & Frankehauser, 1964; Patkai, Johansson, & Post, 1971). There is even some question about a differential effect of effects of altered rhythms based on sex, though the nature and extent of the differences between men and women are unclear (cf. Akerstedt, 1979). Shift work, in general, badly disrupts circadian rhythmicity, and unless an adequate opportunity for entrainment is allowed to occur, significant and chronic problems can result (Ackerstedt, 1976; Aschoff, 1975, 1976; Froberg, Karisson, & Levi, 1972; Kolomodin-Hedman & Swensson, 1975; Walsh, Stock, & Tepas, 1978; Weitzman, Kripke, Goldmacher, McGregor, & Nogeire, 1970).

The etiologies of the endogenous sleep-phase disturbances are not known. These disturbances seem to reflect a shift in the phase of the circadian cycle that does not entrain to the environmental synchronizers. This type of disturbance is common in the blind, for example (Miles, Raynal, & Wilson, 1977). Those who suffer from either the delayed or the advanced sleep phase syndrome are chronically out of synchrony with the environment and experience many of the problems of individuals with jet lag, waking much too early in the morning or feeling sleepy in the late afternoon or early evening (Dement & Guilleminault, 1979). Then there are individuals who experience very little rhythmicity at all in their wake–sleep cycle, or who experience a cycle that has a different period than that of the environment. In both of these cases some basic dysfunction of the circadian pacemakers is probable, but the actual etiology is unknown (Dement & Guilleminault, 1979; Kokkoris, Weitzman, Pollack, Spielman, Czeisler, Bradlow, 1978; Webb & Agnew, 1974).

The circadian rhythm disorders are good candidates for behavioral intervention and do not respond well to medical treatment. The treatment of choice is sleep scheduling in which individual are instructed to establish and maintain a standard waking time and to avoid any unnecessary napping during the day until the biological rhythms entrain themselves (cf. Akerstedt, 1979). Unfortunately, very little can be done for individuals whose rhythms do not entrain even after prolonged sleep-scheduling treatment. Education about the disorders and acceptance of them are needed in these instances to prevent needless anxiety or pharmacotherapy. Drug-related insomnia could easily arise from these kinds of transient disturbances. Chronic napping is also a common result of these kinds of disturbance. The effect of chronic, habitual napping is not yet fully understood, however, and alternatives to this tendency should be encouraged (Akerstedt, 1979; Johnson, Tepas, Colquhoun, & Colligan, 1981).

For a more comprehensive discussion of the influences on and effects of the circadian rhythms on human performance and health, the reader is referred to Johnson, Tepas, Colquhoun, and Colligan (1981).

Aging

The amount, quality, and architecture of sleep changes gradually with maturation. Infants can spend up to 15 hours a day sleeping, of which about 40–50% is REM sleep. In young children, the amount of sleep and relative proportions of NREM and REM sleep change markedly. Total sleep time drops to about 10 hours a day and the percentage of REM sleep to about 18%. The popular notion of sleeping 8 hours a night does not occur until about age 20 (Roffwarg, Muzio, & Dement, 1966). What is usually not considered by either practitioners or patients is that the amount and structure of sleep continues to change from adulthood through to old age. People who are at least 60 years old often sleep no more than 6–7 hours a night and their REM percentage has dropped off to about 13–15%. Moreover, the sleep of the elderly is characterized by substantially less Stage-3 and Stage-4 sleep, compensatory amounts of Stages 1 and 2, frequent nocturnal arousals, longer sleep-onset latencies, and earlier morning waking (Carskadon, van den Hoed, & Dement, 1981; Prinz & Halter, 1982, 1983; Prinz, Peskind, Raskind, Elsdorfer, Zemcuznikov, & Gerber, 1982; Roffwarg *et al.*, 1966).

Complaints of poorer sleep also increase with age. Lighter sleep, more restless sleep, and the symptoms already mentioned are the chief complaints of older individuals. Approximately 67% of the users of medically prescribed hypnotics are between the ages of 45 and 75 (Balter & Bauer, 1975), with the largest percentage of this group over 65 (Mendelson, 1978, 1980). The problems mentioned with the exclusive use of pharmacotherapy for insomnia are compounded with old age. The biological activity of the drugs, for example, is prolonged as metabolism slows. The side effects of many of the agents, including hypotension, tachycardia, arrhythmia, and cerebrovascular insufficiency are significant considerations for the elderly (Freeman, 1978; Salzman, Shader, & Van Der Kolk, 1976). Moreover, the inherent REM-suppressing effects of the sedative-hypnotics functionally eliminate what little REM sleep the elderly still have and add the additional problems associated with REM rebound to the list of contraindications for pharmacotherapy (Kales & Cary, 1971; Kales & Kales, 1973; Oswald & Priest, 1965).

Personality changes in old age compound the problem. Th elderly are more likely to "take their problems to bed with them," thus associating the bed with these problems (Karacan, Thornby, Holzer, Warhelt, Schwab, & Williams, 1976); depression and hypochondriasis are more common (Kales, Caldwell, Preston, Healy, & Kales, 1976); and stress is more likely to be internalized (Gilberstadt & Duker, 1965; Roth, Kramer, & Lutz, 1976; Swenson, Pearson, & Osborn, 1973). Thus, the insomniac personality pattern described earlier also exists in old age, but possibly to a greater extent and with wider and more serious ramifications.

Despite the reduced and fragmented sleep experienced by the elderly, surveys indicate that they actually spend more time in bed per day than younger individuals (Tune, 1968). Their sleep efficiency, therefore, is very low in comparison to that of younger people (Carskadon *et al.*, 1981). Some assume, therefore, that sleep need is lower among older individuals (Best & Taylor, 1952), but when the naps and earlier retiring are also considered, the total amount of sleep the elderly achieve per day is about the same as that of younger people (Tune, 1968)., A polycyclic pattern is what seems best to describe the overall sleep pattern of the elderly, suggesting that the circadian rhythms become somewhat less distinct (Akerstedt, 1979; Gilberstadt & Diker, 1965; Prinz, 1976; Prinz, Vitello, Schoen, & Halter, 1981; Roth *et al.*, 1976).

Significant hormonal changes also occur that affect the quality of sleep in the aged. Growth hormone, for example, which is secreted in a large pulse at sleep onset in young people, is significantly reduced or absent in older individuals (Prinz, Blenkarn, Linnoila, & Weitzman, 1976; Prinz *et al.*, 1981). Plasma NEPI concentration is generally higher in older individuals than in younger ones, suggesting greater sympathetic activity in the aged. This degree of increased NEPI correlates well with the degree of sleep disturbance reported, suggesting that some form of physiological arousal may account for some of the sleep-disruption (Roth *et al.*, 1976).

Finally, a general aggravation of all the other biologically based sleep complaints already discussed occurs in the older population. Thus, breathing-related disturbances (Guilleminault & Dement, 1978a,b; Guilleminault *et al.*, 1975; Guilleminault, Tilkian, & Dement, 1976; Lugaresi, Coccagna, Mantovani, & LeBrun, 1972; Prinz *et al.*, 1981) neurological disturbances, and chronic pain (Feinberg, 1968, Nowlin, 1965) are more common.

Much of the problem appears to lie in the misinformation about the normal age-related changes in sleep. Most people and practitioners judge the quality of sleep based on middle-aged or young-adult norms and consider any sleep not meeting those criteria to be disrupted. If the norms are not understood, or in some cases not accepted, useless and potentially dangerous treatments may be tried and further frustration then occurs when these treatment eventually fail. These treatment failures and frustrations can initiate a vicious cycle transforming an essentially normal sleeping pattern into a disordered one. Education and direct treatment of any biological contributions to unsatisfactory sleep are probably the best ways to manage sleep complaints in the elderly. Additionally, however, because the elderly are generally less active, spend more time in bed not sleeping or occupied with some other activity, and often have negative associations with the bed for a variety of reasons (poor sleep, unsatisfactory sex life, illness), the stimulus-control procedures could be very useful (Bootzin, 1972; Bootzin & Nicassio, 1978; Prinz *et al.*, 1976). The problems in diagnosing and treating sleeping disorders among the aging are significant and warrant even more careful attention thatn the problems of younger clients and patients. The percentage of biologically based problems is greater, however, and therefore much more caution and careful diagnosis of the actual sleep complaint are essential with older patients.

Nocturnal Myclonus and Restless Legs

Many people experience a crawling sensation deep within their legs while they try to fall asleep. When this sensation becomes sufficiently annoying or relentless, sleep can be disrupted. The DCSAD (1979) notes that although these sensations occur whenever sufferers sit or lie down, and although they are usually not painful, they can be constant and obvious enough to produce an overwhelming desire to move the legs, producing sleep disruption. Often people will attempt to relieve these sensations by vigorous exercise. Relief is obtained only during the exercise, however, and the sensations return almost immediately thereafter (cf. Akerstedt, 1979; Bixler, Kales, Vela-Bueno, Jacoby, & Scarone, 1982).

Almost all individuals who experience "restless legs" show nocturnal myocloic activity of the legs as well (Lugaresi *et al.*, 1972). This myclonic activity consists of sudden, unintentional contractions of various leg muscles that literally jerk the sufferer out of sleep. Because these contractions are not usually associated directly with the sensations of restless legs, it is assumed that the two are separate but related phenomena (Lugaresi *et al.*, 1972).

About 10% of the insomniac population shows myoclonic activity (Kales *et al.*, 1982). Kales *et al.* (1982) and Bixler *et al.* (1982) have demonstrated that about the same percentage of noninsomniacs show the same kind and number of occurrences of this activity as well. The insomniacs showed substantially more indications of psychopathology based on MMPI assessments, however, and it is assumed that the psychological tendency for the insomniacs to focus on the sensations and myoclonic activity and to "suffer in silence" is what disrupts their sleep, and not the contractions *per se* (Kales & Kales, 1984).

These phenomena should be distinguished from the bedtime leg cramps many people experience, especially after a strenuous day of walking or running, and from the sensations, akin to a limb falling asleep, produced by insufficient or occluded blood flow to the legs created by either internal vascular disturbances or awkward postures. Restless sensations are also common among growing children, reflecting a sort of "growing pain" (Lugaresi *et al.*, 1972). As such, they should not be overreacted to or be the cause of expensive and often unnecessary testing and medication. These problems are also common among the aged (Kales & Kales, 1984).

Additional Considerations

As we have mentioned, a host of other biologically related conditions can produce significant sleep disturbances and result in a presenting problem of sleep disturbance instead of the underlying problem. Among those not covered in this chapter are various neurological disturbances, especially seizure disorders (Freeman, 1978), endogenous depression (Kupfer & Foster, 1978), schizophrenia (Feinberg & Hiatt, 1978), and various surgical conditions (Williams, 1978). The sleep disturbances produced by these kinds of pathology are usually secondary and not considered the primary pathology. Nonetheless, the possibility of one or more of these primary conditions should be ruled out before a diagnosis and treatment recommendations are made.

As noted in the introduction, a major problem facing insomnia research and treatment has been, and still is, the tendency for researchers and clinicians to focus narrowly on some specific etiology or characteristic of insomnia, or on a limited population of insomniacs. Such focusing congested the literature with clinically irrelevant information and has led to considerable confusion in the development and implementation of efficacious treatments. What is needed is a guiding theoretical conceptualization of insomnia based not only on the existing data on the biological, psychological, and sociological factors in insomnia, but also on the other relevant fields of human research. Such a conceptualization, drawing from theories of development, cognition, and information processing, to name a few, would be concerned with the whole individual, not just the factors immediately pertinent to that individual's insomnia. A psychophysiological conceptualization that incorporates many of these considerations recently has been forwarded by de la Pena (1979).

De la Pena's psychophysiological model is based on the assumption that the individual human brain requires and processes a certain optimal level of information during a normal 24-hour day. This processing is distributed across the states of waking and sleeping and is regulated within each of these states as well. When an individual receives and processes his or her optimal level of information on a given day, the sleep–waking cycle is also optimal, with feelings of relaxed well-being during the day and restful, uninterrupted sleep at night. When a mismatch between the optimal and actual levels of stimulation and information processing occur, however, the sleep–waking cycle is disturbed. If the amount of mismatch is relatively low, it is compensated for by changes within the waking or sleeping components of the cycle, feelings of drowsiness or restlessness during waking, and increases in REM or NREM activity during sleep. This degree of mismatch would occur, for example, in situations that provoke low-level, long-lasting arousal (studying for tests, anticipating an important date, engaging in physically demanding exercise, and the like), or noticeable boredom (being bedridden with an illness, watching television all day, traveling for a long period with little to do). If substantial mismatch occurs, however, the sleep–waking cycle itself can be disrupted. This degree of mismatch would occur after some major stress (death of a loved one, waiting for Christmas morning to come, a sudden major change in health). In these cases sleep loss or some form of insomnia often results (cf. de la Pena, 1979).

This conceptualization takes into account the biopsychosocial parameters relevant to sleep as well as a host of considerations from the cognitive and developmental literatures. Factors related to aging, health, social status, personality, intelligence and education, the environment, and so on are therefore considered. Moreover, the implications for treating insomnia from this model are significant. The individual biopsychosocial factors emphasized in this chapter become essential in a functional diagnosis of the problem. The range of these biopsychosocial factors, however, is expanded to consider more than just health, age, psychopathology, and socioeconomic level.

Recommendations

Adequate diagnosis and treatment of insomnia must include substantially more than the subjective complaint of disrupted sleep. Moreover, the implications of a misdiagnosed insomnia can be greater than simply continued distress from disrupted sleep; many of the conditions described in this chapter could be fatal if left undiagnosed. What is needed, therefore, is a more comprehensive approach to understand an individual's complaint of poor or inadequate sleep. Furthermore, a more flexible attitude on the part of the practitioners to inform themselves and their clients or patients about the relevant parameters (manifestations, norms, etiologies) of the various sleep disturbances and the implications and effects of the available treatments for these disturbances should be encouraged.

For a working diagnosis to be complete, in addition to a comprehensive and detailed sleep history, a recent and complete medical and drug history is also important. Moreover, a psychiatric or personality assessment may clarify any questions the medical and sleep histories do not. Finally, an analysis of the client's sleeping environment, expectations, and beliefs about sleep cover most of the ground necessary to establish a working diagnosis.

Once the diagnosis has been determined, treatment should focus on the most obvious etiological factors. Often the symptoms of insomnia abate once the underlying medical or psychiatric disturbances have been remedied. The psychosocial factors (sick role, family and job situations, for example) should not be neglected in any circumstances, and adjunctive services may be required to complete the treatment. Once the immediate problem has been ameliorated, several general measures to maintain an optimal sleep–waking balance should be instituted. These include establishing a regular, satisfying sleep schedule, improving the general sleep environment, establishing a schedule of proper nutrition and exercise, managing individual stress, and avoiding excesses (moderation in living) (cf. de la Pena, 1979; Kales & Kales, 1984). It is no longer justifiable or acceptable merely to dismiss complaints of insomnia as manifestations of simple tension, stress, or environment. Each complaint should be treated as any other potentially serious medical or psychological problem. Unidimensional diagnoses and treatments of insomnia are usually uninformative and ineffective. Such an approach can also be dangerous in many circumstances.

References

Akerstedt, T. (19767). Interindividual differences in adjustment to shift work. In *Proceedings of the 16th Congress of the International Ergonomics Association,* (pp. 510–514). Santa Monica, CA.

Akerstedt, T. (1979). Altered sleep/wake patterns and circadian rhythms. *ACTA Physiologica Scandinavia Supplement, 469,* 1–48.

Arand, D., Kramer, M., Czaza, J., & Roth, T. (1972). Attitudes toward sleep and dreams in good versus poor sleepers. *Sleep Research, 1,* 130.

Armstrong, R. H., Burnap, D. B., Jacobson, A., Kales, A., Ward, S., & Golden, J. (1965). Dreams and gastric secretions in duodenal ulcer patients. *The New Physician, 14,* 241–243.

Ascher, L. M., & Efran, J. S. (1978). Use of paradoxical intention in a behavioral program for sleep onset insomnia. *Journal of Consulting and Clinical Psychology, 46,* 547–550.

Ascher, L. M., & Turner, R. M. (1979). Paradoxical intention and insomnia: An experimental investigation. *Behavior Research Therapy, 17,* 408–411.

Ascher, L. M., & Turner, R. M. (1980). A comparison of two methods for the administration of paradoxical intention. *Behavior Research and Therapy, 18,* 121–126.

Aschoff, J. (1969). Desynchronization and resynchronization of human circadian rhythms. *Aerospace Medicine, 40*, 844–849.

Aschoff, J., Hoffman, K., Pohl, H., & Wever, R. (1975). Re-entrainment of circadian rhythms after phase-shifts of the zeitgeber. *Chronobiologia, 2*, 23–78.

Baker, C. E. (1983). *Physician's desk reference (PDR)*, Oradell, NJ: Litton.

Balter, M. B., & Bauer, M.L. (1975). Patterns of prescribing and use of hypnotic drugs in the United States. In A.D. Clift (Ed.), *Sleep disturbance and hypnotic drug dependence*. Amsterdam: Excerpta Medica.

Barlow, P., Bartlett, D., Hauri, P., Hellekson, C., Nattle, E., Remmers, J., & Schmidt, N. (1980). Idiopathic hypoventilation syndrome: Importance of preventing hypoxia and hypercapnia. *American Review Respiratory Disease, 121*, 141–145.

Benson, T. X., & Hahn, K. W. (1963). Hypnotic induction and "relaxation": An experimental study. *Archives of General Psychiatry, 8*, 295–300.

Bernstein, D. A., & Borkovec, T. D. (1973). *Progressive relaxation training: A manual for the helping professions*. Champaign, IL: Research Press.

Best, C. H., & Taylor, N. B. (1952). *The living body*. London: Holt.

Better, S. R., Fine, P. R., Simison, D., Doss, G. H., Walls, R. T., & McLaughlin, D. E. (1979). Disability benefits as disincentives to rehabilitation. *Milbank Memorial Fund Quarterly, 57*, 412–417.

Bixler, E. O., Kales, A., & Soldatos, C. R. (1979). Sleep disorders encountered in medical practice: A national survey of physicians. *Behavioral Medicine, 6*, 1–6.

Bixler, E. O., Kales, A., Soldatos, C. R., Healey, S. (1979). Prevalence of sleep disorders in the Los Angeles metropolitan area. *American Journal of Psychiatry, 136*, 1257–1262.

Bixler, E. O., Kales, A., Vela-Bueno, A., Jacoby, J. A., & Scarone, S. (1982). Nocturnal myoclonus and nocturnal myoclonic activity in a normal population. *Research Communications in Chemical Pathology and Pharmacalogy, 36*, 129–140.

Bootzin, R. R. (1972). Stimulus control treatment for insomnia. *Proceedings of the 80th Annual Convention of the American Psychological Association, 7*, 395–396.

Bootzin, R. R., Nicassio, P. M. (1978). Behavioral treatments for insomnia. In Hersen, Eisler, & Miller (Eds.), *Progress in behavior modifications* (Vol. 7., pp. 1–47). New York: Academic Press.

Borkovec, T. D.: Insomnia. *Journal of Consulting and Clinical Psychology, 50*, 880–895.

Borkovec, T. D., Grayson, J. B., O'Brien, G. T., & Weerts, T. C. (1979). Relaxation treatment of pseudoinsomnia and idiopathic insomnia: An electroencephalographic evaluation. *Journal of Applied Behavioral Analysis, 12*, 37–54.

Broughton, R. (1971). Neurology and sleep research. *Canadian Psychological Association Journal, 16*, 283–292.

Bruhova, S., Nevsimal, O., Ourednik, A., & Stepanek, J. (1969). Pickwickian syndrome: The clinical and polygraphic findings and the influence of weight reduction. *Electroencephalography and Clinical Neurophysiology, 26*, 230–231.

Burwell, C., Robin, E., & Whaley, R. (1956). Extreme obesity associated with alveolar hypoventilation: A pickwickian syndrome. *American Journal of Medicine, 21*, 811–818.

Butler, J. (1974). Clinical problems of disordered respiratory control. *American Journal Respiratory Diseases, 110*, 695–698.

Carskadon, M. A., van den Hoed, A. J., & Dement, W. C. (1981). Insomnia and sleep disturbances in the aged. *Journal of Geriatric Psychiatry, 14*, 135–151.

Cluff, L. E. (1981). Chronic disease, function and the quality of care. *Journal Chronic Diseases, 34*, 299–304.

Conroy, R. T., & Mills, J. N. (1970). *Human circadian rhythms*. London: Churchill.

Cramer, H., & Kuhlo, W. (1967). Effets des inhibiteurs de la mono-aminoxidase sur le sommeil et l'electroencephalogramme chez l'homme. *Acta Neurologica Belgium, 67,* 658–669.

Crisp. A. H. (1980). Sleep, activity, nutrition, and mood. *British Journal of Psychiatry, 137,* 1–7.

Crisp, A. H., & Stonehill, E. (1970). Sleep patterns, daytime activity, weight changes, and psychiatric status: A study of three obese patients. *Journal of Psychosomatic Research, 14,* 353–358.

Crisp, A. H., Stonehill, E., & Fenton, G. W. (1971). The relationship of sleep, nutrition, and mood: A study of patients with anorexia nervosa. *Post-Graduate Medicine, 47,* 207–213.

Daly, R. J., & Hassall, C. (1970). Reported sleep on maintenance haemodialysis. *British Journal Medicine, 2,* 508–509.

Davidson, R. T., & Schwartz, G. E. (1976). The psychobiology of relaxation and related states: a multiprocess theory. In D. I. Mostofsky (Ed.), *Behavioral control and modification of physiological activity* (pp. 399–442). Englewood Cliffs, NJ: Prentice-Hall.

de la Pena, A. (1979). Toward a psychophysiologic conceptualization of insomnia. In R. L. Williams & I. Karacan, (Eds.), *Sleep disorders: Diagnosis and treatment* (pp. 101–144). New York: Wiley.

Dement, W. C. (1972). *Some must watch while some must sleep.* Stanford, CA: Stanford Alumni Association.

Dement, W. C., & Guilleminault, C. (1979). Diagnostic classification of sleep and arousal disorders (DCSAD). *Sleep, 2,* 1–6.

Dexter, J. D., & Weitzman, E. D. (1970). The relationship of nocturnal headaches to sleep stage patterns. *Neurology, 20,* 513–518.

Duffy, E. (1962). *Activation and behavior.* New York: Wiley.

Dunleavy, D. L., Brezinova, V., Oswald, I., Maclean, A. W., & Tinker, M. (1972). Changes during weeks in effects of tricyclic drugs on the human sleeping brain. *British Journal of Psychiatry, 120,* 663–672.

Dunleavy, D. L., Oswald, I., Brown, P., & Strong, J. A. (1974). Hyperthyroidism, sleep, and growth hormone. *Electroencephalography and Clinical Neurophysiology, 36,* 259–263.

Duron, B. (1972). La fonction respiratoire pendent le sommeil physiologique. *Bulletin of the Physiopathology of Respiration, 8,* 1277–1288.

Feinberg, I. (1968). The ontogenesis of human sleep and the relationship of sleep variables to intellectual functioning in the aged. *Comprehensive Psychiatry, 9,* 138–147.

Feinberg, I., & Hiatt, J. F. (1978). Sleep patterns in schizophrenia: A selective review. In R. L. Williams & I. Karacan (Eds.), *Sleep disorders: Diagnosis and treatment* (p. 205–232) New York: Wiley.

Frankl, V. E. (1960). Paradoxical intention: A logotherapeutic technique. *American Journal of Psychotherapy, 14,* 520–535.

Freeman, J. T. (1978). Body composition in aging. In J. T. Freeman (Ed.), *Clinical features of the older patient.* Springfield, IL: Charles C. Thomas.

Freemon, F. R. (1978). Sleep in patients with organic diseases of the nervous system. In R. L. Williams & I. Karacan (Eds.), *Sleep disorders: Diagnosis and treatment,* (pp. 261–285). New York: Wiley.

Froberg, J., Karlsson, C. G., & Levi, L. (1972). Shift work: A study of catecholamine excretion, self-ratings, and attitudes. *Studia Laboris et Salutis, 11,* 10–20.

Froberg, J., Karlsson, C. G., Levi, L., & Lidberg, L. (1975a). Circadian variations of catecholamine excretion, shooting range performance and self-ratings of fatigue during sleep deprivation. *Biological Psychiatry, 2,* 175–188.

Froberg, J., Karlsson, C. G., Levi, L., & Lidberg, L. (1975b). Psychobiological circadian rhythms during a 24-hr vigil. *Forsvarsmedicin, 11,* 192–201.

Gastaut, H., Duron, B., Papy, J., Tassinari, C., & Waltregny. A. (1967). Comparative polygraphic study of the 24-hr cycle in pickwickians, the obese, and narcoleptics. *Electroencephalography and Clinical Neurophysiology, 23,* 283.

Gilberstadt, H., & Duker, J. (1965). *A handbook of clinical and actuarial MMPI interpretation.* Philadephia: Saunders.

Glenn, W., Phelps, M., Gersten, L. M.: Diaphragm pacing in the management of central alveolar hypoventilation. In C. Guilleminault & W. C. Dement (Eds.), *Sleep apnea syndromes.* New York: Liss.

Goodman, L. S., & Gilman, A. (1969). *The pharmaceutical basis of therapeutics,* (3rd Ed). New York: MacMillan.

Guilleminault, C., & Dement, W. C. (1978a). *Sleep apnea syndromes* New York: Liss.

Guilleminault, C., & Dement, W. C. (1978b). Sleep apnea syndromes and related sleep disorders. In R. L. Williams & I. Karacan (Eds.), *Sleep disorders: Diagnosis and treatment* (pp. 9–28). New York: Wiley.

Guilleminault, C., Eldridge, R., & Dement, W. C. (1973). Insomnia with sleep apnea: A new syndrome. *Science, 181,* 856–858.

Guilleminault, C., Dement, W. C., & Holland, J. V. (1974). Sleep apnea and sleep disturbances. In P. Levin & D. P. Koella (Eds.), *Sleep: Instinct, neurophysiology, endocrinology, episodes, dreams, epilepsy, and intracranial pathology* (pp. 447–450). Basel: Karger.

Guilleminault C., Phillips, R., & Dement, W. C. (1975). A syndrome of hypersomnia with automatic behavior. *Electroencephalography and Clinical Neurophysiology, 38,* 403–413.

Guilleminault, C., Tilkian, A., & Dement, W. C. (1976). The sleep apnea syndromes. *Annual Review of Medicine, 27,* 465–485.

Hartmann, E. (1968). Amitriptyline and Imipramine: Effects on human sleep. *Psychophysiology, 5,* 207–212.

Hartmann, E. (1968). Longitudinal studies of sleep and dream patterns in manic-depressive patients. *Archives of General Psychiatry, 19,* 312–320.

Hartmann, E. (1969). Antidepressants and sleep: Clinical and theoretical implications. In A. Kales (Ed.), Sleep: *Physiology and pathology.* Philadelphia: Lippincott.

Hartmann, E. (1973). Long sleepers, short sleepers, variable sleepers, and insomniacs. *Psychosomatics, 14,* 95–103.

Hauri, P. (1976). Sleep disorders. In H. S. Abram (Ed.), *Basic psychiatry for the primary care physician* (pp. 137–158). New York: Little, Brown & Co.

Hauri, P. (1979). Biofeedback techniques in the treatment of chronic insomnia. In R. L. Williams & I. Karacan (Eds.), *Sleep disorders: Diagnosis and treatment* (pp. 145–162). New York: Wiley.

Hauri, P. (1981). Treating psychophysiological insomnia with biofeedback. *Archives of General Psychiatry, 38,* 752–758.

Haynes, S. N., Follingstad, D. R., & McGowan, W. T. (1974). Insomnia, sleep patterns and anxiety level. *Journal Psychosomatic Research, 18,* 69–74.

Hill, M., Simmons, F., & Guilleminault, C. (1978). Tracheostomy and sleep apneas. In C. Guilleminault & W. C. Dement (Eds.), *Sleep apnea syndromes.* New York: Liss.

Johnson, L. C., Tepas, D. I., Colquhoun, W. P., & Colligan, M. J. (1981). *Biological rhythms, sleep, and shift work.* New York: SP Medical & Scientific Books.

Jones, H. S., & Oswald, I. (1968). Two cases of healthy insomnia. *Electroencephalography and Clinical Neurophysiology, 24,* 378–380.

Jordon, J. B., Hauri, P., & Phelps, P. J. (1976). The sensorimotor rhythm (SMR) in insomnia. *Sleep, 5,* 175.

Kales, A., & Cary, G. (1971). *Insomnia: Evaluation and treatment.* In E. Robins (Ed.), *Psychiatry* (Supplement to Medical World News), 55–56.

Kales, A., & Kales, J. D. (1970). Evaluation, diagnosis, and treatment of clinical conditions related to sleep. *Journal of the American Medical Association, 213*, 2229–2235.

Kales, A., Kales, J. D. (1984). *Evaluation and treatment of insomnia*. New York: Oxford University Press.

Kales, A., Heuser, G., Jacobson, A., Kales, J., Hanley, J., Zweizig, J. R., & Paulson, M. J. (1967). All-night sleep studies in hypothyroid patients, before and after treatment. *Journal of Clinical Endocrinology and Metabolisim, 27*, 1593–1599.

Kales, A., Caldwell, A. B., Preston, T. A., Healy, S., & Kales, J. D. (1976). Personality patterns in insomnia. *Archives of General Psychiatry, 33*, 1128–1134.

Kales, A., Bixler, E. O., & Kales, J. D. (1977). Comparative effectiveness of nine hypnotic drugs: Sleep laboratory studies. *Journal of Clinical Pharmacology, 17*, 207–213.

Kales, A., Bixler, E. O., Soldatos, C. R., Vela-Bueno, A., Caldwell, A. B., & Cadieux, R. J. (1982). Biopsychobehavioral correlates of insomnia, I: Role of sleep apnea and nocturnal myoclonus. *Psychosomomatics, 23*, 589–600.

Kales, A., Caldwell, A. B., Soldatos, C. R., Bixler, E. O., & Kales, J. D. (1983). Biopsychobehavioral correlates in insomnia. II: MMPI pattern specificity and consistency. *Psychosomatic Medicine, 45*, 341–356.

Kales, J. D., & Kales, A. (1973). Recent advances in the diagnosis and treatment of sleep disorders. In Usdin (Ed.), *Sleep research and clinical practice* New York: Bruner-Mazel.

Kales, J. D., Kales, A., Bixler, E. D., & Soldatos, C. R. (1980). Sleep disorders: What the primary-care physician needs to know. *Post-graduate Medicine, 67*, 213–217.

Karacan, I., & Williams, R. L., (1970). Current advances in theory and practice relating to postpartum syndromes. *Psychiatric Medicine, 1*, 307–328.

Karacan, I., Williams, R. L., Bose, J., Hursch, C. J., & Warson, S. R. (1972). Insomnia in haemodialytic and kidney transplant patients. *Psychophysiology, 9*, 137.

Karacan, I., Thornby, M. A., Holzer, C. E., Warheit, G. J., Schwab, J. J. & Williams, R. L. (1976). Prevalence of sleep disturbance in a primarily urban Florida County. *Social Science and Medicine, 10*, 239–244.

Kazarian, S. S., Howe, M. G., & Csapo, K. G. (1979). Development of the sleep behavior self-rating scale. *Behavior Research and Therapy, 10*, 412–417.

Klein, K. E., & Wegman, H. M. (1975a). Das verhalten des menschlichen organismus beim zeitzonenflug. 1. Die circadiane rhytmik und ihre desynchronisation. *Fortschritte Der Medizin, 93*, 1407–1414.

Klein, K. E., & Wegman, H. M. (1975b). Das verhalten des menschlichen organismus beim zeitzonenflug 2. Die folgen die desynchronisation. *Fortschritte Der Medizin, 93*, 1497–1507.

Knowles, J. B., Laverty, S. G., Keucher, H. A. (1968). The effects of alcohol on REM sleep. *Quarterly Journal on the Study of Alcohol, 29*, 342–349.

Kokkoris, C. P., Weitzman, E., Pollak, C. P., Spielman, A. J., Czeisler, C. A., & Bradlow, H. (1978). Long-term ambulatory temperature monitoring in a subject with hypernycthermal sleep-wake cycle disturbance. *Sleep, 1*, 177–190.

Kolomodin-Hedman, B., & Swensson, A. (1975). Problems related to shift work: A field study of Swedish railroad workers with irregular work hours. *Scandinavian Journal of Work, Environment and Health, 1*, 254–262.

Kuban, K. (1978). Recurrent hypersomnia secondary to sleep apnea. *Archives of Neurology, 35*, 772–773.

Kupfer, D. J., & Foster, F. G. (1978). EEG sleep and depression. In R. L. Williams & I. Karacan (Eds.), *Sleep disorders: Diagnosis and treatment*, (pp. 163–204). New York: Wiley.

Kurt, D., & Krieger, J. (1978). Analysis of apnea in sleep apnea. In C. Guilleminault & W. C. Dement (Eds.), *Sleep apnea syndromes*. New York: Liss.

Lacey, J. H., Crisp, A. H., Kalucy, R. S., Hartmann, M. K., & Chen, C. N. (1975). Weight gain and the sleeping electroencephalogram: Study of 10 patients with anorexia nervosa. *British Medical Journal, 4,* 556–558.

Lacey, J. I. (1967). Somatic response patterning and stress: Some revisions of activation theory. In M. H. Appley & R. Trumball, (Eds.) *Psychological stress,* (pp. 14–45). New York: Appleton-Century-Crofts.

Lugaresl, E., Coccagna, G., Mantovani, M., & LeBrun, R. (1972). Some periodic phenomena arising during drowsiness and sleep in man. *Neurophysiology, 32,* 701–705.

Lugiani, R., & Whipp, B. (1979). Doxapram hydrochloride: A respiratory stimulant for patients with primary alveolar hypoventilation. *Chest, 76,* 414–419.

Markland, O. N., & Dyken, M. L. (1976). Sleep abnormalities in patients with brainstem lesions. *Neurology, 26,* 769–776.

McFarland, R. A. (1975). Air travel across time zones. *American Scientist, 63,* 23–30.

Mendelis, J., Hawkins, D. (1967). Sleep and depression: A controlled EEG study. *Archives of General Psychiatry, 16,* 344.

Mendelson, W. B. (1980). *The use and misuse of sleeping pills.* New York: Plenum Press.

Mendelson, W. B., Gillin, R. J., & Wyatt, R. J. (1977). *Human sleep and its disorders.* New York: Plenum Press.

Mechanic, D., & Volkart, E. (1961). Stress, illness behaviors and sick role. *American Sociological Review, 26,* 51–58.

Mills, J. N. (1973). Transmissions processes between clock and manifestations. In J. N. Mills (Ed.), *Biological aspects of circadian rhythms* (pp. 27–84). London: Plenum Press.

Mills, J. N., Minors, D. S. & Waterhouse, J. M. Exogenous and endogenous influences on rhythms after a sudden time shift. *Ergonomics, 21,* 192–201.

Miles, L. M., Raynal, D. M., & Wilson, M. A. (1977). Blind man living in normal society has circadian rhythms of 24.9 hours. *Science, 198,* 421–423.

Monroe, L. J. (1967). Psychological and physiological differences between poor and good sleepers. *Journal Abnormal Psychology, 72,* 255–264.

Neff, N. H., & Yang, H. Y. T. (1974). Another look at the monoamine oxidase and the monoamine oxidase inhibitor drugs. *Life Sciences, 14,* 2061–2074.

Neil, J. F., Merikangas, J. R., Foster, F. G., Merikangas, K. R., Spiker, D. G., & Kupfer, D. J. (1980). Waking and all-night sleep EEG's in anorexia nervosa. *Clinical Electroencephalography, 11,* 9–15.

Nowlin, J. B. (1965). The association of nocturnal angina pectoris with dreaming. *Annals of Internal Medicine, 63,* 1040–1046.

Orr, W. C., Hall, W. H., Stahl, M. L., Durkin, M. G., & Whitsett, T. L. (1976). Sleep patterns and gastric acid secretion in duodenal ulcer disease. *Archives of Internal Medicine, 136,* 655–660.

Oswald, I. (1969). Sleep and dependence on amphetamines and other drugs. In A. Kales (Ed.), *Sleep: Physiology and pathology.* Philadelphia: Lippencott.

Oswald, I. (1974). Pharmacology of sleep. In O. Petrie-Quadens & J. D. Schlag (Eds.), *Basic sleep mechanisms* (pp. 297–306). New York: Academic Press.

Oswald, I. & Priest, R. G.: Five weeks to escape the sleeping-pill habit. *British Medical Journal, 2,* 1093–1095.

Oswald, I., Jones, H. S., & Mannerheim, J. E. (1968). Effects of two slimming drugs on sleep. *British Medical Journal, 1,* 796.

Parsons, T. *Social systems.* New York: Free Press.

Patkai, P., & Frankenhaeuser, M. (1964). Constancy of urinary catecholamine excretion. *Perceptual and Motor Skills, 19,* 789–790.

Patki, P., Johansson, G., & Post, B. (1971). *Variations in physiology and psychological functions during the menstrual cycle.* (Report No. 340). University of Stockholm, Stockholm: Psychological Laboratory.

Post, R. M., Gillin, J. C., Goodwin, F. K., Wyatt, R. J., & Snyder, F. (1972). The effect of orally administered cocaine on sleep of depressed patients. *Sleep Research, 1,* 72.

Prinz, P. N.: EEG during sleep and waking states. In Eleftheriou & Elias, *Special annual review of experimental aging research* (pp. 135–136). Bar Harbor, ME: EAR.

Prinz, P. N., & Halter, J. (1982). Sleep disturbances in the aged: Some hormonal correlates and newer therapeutic considerations. In Fann & Elsdorfer (Eds.), *Treatment of psychopathology in the aging* (pp. 43–69). New York: Springer.

Prinz, P. N., & Halter, J. B. (1983). Sleep disturbances in the elderly: Neurohumoral correlates. In Chase & Weitzman (Eds.), *Sleep disorders: Basic and clinical research* (pp. 463–488). New York: Spectrum.

Prinz, P. N., Blenkarn, D., Linnoila, M., & Weitzman, E. (1976). Growth hormone levels during sleep in elderly males. *Sleep Research, 5,* 187.

Prinz, P. N., Vitello, M. V., Schoen, R. B., & Halter, J. B. (1981). Sleep/waking patterns and plasma norepinephrine in young and aged men. *Sleep Research, 10,* 70.

Prinz, P. N., Peskind, E., Raskind, M., Eisdorfer, C., Zemcuznikov, T., & Gerber C. (1982). Changes in the sleep and waking EEG in nondemented and demented elderly. *Journal of the American Geriatric Society, 30,* 86.

Read, D. J., Williams, A. L., Hensley, W., Edwards, M., & Beal, S. (1979). Sudden infant deaths; some current research strategies. *Medical Journal of Australia, 2,* 236–238, 240–241, 244.

Relinger, H., & Bornstein, P. H. (1979). Treatment of sleep onset insomnia by paradoxical instruction. *Behavior Modification, 3,* 203–222.

Reidy, R., Husley, R., Bachus, B., Dahl, D., & Levine, B. (1979). Sleep apnea syndrome: Practical diagnostic method. *Chest, 75,* 81–83.

Roffwarg, H. P., Muzio, J. N., & Dement, W. C. (1966). Ontogenetic development of human sleep-dream cycle. *Science, 152,* 604–619.

Ross, J. J., Agnew, H. W., Williams, R. L., & Webb, W. B. (1968). Sleep pattern in preadolescent children: An EEG-EOG study. *Pediatrics, 42,* 324–335.

Roth, T., Kramer, M., & Lutz, T. The nature of insomnia: A descriptive summary of a sleep clinic population. *Comprehensive Psychiatry, 17,* 217–220.

Sackner, M., Landa, J., Forrest, T., & Greeneltch, D. (1975). Periodic sleep apnea. Chronic sleep deprivation related to intermitteant upper airway obstruction and central nervous system disturbance. *Chest, 67,* 164–171.

Salzman, C., Shader, R. I., & Van Der Kolk, B. A. (1976). Clinical psychopharmacology and the elderly patient. *New York State Journal of Medicine, 76,* 71–77.

Schultz, J. H., & Luthe, W. (1959). *Autogenic training.* New York: Grune & Stratton.

Schultz, M. A., Schulte, F. J., Akiyama, Y., & Parmelee, A. H. Jr. (1968). Development of electroencephalographic sleep phenomena in hypothyroid infants. *Electroencephalography and Clinical Neurophysiology, 25,* 351–358.

Schwartz, B., Seguy, M., & Escande, J. (1967). EEG, respiratory, ocular, and myographic correlations in the pickwickian syndrome and other apparently related conditions: A proposal for a hypothesis. *Electroencephalography and Clinical Neurophysiology, 23,* 386–400.

Schweiger, M. S. (1972). Sleep disturbance in pregnancy: A subjective survey. *American Journal of Obstetrics and Gynecology, 114,* 879–882.

Simmons, F., & Hill, M. (1974). Hypersomnia caused by upper airway obstruction. *Annals of Otology, 83,* 670–673.

Spiro, H., & Scheinberg, P. (1978). Reply to Kuban. *Archives of Neurology, 35,* 772–773.

Steinschneider, A. (1972). Prolonged apnea and the sudden infant death syndrome: Clinical and laboratory observations. *Pediatrics, 50*, 646–654.
Sterman, M. B., Howe, R. C., & MacDonald, L. R. (1970). Faciliatation of spindleburst sleep by conditioning electroencephalographic activity while awake. *Science, 18*, 44–48.
Swenson, W. M., Pearson, J. S., & Osborne, D. (1973). *An MMPI source book*. Minneapolis, MN: University of Minnesota Press.
Tan, T. L., Kales, J. D., Kales, A., Soldatos, C. R., & Bixler, E. O. (1981). Biopsychobehavioral correlates of insomnia. IV: Diagnosis based on DSM-III. *American Journal of Psychiatry*.
Taub, J. M. (1979). Effects of habitual napping on psychomotor performance. memory, and subjective states. *International Journal of Neuroscience, 9*, 97–112.
Tune, G. S. (1968). Sleep wakefulness in normal human adults. *British Medical Journal, 2*, 269–271.
Van Oot, P. H., Lane, T. W., & Borkovec, T. D. (1984). Sleep disturbances. In H. Adams & P. B. Sutker (Eds.), *Comprehensive handbook of psychopathology* (pp. 683–724). New York: Plenum Press.
Walsh, J. K., Stock, C. G., Tepas, D. I. (1978). The EEG sleep of workers frequently changing shifts; in Chase, Mitler, Walter, *Sleep research*(Vol. 7., pp. 314–325). Los Angeles: Brain Information Services.
Webb, W. B., & Agnew, H. W. Sleep and waking in a free-time environment. *Aerospace Medicine, 45*, 617–622.
Weitzman, E., Kripke, D., Goldmacher, D., McGregor, P., & Nogeire, C. (1970). Acute reversal of the sleep-waking cycle in man. *Archives of Neurology, 22*, 483–489.
Williams, H. L., & Salamy, A. (1972). Alcohol and sleep. In Kissen & Begleiter (Eds.), *The biology of alcoholism*, pp. 435–483. New York: Plenum Press.
Williams, R. L. (1978). Sleep disturbances in various medical and surgical conditions. In R. L. Williams & I. Karacan (Eds.) *Sleep disorders: Diagnosis and treatment* (pp. 285–302). New York: Wiley.
Williams, R. L., & Karacan, I. (1978). *Sleep disorders: Diagnosis and treatment*. New York: Wiley.
Williams, R. L., Karacan, I., & Hursch, C. J. (1974). *Electroencephalography of human sleep: Clinical implications*. New York: Wiley.
Wyatt, R. J., Chase, T. N., Scott, J., Snyder, F., & Engelman, K. (1970). Effect of L-DOPA on the sleep of man. *Nature, 228*, 999–1001.
Wyatt, R. J., Fram, D., Buchbinder, R., & Snyder, F. (1971). Treatment of intractable narcolepsy with a monoamine oxidase inhibitor. *New England Journal of Medicine, 285*, 987–991.
Zwart, C. A., & Lisman, S. A. (1979). Analysis of stimulus control treatment of sleep-onset insomnia. *Journal of Consulting and Clinical Psychology, 47*, 113–118.
Zwillich, C., Sutton, F., Pierson, D., Creagh, E., & Weil, J. (1975). Decreased hypoxic ventilation drive in the obesity-hypoventilation syndrome. *American Journal of Medicine, 59*, 343–348.
Zung, W., Wilson, W., & Dodson, W. (1964). Effect of depressive disorders on sleep EEG responses. *Archives of General Psychiatry, 10*, 439.

CHAPTER 6

Self-Regulation and Type A Behavior

Nanette M. Frautschi and Margaret A. Chesney

The Type A behavior pattern as a syndrome was identified by Rosenman and his associates (Rosenman *et al.*, 1964) to be characteristic of patients with coronary heart disease (CHD). This syndrome is manifested by competitiveness, a hard-driving orientation toward achievement, easily aroused anger, loud, rapid, accentuated speech patterns, a heightened pace of living, and impatience with slowness and delays. These behaviors were viewed by Friedman and Rosenman (1974) as reflecting a "chronic, incessant struggle" on the part of these individuals "to achieve more and more in less and less time, and if required to do so against the opposing efforts of other things or other people" (p. 67). However, the Type A pattern was not considered a personality trait but rather a set of observable behaviors elicited in susceptible individuals by a challenging situation. Individuals who respond to challenge with the fully developed Type A pattern are classified as Type A_1; those who do not respond to similar challenges with Type A behavior are classified as B_4. Those who show less consistent or incomplete Type A or B behavior patterns are classified as A_2 and B_3, respectively.

Subsequent prospective studies confirmed the role of the Type A pattern as a CHD risk factor. The first evidence of the causal relationship

---

Nanette M. Frautschi • Outpatient Behavioral Medicine, Southern California Permanente Medical Group, Los Angeles, California 90027. *Margaret A. Chesney* • Department of Behavioral Medicine, Stanford Research Institute, Menlo Park, California 94025.

between the Type A behavior pattern and CHD was provided by the Western Collaborative Group Study (WCGS) (Rosenman *et al.*, 1975). In this study, subjects identified as displaying Type A behavior at intake into the study later showed approximately twice the CHD rate as that experienced by Type B's. Other prospective studies in Belgium and at Framingham confirmed this twofold risk (Haynes, Feinleib, & Kannel, 1980, Kornitzer *et al.*, 1982). Furthermore, since the initial study, the Type A pattern has been found to correlate with severity of coronary atherosclerosis observed at autopsy (Friedman, Rosenman, Straus, & Kositcheck, 1968) and in angiographic studies (Blumenthal, Williams, Kong, Schanberg, & Thompson, 1978; Frank, Heller, Kornfeld, Sporn, & Weiss, 1978; Zyzanski, Jenkins, Ryan, Flessas, & Everist, 1976). Not all prospective or angiographic studies have confirmed the association between Type A behavior and CHD (Dimsdale, Hackett, Hutter, Block, & Catanzano, 1979; Shekelle *et al.*, 1985). However, after a thorough survey of the literature, weighting the accumulated evidence, Matthews and Haynes (1986) concluded that the studies failing to show an association between Type A and CHD are either flawed or focus on special populations and, in balance, are not sufficient to call the status of Type A as a CHD risk factor into question. This conclusion is consistent with that of the critical review panel convened by the National Heart, Lung, and Blood Institute which recognized Type A behavior as an independent risk factor for coronary heart disease of equal magnitude as the increased risk imposed by age, blood pressure, serum cholesterol, and smoking (Review Panel on Coronary-Prone Behavior and Coronary Heart Disease, 1981).

Recognition of the CHD risk associated with Type A behavior has fostered considerable interest in methods of modifying the pattern. A modest number of intervention studies have been reported (Suinn, 1982). Although these studies suggest that the behavior pattern is amenable to change, they also indicate that there are high rates of attrition of Type A's in treatment and that elements of the behavior pattern resist modification. After a brief examination of attrition and outcome data of the largest clinical intervention trial conducted to date, a self-regulatory model of Type A behavior is presented that provides a conceptual framework for understanding the resiliency of the behavior pattern. Empirical research demonstrating physiological, behavioral, and cognitive self-regulatory mechanisms is discussed. Following this, the model's implications for treatment of Type A is considered and recommendations are made for further research.

Preliminary Findings of the Recurrent Coronary Prevention Project: Attrition and Outcome Data

Comparative Type A intervention studies are limited in number, with few studies of Type A modification in cardiac patients and fewer still that report morbidity and mortality data as well as behavioral outcome measures (Suinn, 1982). The Recurrent Coronary Prevention Project perhaps best exemplifies the painstaking and long-term research required to assess the effectiveness of treatment interventions for Type A in a clinical population (Friedman *et al.*, 1982; Friedman *et al.*, 1984). Preliminary reports of this major clinical trial assessing the effects of Type A intervention on the rate of recurring coronary events indicate rates of subject attrition to be 18% in the 1st year of the project and 34% by the 3rd year (Friedman *et al.*, 1982; Friedman *et al.*, 1984). Moreover, their findings showed that those who dropped out were rated as more extreme Type A's than those who continued treatment, suggesting that those individuals most in need of treatment are the least likely to avail themselves of it.

The findings of the Recurrent Coronary Prevention Project also suggest that long-term treatment may be necessary for successful interventions with post–myocardial infarction patients. Cardiac patients in the Recurrent Coronary Prevention Project underwent cognitive-behavioral training sessions weekly for 2 months, biweekly for 2 months, and monthly for the remainder of a 3-year period. After 1 year of treatment, they exhibited approximately a 14% change in Type A behavior, as assessed through self-report and the reports of spouses and work colleagues, and a 30% change as assessed by the Type A Structured Interview (Friedman *et al.*, 1982). By the 3rd year, this increased to approximately a 22% reduction in Type A behavior as assessed by self-report and a 39% change as assessed by the Structured Interview (Friedman *et al.*, 1984). Recent research with both cardiac patients and healthy individuals suggests that briefer psychological intervention (5–14 sessions) can promote statistically significant reductions in Type A behavior (see Suinn, 1982, for review). However, the absence of *consistent* reductions in CHD risk factors following these interventions and the relative paucity of information regarding the maintenance of these changes bring into question the clinical significance of brief interventions.

Although the preliminary findings of the Recurrent Coronary Prevention Project underscore the difficulty of changing Type A behavior, they also emphasize the importance of continued Type A intervention. A nearly twofold reduction was reported in the percentage of recurrence of coronary incidents in cardiac patients receiving both Type A modification and medical information in comparison with a group receiving medical information only (Friedman *et al.*, 1984). These promising findings may serve as an impetus to research directed toward clarifying those self-regulatory mechanisms in Type A behavior that impede change.

A Model of Self-Regulation and Type A Behavior

Type A behavior can be conceptualized as a complex psychobiological or self-regulatory system as described by Wolfgang Linden in Chapter 1. To the extent that this system is pathogenic, it is dysfunctional. In an eloquent review of Type A literature, Krantz and Durel (1983) present such a model. Specifically, they argue that Type A behavior not only may emerge as an interaction between the person and environment resulting in enhanced cardiovascular and neuroendocrine response but may also be the result of a constitutionally excessive sympathetic responsiveness in Type A's to perceived stress. In this chapter, this interactive psychobiological model is extended to incorporate the role of positive feedback in reinforcing the association between Type A behavior and physiological arousal, and greater attention is given to the role of attentional and attributional mechanisms in the maintenance of the behavior pattern.

A dysfunctional self-regulatory model would suggest that although Type A individuals experience excessive physiological arousal, rather than engage in behavior to reduce this arousal, they behave in ways that maintain it. Thus, self-regulation serves to maintain Type A behavior and its associated physiological arousal, despite evidence that this pattern may be pathogenic. It may be, as Krantz and Durel propose, that Type A's are constitutionally inclined to excessive cardiovascular responsivity and that Type A behaviors, including rapid and accelerated movements, are engendered by this arousal. On the other hand, it may be that Type A's respond to environmental stress or challenge with increased arousal. Once aroused, Type A's do not "down-regulate" this arousal. Perhaps they perceive the arousal as a central part of an integrated biobehavioral response that is associated with activity and achievement, conditions they value. Type A adults report more rapid career advancement than Type B's; they are better educated (Waldron, Zyzanski, Shekelle, Jenkins, & Tannenbaum, 1977), attain higher occupational status (Mettlin, 1976; Waldron, 1978), and receive more rewards from their work (Matthews, Helmreich, Beane, & Lucker, 1980; Mettlin, 1976; see Zyzanski, 1978 for review). The behavior and associated arousal are repeatedly paired with rewards, providing the basis for a classically conditioned preference for physiological arousal and the environments that elicit it.

Physiological Mechanisms in Type A Behavior

There is evidence that the association between Type A behavior and physiological arousal, although not universally observed in laboratory studies, is well established (Houston, 1983). Inconsistencies in the findings of studies of physiological reactivity and Type A appear related to the differential utility of Type A measures, as well as differences in the physiological measures used and situational parameters of experimental tasks (Contrada, Wright, & Glass, 1985). A greater consistency of association between Type A and physiological reactivity is found when the behavior pattern is assessed using the Structured Interview (SI) rather than paper-and-pencil questionnaires such as the Jenkins Activity Survey (JAS). In contrast to the JAS, the Structured Interview is designed to provide an opportunity to elicit and observe Type A behavior, perhaps explaining its greater utility in predicting differences between Type A's and Type B's in reactivity to stress.

Enhanced physiological responsiveness in Type A's compared to Type B's has been found more frequently in studies in which systolic blood pressure and plasma epinephrine are used as dependent measures than in studies focusing on effects on heart rate, diastolic blood pressure, and plasma norepinephrine. However, because these measures are differentially affected by sympathetic innervation, the inconsistency in findings does not necessarily weaken support for an association between Type A and heightened sympathetic responsiveness (Contrada *et al.*, 1985). In addition to the influence of the dependent measures on the observation of reactivity differences between Type A's and Type B's, differential reactivity to stressors is most often detected when experimental tasks are moderately difficult, external incentives are not high, and subjects are exposed to harassment (Blumenthal *et al.*, 1983; Dembroski, MacDougall, Herd, & Shields, 1979; Gastorf, 1981; Glass, *et al.*, 1980, Experiment 1).

Recent reports of differences between Type A's and Type B's in cardiovascular reactivity in the absence of experimental laboratory manipulation indicate that perception or cognitive appraisal of stress is not essential. For example, the physiologial arousal of Type A's to stressors has been observed to occur during anesthesia, indicating that the arousal may not require cognitive mediation (Krantz & Durel, 1983). Studies in which arousal was pharmacologically blocked by a beta-blocking agent such as Atenolol provide further evidence of the tight bond between Type A behavior and physiological arousal. Along with the expected reductions in sympathetic activity with beta blockade, these studies showed reductions in the intensity of Type A behaviors (Schmieder, Friedrich, Neus, Rudel, & Von Eiff, 1983). As Krantz and Durel (1983) suggest, these data may indicate that the arousal is inherent. It also may be conditioned by repeated association or pairing with stressors.

Regardless of the source, be it constitutional or conditional, Type A behavior has been associated with increased sympathetic arousal, a proposed mechanism by which the behavior pattern is thought to increase CHD risk (Kranz & Manuck, 1984). These findings acquire greater significance when considered in the light of evidence showing that Type A's not only respond to environmental stressors with greater responsiveness than Type B's, but that they have longer recovery times from states of sympathetic arousal (Hart & Jamieson, 1983; Jorgenson & Houston, 1981) and that chronic arousal of the affected systems may lead to structural changes in the cardiovascular system (Henry & Stephens, 1977). It also should be noted that early research, in addition to demonstrating greater sympathetic responsiveness among Type A's and Type B's, also indicates an association between Type A and increased reactivity of the pituitary-cortical system (Friedman, 1978a). Like the catecholamines, cortisol, has been implicated in the etiology of coronary heart disease (Henry, 1983; Williams, 1985).

Behavioral Self-Regulatory Mechanisms in Type A: Seeking Out Challenge

Once heightened arousal is established, a dysfunctional self-regulatory model of Type A behavior would predict that arousal will be maintained through the interaction of Type A's with their environment. The pairing of the behavior pattern with both physiological arousal to challenge and the reinforcing perception of accomplishment may foster a preference on the part of Type A's for challenging situations and the arousal they engender. Research on employed adult males indicates that the work habits of Type A's are consistent with this model. For example, despite being less well-satisfied with their jobs, Type A managers report working more hours per week and traveling more days per year than their Type B counterparts (Howard, Cunningham, & Rechnitzer, 1977). Also reflecting a Type A preference for challenge, Frankenhaeuser,

Lundberg, and Forsman (1980a) showed that Type A males and females selected a faster work pace on a task than Type B males and females. Although the faster pace resulted in a greater total work load, the Type A's performed better than did the Type B's, while reporting the same magnitude of increase in effort and in sympathetic-adrenal and pituitary-adrenal activation over the task as the Type B's. Frankenhaeuser (1983) concluded that "the Type A person, when in control of the situation, sets his or her standards high, copes effectively with self-selected heavy load, and does so without mobilizing excessive physiological resources" (p. 97). Thus, Type A behavior might be considered to be productive and reinforcing in terms of work accomplished without added subjective or physiological stress under some conditions.

The self-regulatory system of the Type A individual becomes one of enhanced pace of activity and, at times, increased effort that is likely to be perceived as productive by the individual as well as by others. This activity is often associated with increased physiological arousal. Once this self-regulatory system is established, the model would predict that disregulation would occur if any one of the elements (e.g., the activity, the arousal) were not present. Confronted with such disregulation, the individual would engage in activities to reestablish self-regulation. In fact, research evidence supports this conclusion. Frankenhaeuser found that Type A's reported and showed as much or more physiological arousal when bored and deprived of work than when given work to do (Frankenhaeuser, Lundberg, & Forsman, 1980b). Type B individuals, on the other hand, reported and showed consistently less arousal under the same conditions (Frankenhaeuser *et al.*, 1980b). Frankenhaeuser suggests that these findings imply that Type A's lack strategies for coping with nonwork situations or with boredom (Frankenhaeuser, 1983). Confronted with such situations, Type A's might be expected to become distressed or modify the situation by initiating activities or by increasing arousal. From a self-regulatory perspective, Type A behavior and its correlates including enhanced physiological arousal would be maintained, and efforts to reduce heart disease risk through modifications of the behavior pattern would be resisted.

Cognitive Self-Regulatory Mechanisms in Type A: Symptom Denial, Selective Attention, and Attributional Biases

The self-regulatory mechanisms that maintain the Type A behavior pattern present obstacles to efforts to modify the pattern. Among these obstacles is a tendency on the part of clients to see few reasons to make major or permanent changes in behavior. This is often because they have not experienced any symptoms of coronary heart disease. On the contrary, the behavior pattern and the physiological arousal that accompanies it are perceived as invigorating and instrumental to achievement and the attainment of desired rewards and goals. This obstacle is encountered most often in the treatment of individuals without documented CHD but is also present in those who have been diagnosed as having clinical CHD, including post–myocardial infarction patients.

The perception of physical symptoms is similar to the perception of emotions because in both a change in physiological arousal must be noted and the symptom must be labeled. There is evidence that Type A persons are not particularly aware of or mislabel physical symptoms including fatigue and chest pain. It has been suggested (Weidner & Chesney, 1985) that in the Type A struggle to achieve, attention to physical symptoms may interfere with productivity and, as a result, symptoms are suppressed. Support for the suppression of symptoms is derived from laboratory research such as that by Carver, Coleman, and Glass (1976) in which Type A and Type B individuals were given treadmill tests. The results indicated that although the Type A's exerted more effort in the task, as measured by oxygen consumption, they reported less fatigue than their counterparts, the Type B's. Since this first study, others have also reported evidence of symptom suppression (Matthews & Volkin, 1981, Stern, Harris, & Elverum, 1981; Weidner & Matthews, 1978); however, such suppression is not always reported. Carmody and his associates (Carmody, Hollis, Matarazzo, Fey, & Conner, 1984), using the Jenkins Activity Survey to assess Type A behavior in a community study of healthy adults, found that Type A's reported more general physical symptoms than Type B's.

The suppression of symptoms observed in some Type A's or individuals who are coronary-prone has been reported in myocardial infarction patients. From clinical observation, Greene, Moss, and Goldstein (1974) reported that Type A's who experienced myocardial infarction delayed reporting early heart attack symptoms and as a result received treatment later than Type B's. This clinical observation was subsequently substantiated by Matthews and her associates (Matthews, Siegel, Kuller, Thompson, & Varat, 1983), who found that Type A's experiencing an acute myocardial infarction experienced less pain, especially if they were engaged in demanding work, and delayed longer in seeking treatment than their Type B counterparts. The most frequent prodromal symptom of myocardial infarction and sudden death is fatigue, and the second most frequent is chest pain (Rissanen, Romo, & Siltanen, 1978). That Type A's have been shown to suppress symptoms such as fatigue may explain why Type A's report later for treatment of myocardial infarction, a delay that may contribute to their higher risk.

Other evidence suggests that, in general, healthy Type A's report symptoms differently than do Type B's. In addition to the research indicating that they report fewer symptoms, there is evidence that they attribute symptoms to different sources that do Type B's. Specifically, Type A's attribute symptoms they may experience to specific environmental factors rather than to illness. Conversely, when considering the source of symptoms experienced by others, Type A's attributed the symptoms to the more intrinsic factor, illness (Jones & Nisbett, 1971; Gastorf, 1980). These findings are important because symptom perception, labeling, and reporting are essential factors in the modifications of Type A behavior. Thus, the specific symptoms that could warn the Type A of an impending problem are among those that are denied or minimized, and processes of self-regulation or seeking treatment are not activated.

Denial and minimization as coping strategies for myocardial infarction have been differently associated with prognosis, depending on the stage of treatment. In the acute phase, these strategies are associated with less distress and anxiety (Doehrman, 1977; Gentry, Foster, & Haney, 1973). However, in the later stages of treatment, there is some evidence that these strategies have been associated with noncompliance with treatment regimens. Specifically, Croog, Shapiro, and Levine (1971) reported that denial was significantly related to nonadherence as well as the failure to initiate treatment. Thus, denial can be viewed as interfering with self-regulation when such regulation involves the effective use of treatment resources.

Selective Attention and Task Orientation

Selective attention and task orientation laboratory experiments shed some additional light on Type A selective attention and denial by examining the behavior of Type A and Type B individuals in response to various tasks or situations. These experiments indicate that when confronted with difficult problem-solving tasks presented in the presence of distractions, Type A's will ignore the distracting, peripheral cues and perform better than their Type B counterparts (Gastorf, Suls, & Sanders, 1980; Glass, 1977, Chapter 7, Experiments 3, 4; Matthews & Brunson, 1979, Experiments 2, 3). Conversely, Type B's outperform Type A's on tasks that require a broad focus of attention (Gastorf *et al.*, 1980; Matthews & Brunson, 1979, Experiment 1). It may be that this selective, task-oriented attentional focus plays a role in the observation that Type A's work more quickly on tasks than Type B's (Burnam, Pennebaker, & Glass, 1975).

When tasks require careful responses with long intervals of waiting between tasks, Type B's outperform Type A's, perhaps suggesting that the selective attending of the more impulsive, time-urgent Type A's is not maintained during long periods of inactivity or waiting. These experiments indicate that the selective attention observed in relation to symptoms is also activated in the service of task performance. To the extent that symptoms are similar to distracting cues, Type A's experiencing cardiovascular symptoms during tasks might be expected to ignore them.

Failure: Personal Responsibility Attributions

The responses of Type A's in laboratory experiments designed to present a failure situation suggest that behavioral responses to failure may have emotional and physiological correlates that increase risk of CHD for Type A's. In terms of self-regulation, these studies point out a pattern of responses that are dysfunctional rather than regulatory. When presented with challenging puzzles, some of which were actually unsolvable, Type A's increased their initial efforts more than Type B's following feedback of failure. However, if the failure continues, the Type A's cease their efforts and give up responding (Brunson & Matthews, 1981; Glass, 1977; Krantz, Glass, & Snyder, 1974; Weidner & Matthews, 1978). Type A's have been found (Brunson & Matthews, 1981) to attribute failure in such experiments to their own lack of ability, whereas Type B's attribute failure to external factors. Perhaps it is their attribution of the failure to their own inability that initially spurs on their efforts and by doing so may maintain their arousal and heighten their risk for CHD.

On the other hand, the mood that is engendered by the laboratory experiments that present prolonged failure might be best described as depressed. Such depression would not be unexpected since Type A's attribute failure to their personal inability. It is of interest that depression has been associated with CHD, that is, extent of atherosclerosis, myocardial infarction, and Type A behavior. Zyzanski *et al.* (1976) found that men with two or more coronary vessels obstructed more than 50% each, as documented by angiography, scored significantly higher than those with less obstruction on depression and anxiety self-report scales as well as on the global Type A scale of the Jenkins Activity Scale. Dimsdale, Hackett, Block, and Hutter (1978) also reported a low but significant relationship between Type A and depressed mood in patients hospitalized for coronary angiography. Moreover, there is evidence that feelings of despair, hopelessness, and depression as well as emotional exhaustion belong to the prodromatas of myocardial infarction and sudden death (Appels, 1983; Elliott & Eisdorfer, 1982; Greene *et al.*, 1974,

Nixon, 1976). In one study of interviews with surviving family members (Greene *et al.*, 1974), sudden death due to CHD was found to be particularly prevalent among men who were described as having been depressed for a week to several months prior to death.

Physiological Consequences of Self-Regulatory Mechanisms

Although the point is conjectural at this time, specific physiological pathways accompanying arousal and depression have been indicated as a possible mechanism by which Type A behavior is associated with increased risk of CHD (Henry & Stephens, 1977; Price, 1982). Sympathetic arousal is engendered by tasks that are perceived as challenging, including tasks that initially provide feedback of failure. This arousal is marked by an excessive release of catecholamines, which have been implicated in the etiology of CHD and sudden death (Herd, 1981; Rosenman & Friedman, 1974). The depressed mood that has been associated with prolonged failure in laboratory experiments and with CHD events may activate the pituitary-adrenal cortical system, resulting in excessive cortisol levels which have also been implicated in the pathogenesis of CHD (Henry, 1983).

In summary, the responses of Type A's to environmental challenge do not reflect healthy self-regulation but rather may activate neuroendocrine systems that have been linked to CHD. On occasions involving challenge without failure, Type A's, more than Type B's, selectively attend to the task, suppress physiological symptoms of fatigue, and yet experienced elevated cardiovascular and catecholamine responses. When initially presented with failure, Type A's, more than Type B's, increase their efforts and would be expected to show parallel responses in terms of selective attention, symptom suppression, and cardiovascular and catecholamine responses. When failure is prolonged, Type A's, more than Type B's, give up their efforts, attribute the failure to their inability, and may become depressed and show elevations in cortical levels. Thus, when presented with stressful or challenging situations Type A's might be characterized as engaging in a primary and perhaps often a singular focus on the task (increasing their efforts) and not attending to peripheral factors, including their own physiological symptoms of arousal and fatigue. Thus, rather than the symptoms signaling the Type A to engage in effective self-regulatory behavior to reduce arousal and risk, the focus on the task activates physiological response systems that are associated with increased risk.

Implications for Treatment

The adoption of a self-regulatory model of Type A has strong implications for treatment intervention. Within this model, cognition, behavior, and physiology interlock within Type A in such a manner as to maintain sympathetic arousal. Temporary fluctuations in physiological reactivity during challenge or failure become frequent, prolonged, and finally pathogenic. The self-regulatory mechanisms that contribute to this state of chronic dysregulation also influence the course of treatment. Reduced motivation and openness to therapeutic change may result from the Type A's inattention to symptom of physical illness and psychological distress. The Type A's approach to therapeutic assignments and interactions with therapists also reflects disregulatory mechanisms. Prescriptions to adopt a hobby so as to reduce vocational demands and the associated arousal may result in the Type A's taking up a competitive sport and practicing it with the same driven, aggressive zeal that characterizes his or her behavior in the office or boardroom. As is show by the research of Frankenhaeuser (Frankenhaeuser *et al.*, 1980b). Type A's may lack strategies for coping with nonwork situations and may show increased physiological arousal when deprived of work or when bored. Homework assignments that limit work activities or involve unstructured leisure time may, paradoxically, increase rather than decrease arousal unless Type A's are trained in alternative coping strategies. Similarly, an initial failure to accomplish an assigned homework task may produce protestations on the part of Type A's that they "can do it" and the setting of increased goals for the next assignment rather than serving as the impetus for reevaluation of the assignment and alternatives for accomplishing it. In short, those aspects of Type A behavior that are associated with heightened arousal and increased risk also reduce the likelihood of successful intervention.

Timing of the Intervention

A primary question faced by a clinician is how to intervene with an individual who does not acknowledge having a problem and is rewarded by society for the pathological behavior. Friedman (1978b) has addressed this issue and has argued that the most successful intervention are timed after the occurrence of a coronary event, such as a myocardial infarction, when the consequences of Type A behavior are most salient to the individual. In support of this point, Suinn was more successful in lowering lipid levels in a sample of post–myocardial infarction patients (Suinn, 1975) than in a nonclinical group (Suinn & Bloom, 1978). However, given the relatively high frequency of dropouts in long-term cardiovascular rehabilitation programs (Friedman *et al.*, 1982), it appears that the awareness of consequences is transitory and in some instances is not in itself capable of sustaining life-style change. Moreover, although interventions for post–myocardial infarction patients may reduce the frequency of recurrent events (Friedman *et al.*, 1984), it is clearly desirable that interventions be directed also toward primary and secondary prevention.

For successful intervention with adults, particularly those who are at increased risk of CHD but have not yet suffered a myocardial infarction, it may be critical to present a convincing "cost–benefit" analysis with respect to treatment (Roskies, 1983). Such an analysis involves assisting the Type A individual to identify the short- and long-term costs and benefits of involvement in a program of life-style change. Although Type A's readily attribute their material or occupational success to their behavior pattern, they may be unaware that this same behavior may reduce their ability to perform on some tasks and may also increase their risk of CHD. Evidence of a shifting ration in favor of Types B's to Type A's at the highest occupational levels (Howard *et al.*, 1977) may stimulate motivation for change. Additionally, defining the goal of a program as assisting Type A's to discriminate when alternative styles may be more useful or efficient rather than eliminating all Type A behavior may increase their willingness to become involved in a therapeutic program. Although a delineation of costs and benefits is imperative in initial sessions, the selective attention that is characteristic of Type A's necessitates repetition of these issues throughout treatment (Friedman, 1978b).

The behavioral and physiological similarities in Type A children and adults (Blaney, 1983; Lawler, Allen, Critcher, & Standard, 1981; Matthews, 1979; Matthews & Angulo, 1980; Matthews & Siegel, in press; Matthews & Volkin, 1981; Murray, Blake, Prineas, & Gillum, 1983), when coupled with evidence that atherosclerosis begins in childhood and adolescence (Enos, Holmes, & Beyer, 1953; McNamara, Molot, Stremple, & Cutting, 1971), provide a strong rationale for early assessment and treatment. Although there are few, if any, intervention studies with children (Suinn, 1982) treatment with children may have an additional advantage in that the pattern may be more malleable early in its development than in the adult years.

Types of Interventions

Systematic interventions for Type A behavior have generally included alteration of environmental elicitors of the behavior pattern as well as intervention in the self-regulatory mechanisms that characterized the pattern (Chesney, Frautschi, & Rosenman, 1985; Suinn, 1982; Friedman *et al.*, 1982). Whereas supportive or dynamic psychotherapy has been used in the treatment of the behavior pattern, cognitive-behavioral interventions have been more frequently reported in the literature (Suinn, 1982). The latter include self-monitoring of arousal and accompanying thoughts and behavior (Friedman *et al.*, 1982; Levenkron, Cohen, Mueller, & Fisher, 1982; Southern & Smith, 1982), a first step in modifying both the selective attention and misattribution that contribute to dysregulation in Types A's. Relaxation training and biofeedback are often components of cognitive-behavioral interventions (Girdano & Girdano, 1977; Suinn & Bloom, 1978, Yarian, 1976). These approaches enhance awareness of symptoms of tension, fatigue, and discomfort and establish these symptoms as cues for arousal reduction. In addition to self-monitoring, cognitive-behavioral interventions typically involve contracting for and reinforcement of changes in thoughts and behavior (Friedman *et al.*, 1982, Levenkron *et al.*, 1982; Southern & Smith, 1982). This allows new associations to be made between relaxation and reward and fosters an increased preference for less challenging environments.

Although it is still too early for firm conclusions, the evidence to date suggests that behavior therapy is somewhat more effective than psychotherapy in modifying Type A behavior (Suinn, 1982). One may speculate that this differential success may reflect a greater effectiveness of behavioral techniques in altering the self-regulatory mechanisms underlying the Type A behavior pattern.

Type A behavior is strongly reinforced within the culture and, as delineated in the self-regulatory model, provides the opportunity for repeated pairings of physiological arousal and reward and the development of preferences in Type A's for challenging environments and the arousal they engender. Additionally, because the behavior pattern is not always associated with successful outcomes and in some circumstances may result in less effective task performance, it is particularly difficult to change (Price, 1982). Partial schedules of reinforcement such as this have been found to produce high rates of targeted behaviors that are relatively resistant to extinction. Moreover, the cues that could allow Type A's to discriminate conditions in which Type A behavior will be successful rather than debilitating are subtle and not easily identified. Assisting Type A's in determining when their behavior is producing excessive arousal or reduced effectiveness and training them to reward themselves for behavior change and arousal reduction may be critical in offsetting the powerful effects of patterns well established by conditioning. Self-reward, particularly self-praise, by virtue of its immediacy as a reinforcer, may bring about change and render a dysfunctional self-regulatory system more functional.

Direct intervention in the attentional and attributional processes of Type A's also appears important in training them to regulate their arousal more effectively. The minimization and misattribution of symptoms of illness of Type A's suggest that health education may be beneficial. Matthews and her associates (Matthews *et al.*, 1983) has recommended work-site health education programs for individuals at increased risk for coronary heart disease in which participants would be taught to recognize prodromal signs of myocardial infarction such as fatigue, depression, and chest pain and seek medical treatment. Such a program would appear to be particularly effective because it is under challenging conditions such as heightened work demands that Type A's are least attentive to physical symptoms.

Behavioral prescriptions or structured homework assignments may be sufficiently challenging so as to elicit the selective attention and attributional biases associated with the behavior pattern and heightened physiological reactivity. They also provide the therapist with abundant opportunities for direct observation of these self-regulatory mechanisms and intervention. For example, the maintenance of a narrow, constricted task focus in carrying out a homework assignment allows this attentional aspect of the Type A pattern to be directly assessed and modified. The use of humor and the modeling of flexibility, moderate pacing of activities, and creativity in response to problems encountered in the performance of homework is also extremely helpful in fostering change.

Failure experiences during the course of homework assignments also are unique opportunities for evaluation and intervention. Brief failures typically result in increases in performance criterion whereas prolonged failure may result in deterioration of problem-solving strategies and a failure to attend to relevant cues. Modeling of acceptance of occasional failure as part of human failibility, the setting of realistic standards, and the continued attention to relevant cues in the face of prolonged failure may be powerful interventions.

Although interventions of this kind are intended to provide Type A's with skills for better self-regulation of physiological reactivity and ultimately to reduce CHD risk, they involve risks as well as benefits. The widening of the Type A's attentional field through self-monitoring of fatigue and tension requires caution, especially when paired with arousal-reducing strategies. Current conceptualizations (Friedman & Rosenman, 1974; Price, 1982) of Type A behaviors as a defense against underlying feelings of insecurity or despondency suggest the possibility of precipitating depressive symptoms during treatment. Although some feelings of discomfort may serve as an impetus for therapeutic change, clinical levels of depression may greatly impede progress. Self-monitoring of relaxed and pleasurable feelings, in contrast to tension, and contracting to increase recreational, artistic, or social activities rather than reduce vocational demands may be a safer intervention strategy. Of course, increases in these positive behaviors will necessitate reduction in negative ones, but without making salient any negative feelings Type A's may be experiencing.

Unless care is taken, interventions may also have an unforeseen impact on the educational, vocational, or economic productivity of Type A's. The behavior pattern is associated with success in these realms and, as Frankenhaeuser's research (Frankenhaeuser *et al.*, 1980a) has shown, not always associated with heightened physiological reactivity. Extensive individual assessment may be required in order to determine in what conditions physiological arousal becomes excessive and the behavior detrimental. The use of physiological indexes (for instance, systolic blood pressure as measured by ambulatory monitors) to differentiate the circumstances associated with heightened arousal can increase the specificity of treatment and reduce the possibility of needlessly restricting adaptive behavior.

In some instances, direct pharmacological intervention in addition to cognitive-behavioral change may be required. When an individual appears unresponsive to behavioral treatment, or it is suspected that underlying structural changes have already resulted from chronic arousal, medication may be a necessary adjunct to treatment. Krantz and Durel (1983) have shown significant reductions in physiological arousal, as well as some behavioral manifestations of the Type A pattern in response to the administration of beta blockers. However, they caution clinicians that although pharmacological intervention may temper the intensity of Type A, it does not convert Type A individuals into Type B's, and they recommend continued efforts in modifying the information-processing and behavioral aspects of the pattern in addition to the physiological components.

Summary and Directions for Future Research

The self-regulatory model of Type A that has been presented in this chapter posits that Type A's, rather than reducing physiologic arousal, behave in ways that maintain responsiveness and increase their risk of coronary heart disease. Type A's prefer and actively seek out challenging or stressful environments and experience as much or more physiological arousal when deprived of work than when given work to do. Their preferences for stimulation and challenge are thought to reflect conditioning secondary to the repeated association of the behavior pattern, the accompanying arousal, and reward.

Attentional and attributional biases also were implicated in the dysfunctional self-regulatory process. Type A's narrow task focus and attribution of performance failure to deficits in their abilities rather than task characteristics are associated with accelerated efforts and sympathetic arousal in response to challenge and initial failure, and reduced responsiveness, depression, and possibly increased adrenal-cortical reactivity with prolonged failure. These neurohormonal responses, particularly the enhanced sympathetic arousal, have been proposed as the mechanisms whereby Type A behavior is thought to increase the risk of coronary heart disease. Moreover, attentional and attributional biases foster a minimization or denial of fatigue and other prodromal signs of myocardial infarction that would alert Type A's to the need for corrective action to bring about arousal reduction.

Given a bidirectional self-regulatory model of Type A, interventions may be focused directly on the physiological reactivity with subsequent reductions in some Type A behaviors. Alternatively, interventions may be focused on the cognitive-behavioral components of the pattern with some reductions in physiological reactivity following.

Several aspects of the self-regulatory model of Type A behavior remain to be clarified in future research. A central concept in the self-regulatory model is that Type A individuals prefer and actively seek out challenging or arousal-producing environments. However, much is still unknown regarding the circumstances in which Type A individuals exhibit enhanced physiological arousal in the naturalistic environment. Situational variables and task characteristics have been identified through laboratory research that elicit differences between Type A and Type B individuals in neurohormonal and cardiovascular reactivity with some consistency. For example, moderately difficult or competitive tasks, tasks involving harassment of participants, and, alternatively, periods of inactivity have been associated with heightened arousal, but these studies do not allow for much specificity in prediction and provide the clinician with little concrete information to guide intervention.

The self-regulatory model of Type A behavior also suggests that through continued exposure to challenging settings, temporary fluctuations in physiological reactivity may become more frequent or prolonged and eventually may become pathogenic. However, the exact mechanisms linking enhanced neurohormonal and cardiovascular reactivity to coronary heart disease are still unknown. Additionally, the intensity, frequency, and duration of the physiological changes necessary for subsequent development of coronary heart disease are unclear.

A second key concept in the self-regulatory model is that, once elicited, arousal is maintained not only through the behavior of Type A's but through their cognitive or information-processing style. Although the model does not address the etiology of cognitive mechanisms, focusing more narrowly on their physiological consequences, a variety of explanations have been offered within the literature (see Matthews, 1982, for review) for the selective attention and attributional biases that characterize the Type A behavior pattern. The most comprehensive research in this area has been conducted by Glass (1977), who conceptualized these behaviors as an attempt by Type A persons to assert and maintain control over stressful or uncontrollable events in their environment. The "uncontrollability" hypothesis, as well as several alternative explanations, have received some support in the research literature (Matthews, 1982). Further research is clearly needed for a full understanding of the etiology of these self-regulatory mechanisms.

References

Appels, A. (1983). The year before myocardial infarction. In T. M. Dembroski, T. H. Schmidt, & G. Blumchen (Eds.), *Biobehavioral bases of coronary heart disease*. New York: Karger.

Blaney, N. T. (1983, August). *Behavioral and cognitive style of Type A children*. Paper presented at the American Psychological Association's annual meeting, Anaheim, CA.

Blumenthal, J. A., Williams, R., Kong, Y., Schanberg, S. M., & Thompson, L. W. (1978). Type A behavior pattern and coronary arteriosclerosis. *Circulation, 58*, 634–639.

Blumenthal, J. A., Lane, J. D., Williams, R. B., McKee, D. C., Haney, T., & White A. (1983). Effects of task incentive on cardiovascular response in Type A and Type B individuals. *Psychophysiology, 20*, 63–70.

Brunson, B. I., & Matthews, K. A. (1981). The Type A coronary-prone behavior pattern and reactions to uncontrollable events: An analysis of learned helplessness. *Journal of Personality and Social Psychology, 40*, 906–918.

Burnam, M. A., Pennebaker, J. W., & Glass, D. C. (1975). Time consciousness, achievement-striving, and the Type A coronary-prone behavior pattern. *Journal of Abnormal Psychology, 84*, 76–79.

Carmody, T. P., Hollis, J. F., Matarazzo, J. D., Fey, S. G., & Conner, W. E. (1984). Type A behavior, attentional style and symptom reporting among adult men and women. *Health Psychology, 3*, 45–61.

Carver, C. S., Coleman, A. E., & Glass, D. C. (1976). The coronary-prone behavior pattern and the suppression of fatigue on a treadmill test. *Journal of Personality and Social Psychology, 33*, 460–466.

Chesney, M. A., Frautschi, N. M., & Rosenman, R. H. (1985). Modifying Type A behavior. In J. C. Rosen & L. J. Solomon (Eds.), *Prevention in health psychology*. Hanover, NH: University Press of New England.

Contrada, R. J., Wright, R. A., & Glass, D. C. (1985). *Journal of Research in Personality, 19*, 12–30.

Croog, S. H., Shapiro, D. S., & Levine, S. (1971). Denial among heart patients. *Psychosomatic Medicine, 33*, 385–397.

Dembroski, T. M., MacDougall, J. M., Herd, J. A., & Shields, J. L. (1979). Effect of level of challenge on pressor and heart rate responses in Type A and B subjects. *Journal of Applied Social Psychology, 9,* 209–228.

Dimsdale, J. E., Hackett, T. P., Block, P. C., & Hutter, A. M. (1978). Emotional correlates of the Type A behavior pattern. *Psychosomatic Medicine, 40,* 580–583.

Dimsdale, J. E., Hackett, T. P., Hutter, A. M., Block, P. C., & Catanzano, D. M. (1979). Type A behavior and angiographic findings. *Journal of Psychosomatic Research, 23,* 273–276.

Doehrman, S. R. (1977). Psychosocial aspects of recovery from coronary heart disease: A review. *Social Science and Medicine, 11,* 199–218.

Elliot, G. R., & Eisdorfer, C. (1982). *Stress and human health: Analysis and implications of research.* New York: Springer.

Enos, W. F., Holmes, R. H., & Beyer, J. (1953). Coronary disease among U.S. soldiers killed in Korea. *Journal of American Medical Association, 152,* 1090–1093.

Frank, K. A., Heller, S. S., Kornfeld, D. S., Sporn, A. A., & Weiss, M. B. (1978). Type A behavior pattern and coronary angiographic findings. *Journal of the American Medical Association, 240*(8), 761–763.

Frankenhaeuser, M. (1983). Sympathetic-adrenal and pituitary-adrenal response to challenge: Comparison between the sexes. In T. M. Dembroski, T. H. Schmidt, & G. B. Lumchen (Eds.) *Biological basis of coronary-prone behavior.* Basel: Karger.

Frankenhaeuser, M., Lundberg, U., & Forsman, L. (1980a). Dissociation between sympathetic-adrenal and pituitary-adrenal responses to an achievement situation characterized by high controllability: Comparison between Type A and Type B males and females. *Biological Psychology, 10,* 79–91.

Frankenhaeuser, M., Lundberg, U., & Forsman, L. (1980b). Note on arousing Type A persons by depriving them of work. *Journal of Psychosomatic Research, 24,* 45–47.

Friedman, M. (1978a). Type A behavior: Its possible relationship to pathogenic processes responsible for coronary heart disease (a preliminary inquiry). In T. M. Dembroski, S. M. Weiss, J. L. Shields, S. G. Haynes, & M. Feinleib (Eds.), *Coronary-prone behavior.* Baltimore: Williams & Wilkins.

Friedman, M. (1978b). Modifying the Type A behavior in heart attack patients. *Primary Cardiology, 11,* 9–13.

Friedman, M., & Rosenman, R. (1974). *Type A behavior and your heart.* New York: Knopf.

Friedman, M., Rosenman, R. H., Straus, R., Kositcheck, R. (1968). The relationship of behavior pattern A to the state of coronary vasculature. *American Journal of Medicine, 44,* 525–537.

Friedman, M., Thoresen, C. E., Gill, J. J., Ulmer, D., Thompson, L., Powell, L., Price, V., Elek, S. R., Rabin, D. D., Breall, W. S., Piaget, G., Dixon, T., Bourg, E., Levy, R. A., & Tasto, D. (1982). Feasibility of altering Type A behavior pattern after myocardial infarction. Recurrent coronary prevention project study: Methods, baseline results and preliminary findings. *Circulation, 66*(1), 83–92.

Friedman, M., Thoresen, C. E., Gill, J. J., Powell, L. H., Ulmer, D., Thompson, L., Price, V. A., Rabin, D. D., Breall, W. S., Dixon, T., Levy, R., & Bourg, E. (1984). Alteration of Type A behavior and reduction in cardiac reoccurrences in postmyocardial infarction patients. *American Heart Journal, 108*(2), 237–248.

Gastorf, J. W. (1980, August). *Type A's and the attribution of illness.* Paper presented at the annual meeting of the American Psychological Association, Montreal.

Gastorf, J. W. (1981). Physiological reaction of Type A's to objective and subjective challenge. *Journal of Human Stress, 7,* 16–20, 27.

Gastorf, J. W., Suls, J., & Sanders, G. S. (1980). Type A coronary-prone behavior pattern and social facilitation. *Journal of Personality and Social Psychology, 38,* 773–780.

Gentry, W. D., Foster, S., & Haney, T. (1973). Anxiety and urinary sodium/potassium as stress indicators on admission to a coronary care unit. *Heart and Lung, 2,* 875–879.

Girdano, D., & Girdano, D. (1977). Performance-based evaluation. *Health Education*, March/April, 13–15.

Glass, D. C. (1977). *Behavior patterns, stress, and coronary disease*. Hillsdale, NJ: Erlbaum.

Glass, D. C., Krakoff, L. R., Contrada, R. J., Hilton, W. F., Kehoe, K., Mannucci, E. G., Collins, C., Snow, B., & Elting, E. (1980). Effect of harassment and competition upon cardiovascular and plasma catecholamine responses in Type A and B individual. *Psychophysiology, 17*, 453–463.

Greene, W. A., Moss, A. J., & Goldstein, S. (1974). Delay, denial and death in coronary heart disease. In R. S. Eliot (Ed.)., *Stress and the heart*. New York: Futura.

Hart, K. E., & Jamieson, J. L. (1983). Type A behavior and cardiovascular recovery from a psychosocial stressor. *Journal of Human Stress, 9*(1), 18–24.

Haynes, S. G., Feinleib, M., & Kannel, W. B. (1980). The relationship of psychosocial factors to coronary heart disease in the Framingham Study: III. Eight-year incidence of coronary heart disease. *American Journal of Epidemiology, 111*, 35–37.

Henry, J. P. (1983). Coronary heart disease and arousal of the adrenal cortical axis. In T. M. Dembroski, T. H. Schmidt, & G. Blumchen (Eds.), *Biobehavioral bases of coronary heart disease*. New York: Karger.

Henry, J. P., & Stephens, P. M. (1977). *Stress, health, and the social environment*. New York: Springer-Verlag.

Herd, J. A. (1981). Behavioral factors in the physiological mechanisms in cardiovascular disease. In S. M. Weiss, J. A. Herd, & B. H. Fox (Eds.), *Perspectives on behavioral medicine*. New York: Academic Press.

Houston, B. K. (1983). Psychophysiological responsivity and the Type A behavior pattern. *Journal of Research in Personality, 17*, 22–39.

Howard, J. H., Cunningham, D. A., & Rechnitzer, P. A. (1977). Work patterns associated with Type A behavior. A managerial population. *Human Relations, 30*, 825–836.

Jones, E. E., & Nisbett, R. E. (1971). *The actor and the observer: Divergent perceptions of the causes of behavior*. Morristown, NJ: General Learning Press.

Jorgenson, R. S., & Houston, B. K. (1981). The Type A behavior pattern, sex differences, and cardiovascular response to and recovery from stress. *Motivation and Emotion, 5*, 201–214.

Kornitzer, M., Magotteau, V., Degre, C., Kittel, F., Struyven, J., & Van Thiel, E. (1982). Angiographic findings and the Type A pattern assessed by means of the Bortner scale. *Journal of Behavioral Medicine, 5*, 313–320.

Krantz, D. S., & Durel, L. A. (1983). Psychobiological substrates of Type A behavior pattern. *Health Psychology, 2*(4), 393–411.

Krantz, D. S., & Manuck, S. B. (1984). Acute psychophysiologic reactivity and risk of cardiovascular disease: A review and methodologic critique. *Psychological Bulletin, 96*, 435–464.

Krantz, D. S., Glass, D. C., & Snyder, M. L. (1974). Helplessness, stress level, and the coronary-prone behavior pattern. *Journal of Experimental Social Psychology, 10*, 284–300.

Lawler, K. A., Allen, M. T., Critcher, E. C., & Standard, B. A. (1981). The relationship of physiological responses to the coronary-prone behavior pattern in children. *Journal of Behavioral Medicine, 4*. 203–216.

Levenkron, J., Cohen, J., Mueller, H., & Fisher, E. (1982). *Modifying the Type A coronary-prone behavior pattern*. Unpublished manuscript.

Matthews, K. A. (1979). Efforts to control by children and adults with the Type A coronary-prone behavior pattern. *Child Development, 50*, 842–847.

Matthews, K. A. (1982). Psychological perspectives on the Type A behavior pattern. *Psychological Bulletin, 91*(2), 293–323.

Matthews, K. A., & Angulo, J. (1980). Measurement of the Type A behavior pattern in children: Assessment of children's competitiveness, impatience–anger and aggressions. *Child Development, 57*, 466–475.

Matthews, K. A., & Brunson, B. I. (1979). Allocation of attention and the Type A coronary-prone behavior pattern. *Journal of Personality and Social Psychology, 37*, 2081–2090.

Matthews, K. A., & Haynes, S. G. (1986). Type A behavior pattern and coronary risk: Update and critical evaluation. *American Journal of Epidemiology, 123*, 923–960.

Matthews, K. A., & Siegel, J. M. (1982). The Type A behavior pattern in children and adolescents: Assessment, development and associated coronary risk. In A. R. Baum & J. E. Singer (Eds.), *Handbook of health and medical psychology* (Vol. 2). Hillsdale, NJ: Erlbaum.

Matthews, K. A., & Volkin, J. I. (1981). Efforts to excel and the Type A behavior pattern in children. *Child Development, 52*, 1283–1289.

Matthews, K. A., Helmreich, R. L., Beane, W. E., & Lucker, G. W. (1980). Pattern A, achievement-striving and scientific merit: Does Pattern A help or hinder? *Journal of Personality and Social Psychology, 39*, 962–967.

Matthews, K. A., Siegel, J. M., Kuller, L. H., Thompson, M., & Varat, M. (1983). Determinants of decisions to seek medical treatment by patients with acute myocardial infarction symptoms. *Journal of Personality and Social Psychology, 44*, 1144–1156.

McNamara, S. S., Molot, M. A., Stremple, J. F., & Cutting, R. T. (1971). Coronary artery disease in combat casualties in Vietnam. *Journal of the American Medical Association, 216*, 1185–1187.

Mettlin, C. (1976). Occupational careers and the prevention of coronary prone behavior. *Social Science and Medicine, 10*, 367–372.

Murray, D. M., Blake, S. M., Prineas, R., & Gillum, R. (1983, August). *Cardiovascular reactivity in Type A children during a cognitive challenge.* Paper presented at the American Psychological Association annual meeting, Anaheim, CA.

Nixon, P. G. F. (1976). The human function curve with special reference to cardiovascular disorders: Part 1. *Practitioner, 217*, 765–770.

Price, V. A. (1982). *Type A behavior pattern: A model for research and practice.* New York: Academic Press.

Review Panel on Coronary-Prone Behavior and Coronary Heart Disease. (1981). Coronary-prone behavior and coronary heart disease: A critical review. *Circulation, 63*(6), 1199–1215.

Rissanen, V., Romo, M., & Siltanen, P. (1978). Premonitory symptoms and stress factors preceding sudden death from ischaemic heart disease. *Acta MedicaScandinavica, 204*, 389–396.

Rosenman, R. H., Brand, R. J., Jenkins, C. D., Friedman, M., Straus, R., & Wurm, M. (1975). Coronary heart disease in the Western Collaborative Group Study: Final follow-up experience of 8½ years. *Journal of the American Medical Association, 233*, 872–877.

Rosenman, R. H., & Friedman, M. (1974). Neurogenic factors in pathogenesis of coronary heart disease. *Medical Clinics of North America, 58*, 269–279.

Rosenman, R. H., Friedman, M., Straus, R., Wurm, M., Kositschek, R., Hahn, W., & Werthessen, N. T. (1964). A predictive study of coronary heart disease. The Western Collaborative Group Study. *Journal of the American Medical Association, 189*, 15–22.

Roskies, E. (1983). Stress management for Type A individuals. In D. Meichenbaum & M. E. Jaremko (Eds.), *Stress reduction and prevention.* New York: Plenum Press.

Schmieder, R., Friedrich, G., Neus, H., Rudel, H., & Von Eiff, A. W. (1983). The influence of beta blockers on cardiovascular reactivity and Type A behavior pattern in hypertensives. *Psychosomatic Medicine, 45*(5), 417–423.

Shekelle, R. B., Hulley, S. B., Neaton, J. D., Billings, J., Borhani, N. D., Gerace, T. A.,

Jacobs, D., Lasser, N., Mittlemark, M., & Stamler, J., for the Multiple Risk Factor Intervention Trial Research Group. (1985). The MRFIT Behavior Pattern Study. II. Type A behavior and incidence of coronary heart disease. *American Journal of Epidemiology, 122*, 559–570.

Southern, S., & Smith, R. (1982). *Behavioral self-management counseling for Type A coronary-prone university students*. Unpublished manuscript.

Stern, G. S., Harris, J. R., & Elverum, J. (1981). Attention to important versus trivial tasks and salience of fatigue-related symptoms for coronary-prone individuals. *Journal of Research in Personality, 15*, 467–474.

Suinn, R. (1975). The cardiac stress management program for Type A patients. *Cardiac Rehabilitation, 5*(4).

Suinn, R. M. (1982). Intervention with Type A behaviors. *Journal of Consulting and Clinical Psychology, 50*(6), 933–949.

Suinn, R., & Bloom, L. (1978). Anxiety management training for Pattern A behavior. *Journal of Behavioral Medicine, 1*, 25–35.

Waldron, I. (1978). The coronary-prone behavior pattern, blood pressure, employment and socio-economic status in women. *Journal of Psychosomatic Research, 22*, 79–87.

Waldron, I., Zyzanski, S., Shekelle, R. B., Jenkins, C. D., & Tannenbaum, S. (1977). The coronary-prone behavior pattern in employed men and women. *Journal of Human Stress, 3*, 2–18.

Weidner, G., & Chesney, M. A. (1985). Stress, Type A behavior, and coronary heart disease. In W. E. Conner & J. B. Bistow (Eds.), *Coronary heart disease: Prevention, complications and treatment*. Philadelphia: J. B. Lippincott.

Weidner, G., & Matthews, K. A. (1978). Reported physical symptoms elicited by unpredictable events and the Type A coronary-prone behavior pattern. *Journal of Personality and Social Psychology, 36*, 1213–1220.

Williams, R. B. (1985). Neuroendocrine response patterns and stress: Biobehavioral mechanisms of disease. In R. B. Williams (Ed.), *Perspectives on behavioral medicine: Neuroendocrine control and behavior*. New York: Academic Press.

Yarian, R. (1976). *The efficacy of electromyographic biofeedback training as a method of deep muscle relaxation for college students displaying either coronary or non-coronary behavior patterns.* Unpublished doctoral dissertation, University of Maryland.

Zyzanski, S. J. (1978). Association of the coronary-prone behavior pattern. In T. M. Dembroski, S. M. Weiss, J. L. Shields, S. G. Haynes, & M. Feinleib (Eds.), *Coronary-prone behavior*. New York: Springer-Verlag.

Zyzanski, S. J., Jenkins, C. D., Ryan, T. J., Flessas, A., & Everist, M. (1976). Psychological correlates of coronary angiographic findings. *Archives of Internal Medicine, 136*, 1234–1237.

Chapter 7

Biopsychological Barriers to the Behavioral Treatment of Hypertension

Wolfgang Linden

This chapter has three objectives:

1. To review briefly review the presently used behavioral modes of treatment for essential hypertension (EH), outline their rationales, and provide a summary of research on their long-term effectiveness.
2. To delineate the physiology of normal and abnormal blood pressure regulation with an emphasis on self-regulatory mechanisms and their interactions.
3. To contrast rationales for presently used treatment modes with the currently available knowledge on pressure regulation mechanisms, noting where rationales are appropriate and sufficient or where they may be inadequate.

As previous authors have provided extensive reviews of physiological regulation mechanisms (Conway, 1984; Dustan, 1982; Folkow, 1982; Guyton, 1980; Kaplan, 1978) and the behavioral treatment of EH (Frumkin, Nathan, Prout, & Cohen, 1978; Linden, 1984; Seer, 1979; Shapiro, Schwartz, Ferguson, Redmond, & Weiss, 1977) only highlights of this work will be described below. Research linking these two domains is

Wolfgang Linden • Department of Psychology, University of British Columbia, Vancouver, British Columbia, Canada V6T 1Y7.

largely nonexistent. The primary focus of this chapter is a discussion of the usefulness of current treatment rationales in light of available knowledge on biological self-regulation mechanisms.

Behavioral Treatments

Although drug treatment for essential hypertension may reduce pressure levels of many hypertensives and is positively affecting the rate of cardiovascular fatality (VA Cooperative Studies, 1970; 1972), there remain numerous drawbacks in its use. Many patients are unaware of their hypertension. Others are aware but do not want to seek treatment. Of those individuals in active treatment, many maintain high pressure levels because of poor compliance with a prescribed regimen and/or the wrong choice or dosage of drug (Kasl, 1978; Wilber & Barrow, 1972). Many patients do not comply because of debilitating side effects (for a review see Weinstein & Stason, 1976). Cost also plays a major role because the drug must be taken for many years, often for the remainder of a patient's life, and continued medical supervision is required. The utility of drug treatment remains in dispute for the largest group of people with elevated cardiovascular risk, those with pressure values only in the borderline and mild EH range (Alderman & Madhavan, 1981).

Independent of the means of reducing blood pressure, however, the payoff for any successful treatment is substantial because a reduction of only 5 mm Hg in resting diastolic pressure has been associated with a 20% reduction in mortality (Hypertension Detection and Follow-up Program Cooperative Group, 1979). Successful treatment has also been noted to reverse left ventricular hypertrophy (Hypertension Detection and Follow-up Program Cooperative Group, 1985).

In addition to the various drug treatments, a wide range of behavioral procedures for reducing elevated blood pressure are available and have been tested in recent years (for a review see Linden, 1984). These procedures possess many advantages over drug treatments including lower cost, lack of negative side effects and reasonably good compliance primarily because of the patient's positive attitude toward behavioral methods based on self-control. Among the behavioral modes of treatment that have been applied most often and are fairly well researched are relaxation techniques such as autogenic training, progressive muscular relaxation, transcendental meditation, and Benson's relaxation response, as well as biofeedback and stress management procedures. The relaxation methods appear to have a number of essential components in common. Benson (1975) identified four common elements: (a) a generally quiet environment and the instruction to keep the eyes closed, (b) a body position which *per se* is associated with low muscle tension, (c) a passive attitude achieved through instructions to push interfering thoughts aside, and (d) use of a mental vehicle, for example, thinking of a certain word or sound, observing an object, or listening to a prerecorded text that is repeated many times and is intended to reduce the awareness of environmental cues. Biofeedback is primarily applied as blood pressure feedback through which subjects are to acquire control over their autonomic functioning in ways similar to the relaxation training procedures but with additional physiological feedback of actual occurring changes. Stress management generally refers to treatment packages that are more comprehensive than either relaxation procedures or biofeedback alone. These packages typically include common elements such as relaxation training, possibly some blood pressure biofeedback, and generally the training of coping skills for a variety of environmental stressors at both behavioral (assertion training) and cognitive levels (cognitive reappraisal of environmental cues). The common objective of all behavioral methods is to reduce sympathetic overarousal based on the rationale that this is the primary dysfunction in essential hypertension. The treatment for these approaches observed in many well-controlled studies have been encouraging so far. All methods lead to significant reductions in blood pressure in the laboratory, generalize to home and work sites, and tend to be maintained for up to 3 years following treatment completion (Agras, 1983; Charlesworth, Williams, & Baer, 1984; Glasgow, Gaarder, & Engel, 1982; Jorgensen, Houston, & Zurawski, 1981; Libo & Arnold, 1983; Luborsky *et al.*, 1982; Southam, Agras, Taylor, & Kramer, 1982). In these and other outcome studies relaxation, biofeedback, and stress management consistently fare better than either no treatment or placebo conditions. Such outcome comparisons revealed blood pressure reductions of 6 to 18 mm SBP and 8 to 15 mm DBP for biofeedback and 4 to 26 mm Hg SBP and 2 to 19 mm Hg DBP for muscular relaxation in the laboratory (Linden, 1984). There are not enough well-controlled studies available yet to give similarly concrete figures for autogenic training or stress management packages. Although outcome data make all these methods look comparable with respect to effectiveness in follow-up, generalization potential, and cost–benefit analysis, relaxation methods and stress management packages are generally favored over biofeedback. Biofeedback is expensive because of equipment needs and individual attention requirements by a well-trained professional. Relaxation can easily be taught in groups. Behavioral treatment methods are mostly applied to patients in the borderline and mild hypertension range, as reductions of 10 mm Hg SPB and DBP on average are sufficient to bring most patients back into the normal ranges and may therefore constitute sufficient treatment for these subgroups. At present, there is no claim made that behavioral treatments may be totally satisfactory modes of intervention for moderate to high EH pressures ranges. It appears clear from this body of literature that behavioral methods are useful and cost-efficient aids in the treatment of essential hypertension, but their rationales appear fairly coarse given the complexity of hemodynamics that underlie the problem. Careful attention directed at understanding abnormal blood pressure regulation mechanisms in EH may possibly lead to suggestions for more effective behavioral treatments. This is the objective of the remainder of this chapter.

Physiological Regulation of Normal and Abnormal Blood Pressure Levels

Blood pressure is a physiological parameter which must be considered a composite or the result of a variety of different physiological processes at the cardiac and vascular levels. Blood pressure is primarily determined by cardiac output and by the resistance that the blood vessels offer to the flow of blood initiated by the heart. Cardiac output in turn is determined by both stroke volume and frequency of the heart beat. If one or more of these variables change in the same direction, blood pressure increases or decreases if other determining variables remain stable. It is, however, possible that no significant change in blood pressure will be evident if one determining variable (e.g., heart rate frequency) increases while another variable, for example, peripheral resistance, decreases to a comparable degree. The determination of blood pressure therefore does not provide comprehensive information about entire cardiovascular activity patterns and does not permit a reliable conclusion as to which physiological events have in fact contributed to this blood pressure value as an end point. In order to gain a comprehensive understanding of cardiovascular activity it is therefore necessary to determine concurrent changes in all those variables involved in blood pressure regulation. This requirement represents enormous problems for the blood pressure researcher.

The understanding of blood pressure control systems is further complicated by the fact that all determining variables interact with each other and are tied to multiple self-regulatory feedback systems (Guyton, 1980). Guyton, Cowley, and Coleman (1972) and Guyton (1980) have described eight distinct feedback systems that contribute to the control of blood pressure levels: (a) the baroreceptor system; (b) the renin-angiotensin vasoconstriction system; (c) the kidney body-fluid system; (d) the chemoreceptor system; (e) the CNS ischemic reaction; (f) the vascular stress-relaxation mechanism; (g) the capillary fluid-mobility mechanism, and (h) the aldosterone feedback system.

The *baroreceptor* system is based on sensible nerve endings that react upon deformation or strain of the blood vessels. When blood pressure increases, due to increased cardiac output, for example, deformation or strain of the vessels activates the baroreceptor endings. This baroreceptor activation leads to an inhibition of the vasomotor discharge by means of the pathway of the sympathetic nervous system (SNS). Decreased vasomotor activity concurrently increases the activity of the cardiac vagus. The resulting vessel dilation and decrease of cardiac activity opposes the increase in blood pressure and leads to a return of normal blood pressure values. The excelling characteristic of a properly functioning baroreceptor system is the rapidity of this control mechanism. Within a 15 seconds the baroreceptor reflex compensates for by far the largest proportion of previous change. The remaining portion of blood pressure change, however, must be compensated for by other more slowly functioning control systems.

The *renin-angiotensin vasoconstriction* system controls against abnormally low blood pressure. When blood pressure decreases, the kidneys secrete renin which in turn results in the formation of angiotensin. Increases in angiotensin lead to a constriction of peripheral blood vessels and blood pressure increases. This mechanism achieves its optimal efficiency after approximately 20 minutes and its is able to compensate for 62% of the acute blood pressure changes (Guyton *et al.*, 1972).

The *kidney body-fluid regulation system* controls elevated blood pressure through a progressive loss of body fluid whereby blood volume and finally blood pressure are reduced. This system requires healthy kidneys and a stable salt-water supply. In addition, it requires several days before reaching optimal efficiency. The kidney body-fluid control system possesses the ability to remain active until *complete compensation* has been achieved and the blood pressure returns to normal values, that is, the value present prior to the strain.

In the *chemoreceptor system* low blood pressure will trigger a decreased activation of peripheral chemoreceptors, thereby stimulating the SNS. The parasympathetic nervous system (PNS) will then be inhibited, with the consequence being a stabilizing rise in blood pressure. The *ischemic reaction of the central nervous system* decreases the blood flow to the lower areas of the brain when blood pressure decreases. This again has a stimulating effect on the sympathetic nervous system and leads to a blood pressure increase. Elevated pressure in the circulatory system activates the *stress-relaxation mechanism* which leads to a slow relaxation of the vessel walls and lower pressure through this mechanism. Inversely, low blood pressure leads to a slow vasoconstriction and thus increases blood pressure.

The *capillary liquid mobility mechanism* influences blood pressure such that, with elevated pressure in the capillaries, fluid from the circulatory system will be drawn into the interstitial tissues. If pressure is very low, fluid from these interstitial tissues will be liberated and again reintroduced into the circulatory system.

The *aldosterone feedback mechanism,* which is activated by a low blood pressure, is a component of the kidney body fluid system. This mechanism triggers a heightened production of aldosterone, thereby leading to increased storage of salt and water in the kidneys.

Guyton (1980) has made the argument that of all blood-pressure-controlling mechanisms only one should truly be called a control mechanism, that is, the renal body-fluid control mechanism. He suggests calling all other mechanisms "damping" or "buffering" mechanisms because, although they facilitate and contribute to the control of blood pressure, they cannot bring blood pressure changes back to their basal levels without the help of other systems. Specifically, it is only the kidney body-fluid system that has a 100% maximum gain that will continuously control the return of pressure to its original value. Other systems are considerably more rapid in their action but not so complete. These highly varying degrees of rapidity versus completeness in feedback gain are displayed in Figure 1, where the amount of gain for different systems is displayed as a function of time.

This graph again stresses the point that all control mechanisms that have rapid but not infinite gain can therefore be considered only moderators or buffers. The only true control system that allows for 100% control or infinite gain is the renal blood-volume pressure control system. On this basis Guyton builds a strong argument that the renal blood-volume pressure control system is possibly the most important in understanding abnormal pressure regulation. The complexity of all regulatory systems involved in the control of blood pressure represents a typical example of the multilevel interactive models described in Chapter 1, where it was mentioned that possibly more than one system can be involved in the control of a particular physiological function and that these multiple systems may have cumulative, accelerating effects or may possibly cancel each other out if the directionality of their effect is of similar magnitude but in opposing directions. Hence, the blood pressure control system

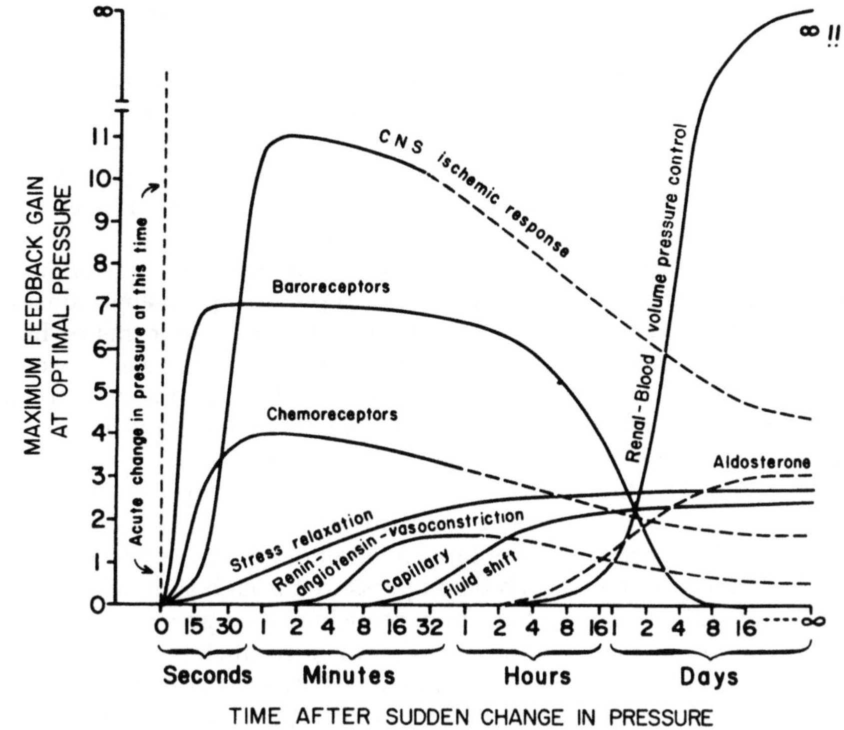

Figure 1. The degree of activation, expressed in terms of feedback gain, of different pressure-control mechanisms following a sudden change in arterial pressure. Note the rapid activation of the nervous mechanisms, the moderately rapid activation of several intermediate pressure control mechanisms, and the slow but extremely powerful activation of the renal body-fluid control mechanism. From *Circulatory Physiology: III. Arterial Blood Pressure and Hypertension* (p. 7) by A. C. Guyton, 1980, Philadelphia: W. B. Saunders. Copyright 1980 by the W. B. Saunders Company. Reprinted by permission.

represents a system with these multilevel, self-regulatory biological mechanisms.

The complexity of blood pressure regulating mechanisms as described above doubtless appears very confusing and represents enormous challenges to the measurement of these simultaneously occurring, interacting processes. However, in light of the multiple objectives that blood pressure regulation must fulfill this complexity appears necessary: namely, it is the function of arterial blood pressure regulation to provide a constant pressure head which can meet the requirements of the pressure regulation system. These requirements include a constant pressure steady and high enough so that any tissue can call for significantly increased blood flow at any time. A steady pressure level also must be maintained so that the blood flow controlling apparatus can always be assured of sufficient blood pressure in demand situations. Finally, pressure is to be prevented from increasing so much that the energy load on the heart is deleterious to long-term survival of the heart muscle itself and lasting damage to the vessels themselves can occur.

In principle, a pathological change or dysfunction in any one of these regulation systems could contribute to blood pressure problems, considering that the other mechanisms do not balance or counter this pathology. That, of course, is exactly the purpose of this complex system, namely, to provide multiple control so that inefficiency in one system can be and will be counterbalanced by other pressure control mechanisms. For example, it is known that people who have entire limbs surgically removed and who therefore experience a dramatic drop in overall peripheral resistance will still have constant blood pressure that becomes balanced within a brief period of time. In addition, it has been found that in earlier attempts to treat high blood pressure through sympathectomy these interventions were successful in reducing blood pressure but only for short periods of time; within a few months pressure levels returned to normal (cf. Smithwick & Robertson, 1973). There are many more examples that could be cited as to how dramatic changes to one control system still have resulted in constant blood pressure which could then be attributed to the proper functioning of other systems.

This introduction to basic mechanisms of blood pressure regulation provides the necessary tools for understanding how high blood pressure can develop and be maintained. A number of the pressure regulation systems mentioned primarily serve to control for abnormally low pressure; for this reason, the chemoreceptor system, the ischemic reaction of the central nervous system, and the aldosterone feedback mechanism are of lesser importance for the understanding of high blood pressure than are the baroreceptors, the renin-angiotensin system, the kidney blood-volume regulation system, and the stress relaxation mechanism. The remainder of this chapter concentrates on those mechanisms principally capable of reducing elevated pressure and, if dysfunctional, represent the most likely "candidates" for explaining sustained pressure elevations.

In order to gain an understanding and establish a perspective on the pathways of the shift from low (or normal) to high blood pressure, we will have to describe how these regulation systems become instable, and, more specifically, we will have to understand how instability can lead to a shift to higher levels that are accepted and maintained by other regulatory systems. How can a change that occurs in one or more systems not become a target of counteraction by other mechanisms? In some ways there has to be either a detachment of various systems or multiple damages within the body of self-regulatory systems. At this point, there has been a fair amount of research, but the conclusions still remain somewhat speculative. The emphasis in these past studies has been on the baroreceptor system, the kidney blood-volume control system, and the notion of sympathetic hyperreactivity which in turn ties in with both regulation systems (Conway, 1984; Dustan, 1982; Guyton, 1980).

With respect to the baroreceptor system, it has been argued that systematic, chronic changes in the system may play a role in the etiology and maintenance of essential hypertension (Shimada, Kitazumi, Sadakane, Ogura, & Ozawa, 1985). Justification for this argument can be derived from the observation that baroreceptors possess variable, adaptive set points which increase when the baroreceptors are exposed to continuous strain and innervation. Numerous studies support this hypothesis. The observation of heightened baroreceptor thresholds in hypertensive animals (Folkow, 1975; McCubbin, Green, & Page, 1956) ties in with the earlier description of the baroreceptor system as a buffering or moderating system but not a true control system. Because baroreceptors will act very rapidly in reducing blood pressure but do not reduce pressure to the original baseline value, repeated activation of the baroreceptor system will set the resulting presumed baseline pressures at a higher level as long as the stimulation of the baroreceptors occurs in sufficiently short intervals so that other control systems (primarily the kidney blood-volume control system) do not come into effect. The baroreceptor of a hypertensive dog, for example, started firing only at a pressure level that in an animal with normal blood pressure would have led to a continuous discharge (Sleight, Robinson, Brooks, & Rees, 1975). Mancia, Ferrari, Gregorini, Ludrovk, and Zanchetti (1978) have further supported this observation of decreased baroreceptor sensitivity in human subjects with elevated blood pressure.

In the search for transformation mechanisms that explain how repeated, acute increases in pressure lead to chronic pathological hypertension it must be demonstrated how short-term elevations affect multiple elements of the pressure control system so that they will maintain pressure at higher levels. It has been observed that during extreme acute arousal there may be excessive secretion of renin and subsequent formation of angiotensin which can cause severe vasospasms in arterioles and small arteries, possibly leading to bulbous enlargements of the vessels between segments of the spasm (cf. Giese, 1976; Goldby & Beilin, 1974).

The bulbous enlargements then may leak almost pure plasma into the vascular wall which in turn leads to the deposition of plasma, proteins, and subsequent vascular fibrosis. If the vessel walls are damaged, any pressure control system involving blood vessel flexibility may be hampered. Furthermore, when arterial pressure becomes extremely high, it has been observed that the usual autoregulation mechanism that protects the capillaries from unusually high intravascular pressure often fails (Walker & Guyton, 1967). There have been observations that if such damage is initiated in the blood vessels, simultaneous progressive renal lesions will tend to decrease all functional capacities of the kidneys, which threatens the facilitation of pressure regulation through the kidney blood-volume controller (Moehring, Moehring, Petri, Haack, & Hackenthal, 1975). The potential damage in the kidney is particularly important since only the kidney blood-volume pressure control system has the unique propensity for infinite gain previously mentioned. This mechanism will be discussed in detail below.

The kidney blood-volume pressure control mechanism that we are about to discuss clearly differs in its propensities from the other mechanisms, such that it has what Guyton (1980) calls a "servocontrol" mechanism, whereas all other pressure regulation systems have only buffering or damping effects. A servocontrol is analogous to what obesity researchers have called the set point theory. Specifically, a servocontroller is defined as a mechanism with two major components. The first is a system that is independently capable of readjusting a controlled variable (in this case blood pressure) back toward a control value whenever the variable strays on either side of that control value. The second component necessary to a true servocontroller is an independent system (or systems) that can alter the control value to which the intrinsic system readjusts the variable. Therefore, the notion of a servocontroller is an excellent prototype of the multiple system approach that we described in Chapter 1. That is, within a certain system there may be functional self-regulation; however, this system again is embedded in another level of systems which may change the set points (or other inherent definition of a target) that the first system attempts to achieve. Whereas other buffering mechanisms, as noted above, have no intrinsic means of determining the correct long-term level of arterial pressure, the kidney blood-volume pressure servocontroller does have such intrinsic properties and will make the necessary adjustments in order to maintain a constant baseline level of arterial pressure on a long-term basis (Guyton, 1980; Guyton *et al.*, 1974). For an understanding of the components and interactions of the kidney blood-volume pressure servocontroller the basic components must be explained and the particular importance of this system for long-term blood pressure control outlined. The key elements of this system are displayed in Figure 2. The function of each element will be explained in more detail in the following section.

Boxes 1, 2, 4, and 5 describe a typical negative feedback control loop. The general characteristics and functions of such a loop have been described elsewhere (Schwartz, 1976). For the present case, an increase in arterial pressure produces an increase in the kidney's output of water and salt (cf. Navar, 1978). Then, as illustrated by the dashed arrow between boxes 2 and 4, the increased output of water and salt leads to a decrease in blood volume. This decrease in blood volume in turn decreases the cardiac output (box 5). A decrease in cardiac output feeds back to box 1 to decrease arterial pressure. Note, however, that the person's fluid intake (see box 3) has a tendency to increase blood volume. Thus, the kidney output of fluid is balanced against the daily fluid intake. When output and intake are exactly equal, arterial pressure will also remain constant. When output is greater than intake, pressure tends to fall progressively until stability is reached. Conversely, if intake is greater than output, blood volume, cardiac output, and, concurrently, arterial pressure will rise (until ultimately the heart fails).

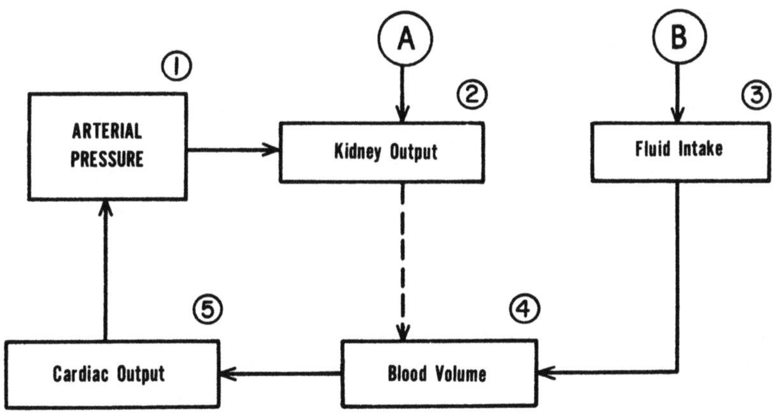

Figure 2. Block diagram of the kidney blood volume pressure servocontroller, the keystone to long-term arterial pressure regulation. Points A and B represent the two unique inputs to this system at which the set point for pressure control can be altered. From *Circulatory Physiology: III. Arterial Blood Pressure and Hypertension* (p. 21) by A. C. Guyton, 1980, Philadelphia: W. B. Saunders. Copyright 1980 by the W. B. Saunders Company. Reprinted by permission.

There is a distinct difference between this servocontrol system and the other buffering systems. Each of the previously discussed mechanisms will bring arterial pressure toward normal by a certain percentage but will not bring it back 100% to its original level; they reach a plateau in their pressure-adjusting effect and do not possess infinite gain capabilities as does the kidney blood-volume pressure servocontroller (as in Figure 1).

This particular advantage of the kidney servocontroller requires further explanation. First, let us consider a healthy individual with initial normal pressure, that is, the long-term baseline control value, and a balanced daily fluid output and intake. What happens when arterial pressure rises slightly above normal? If there is no commensurate increase in intake, then there will be more output than intake and the blood volume will decrease. Furthermore, blood volume will continue to decrease indefinitely until the kidney output decreases back to its original value and again equals fluid intake. However, kidney output will not return to its original value until the arterial pressure also returns to its original or baseline value, its set point. Therefore, the effects of the feedback loop described in boxes 1, 2, 4, and 5 are evident until such time that arterial pressure returns to its set point or original baseline value.

When the arterial pressure falls below normal the kidney output decreases below the level of the fluid intake. As a result, blood volume, cardiac output, and arterial pressure continue to rise until the kidney output comes back into equilibrium with the fluid intake. When this has been achieved, the arterial pressure also has returned to the original control value. Thus, if the kidney blood-volume pressure servocontroller is left entirely alone without other factors besides pressure itself affecting either kidney output or fluid intake, this mechanism will always return arterial pressure to its original level. However, it does not do this instantaneously because the cumulative effect of this control mechanism requires minutes, hours, or sometimes even weeks to develop fully. Therefore, this mechanism is not of significant value as a short-term arterial pressure buffering system but has its value as the keystone of long-term regulation of arterial pressure control. For an illustration of this point, the reader may refer again to Figure 1, which displays the degree of gain of which various control systems are capable and the amount of time required to achieve it.

Now that a basic model of the servocontroller and its first component, readjustment to the control value, has been described, we can proceed to illustrate the second component and the manner in which it may possibly relate to developing high blood pressure. Namely, we must understand how the set point is defined and how possibly it can be altered. Specifically, the intrinsic control system as displayed in Figure 2 can be altered at two different points, *A* and *B*, to change the control value to which the arterial pressure is regulated. At point *B* it is easy to understand that one can change the daily level of fluid intake by drinking more. This obviously will change the kidney output required to balance the fluid intake and it will also modify the level of arterial pressure required to give that amount of kidney output. Thus, the change in fluid intake alters the control pressure level, that is, the set point, to which the servosystem as shown in Figure 2 will adjust the arterial pressure.

The servocontroller can also change the set point at point *A*. When the kidneys are operating normally and are not disturbed in any way, they have a predictable long-term response to arterial pressure changes: a given pressure triggers a certain kidney output and a given increase in pressure gives a certain increase in kidney output. However, other factors besides arterial pressure affect the response of kidney output to arterial pressure. These factors include salt intake, the level of hormones, such as catecholamines, angiotensin, antidiuretic hormone (ADH), and aldosterone; as well as the degree of neural stimulation of the kidney. A change in any one of these factors will therefore change the level of kidney output at a given arterial pressure. Therefore, the control pressure level to which the arterial pressure is regulated may also change.

This information provides important clues for understanding the maintenance and etiology of hypertension. As the kidney blood-volume pressure servocontroller is the only system that possesses infinite gain characteristics, ultimately some kidney dysfunction is necessary (and possibly a sufficient component) in determining high blood pressure. However, the factors that induce a healthy kidney with a low set point and a functioning servocontroller to shift its activity levels to a higher level and maintain it there must be explained for a complete understanding of the development of essential hypertension. Generally, the sympathetic nervous system is considered to play an important role here, and a brief review of research on such effects is presented next.

There is clear consensus in major literature reviews (Conway, 1984; Dustan, 1982; Guyton, 1980) that changes in sympathetic tone are characteristic of many hypertensives, in particular those in the borderline and low EH range and those with labile pressure. These individuals often show increased pressor responses to psychological stressors which may occur before hypertension has developed and may characterize those individuals who are genetically susceptible. Numerous studies demonstrate the involvement of elevated sympathetic tone in borderline hypertension. Some of these are based on orthostatic manipulations (Frohlich, Tarazi, Ulrych, Dustan, & Page, 1967; Louis, Doyle, & Anavekar, 1973).

The results of investigations by Julius, Esler, and Randall (1975) indicated that young people with borderline hypertension tend to have increased adrenergic activity. Further studies by Falkner, Onesti, Angelakos, Fernandes, and Langman (1979) have shown exaggerated pressor responses to mental arithmetic in normotensive young people with powerful hypertension. This hyperreactivity was not accounted for by either intrinsic disturbances of contractility or by increased central blood volume, thus supporting the notion of SNS hyperactivity. Chobanian and his coworkers (1978) further underlined that for the borderline EH subject it was SNS reactivity to strain rather than resting tone that was elevated. In addition, there is evidence that peripheral sympathetic system activity may also be excessive; in patients with the hyperdynamic syndrome increased heart rate responses to isoproterenol infusions were found (Frohlich, Tarazi, & Dustan, 1969). The success of beta-blocker treatment further supports the hypothesis of sympathetic hyperarousal in hypertensives even though the action mechanisms for beta blocker themselves are poorly understood. Unfortunately, changes in sympathetic tone in humans can be measured only with great difficulty and typically only by indirect means. An elevation in plasma norepinephrine or epinephrine can, with reservation, be taken to indicate increases in sympathetic activity. Conway in his review (1984) suggested that at least some hypertensives have clearly elevated plasma norepinephrine concentration whereas others may have elevated epinephrine levels. Some additional clarification of the notion of heightened sympathetic tone has been provided in a series of two recent studies by Fredrikson, Dimberg, Frisk–Holmberg, and Stroem (1985) and Fredrikson and Engel (1985). In both studies, stress responsivity of hypertensives and normotensive controls was studied on a variety of sympathetic parameters of which some were cardiovascular in nature (blood pressure, blood flow, heart rate) and one not directly related to cardiovascular systems (electrodermal response). Whereas hypertensives displayed consistent hyperarousal on cardiovascular measures, they did not show differential responsivity on noncardiovascular arousal indices. These researchers suggested that sympathetic hyperactivity of hypertensives is specific only to the cardiovascular system but not part of generalized sympathetic nervous system arousal.

The missing link in identifying sympathetic hyperreactivity as a predictor or precursor of high blood pressure is, of course, the demonstration that individuals with cardiovascular hyperresponses are in fact at significantly higher risk for the long-term development of chronic high blood pressure. Unfortunately, there are few longitudinal studies available to substantiate this point. Four studies provide some evidence that this hypothesis may be correct. Wilson and Meyer (1981), in a large sample of 3,395 men and 425 women, found excessive response to an exercise stressor to be generally predictive of subsequently elevated resting pressures when measured two years following the initial testing. Another prospective study supporting the same point was executed by Keys *et al.* (1971), who reported that cardiovascular reactivity, specifically diastolic blood pressure response to a cold stressor, was a significant predictor of subsequent coronary heart disease.

A third pertinent study provides a 45-year follow-up of subjects exposed to the cold pressor test in 1934 (Wood, Sheps, Elveback, & Schirger, 1984). At follow-up in 1979 hypertension had occurred in 71% of the initial hyperreactors but only in 19% of the initial normoreactors. Despite its laudable sample size, however ($N=142$ in 1979), the findings must be interpreted with some reservation since about half of the original sample ($N=300$) were not available at follow-up. Finally, a fourth study with monkeys provides some additional related prospective evidence. Manuck, Kaplan, an Clarkson (1983) measured individual differences in acute heart rate responses to a discrete stressor. Monkeys on a moderately atherogenic diet were exposed to a threatening stimulus (operationalized as a glove used to capture the animal) which consistently elicited very large heart rate changes. Animals were divided into low mean (61% over resting) and high mean (88% increases) heart rate reactors. Necropsy results clearly indicated that high heart rate reactors had significantly greater coronary and aortic atherosclerosis then did low heart rate reactive animals. These four studies together provide some tentative support for the hypothesis that cardiovascular (that is, heart rate) responsiveness under psychological strain is a marker in the development of heart disease. Only two of these, Wilson and Meyer (1981) and Wood *et al.* (1984), directly relate to elevated resting blood pressure as the long-term outcome in hyperreactive individuals.

Finally, it has been argued above that there may be multiple interactions between the baroreceptor, the kidney blood-volume servo-controller, and the sympathetic nervous system. A recent study by Light, Koepke, Obrist, and Willis (1983) provides empirical evidence for such a link by presenting data on responses to competitive mental tasks in young men with one or two hypertensive parents and/or with borderline hypertension. In this study, blood pressure, heart rate, and urinary sodium and fluid excretion were measured. In the high risk group (defined as individuals with hypertensive parents), the degree of retention was directly related to the magnitude of heart rate increase during stress, thereby suggesting common mediation by way of the sympathetic nervous system. Thus, psychological stress appears to induce changes in renal excretory functions which in individuals at risk may play a critical role in long-term blood pressure regulation.

From this review of the literature it appears that there are multiple pathways linking behavioral and cognitive factors and the development and maintenance of essential hypertension, all of which somehow involve the kidney. Specifically, we were looking for explanations as to how the set point of the kidney servocontroller could be modified so that the system then maintains the elevated pressure.

One such pathway is comprised of genetically predisposed dysfunctional kidneys which fail to adapt to the high salt intake typical of the present diet in Western society. Continued high salt consumption combined with a deficient kidney leads to servocontroller resetting and elevated blood pressure. Another pathway is more complex and involves multiple components of the self-regulation mechanism that involve the kidney and resetting of the renal function curve, that is, the servocontroller threshold. The presumed common denominator in this pathway is heightened SNS reactivity due either to a genetic predisposition for hyperreactivity or to poor cognitive-behavioral coping skills in response to high and/or repeated environmental demands. The coexistence of both genetic predisposition and poor coping is likely to have additive, negative effects on sympathetic reactivity. Next, frequent and excessive SNS arousal may directly and negatively affect kidney functioning or it may do so indirectly in a number of ways. These include damage to the blood vessels, both on a systemic level and within the renal vasculature itself, due to acute, extreme bursts of SNS activity. Lastly, sympathetic hyperreactivity may lead to resetting of the baroreceptor threshold, which may contribute to maintenance of elevated arterial pressure and in turn may lead to slow but cumulative structural changes in the vasculature, that is, loss of flexibility. This loss of flexibility heightens vascular resistance, which again will provoke shifts in the renal function curve.

Unfortunately, one can not unequivocally assert at this time that any one, or even all, of the pathological processes described above are necessary and sufficient conditions for provoking and maintaining essential hypertension. Knowledge of the gain propensities of various self-regulatory systems, however, would logically dictate that kidney dysfunction must play a role.

Although the known interactions of various self-regulatory mechanisms in arterial pressure have already required a fairly complex discussion, the matter is further complicated by the fact that a variety of subtypes of essential hypertension have been identified. We have already distinguished early essential hypertension with elevated cardiac output (primarily arising from excessive SNS activity) and normal peripheral resistance for chronic EH with normal or even abnormally low cardiac output but significantly elevated peripheral resistance. Further important distinctions are the salt-sensitive versus salt-resistant type and the low versus high plasma renin distinction.

High salt intake has long been suspected to be a general contributor to hypertension and coronary artery disease, but it now appears clear that salt intake in the general population and blood pressure are not strongly related (Holden, Ostfeld, Freeman, & Hellenbrand, 1983; Swales, 1980) Many hypertensives, however, react adversely to high sodium intake (Fujita, Noda, & Ando, 1984; Kawasaki, DeLea, Barter, & Smith, 1978). Fujita and his colleagues found an elevated cardiac index and higher epinephrine and norepinephrine and plasma renin activity, relative to normotensive controls, in borderline hypertensives after a sodium load. Treatment with antidiuretic medication (Fujita *et al.*, 1984) or salt restriction (Ambrosioni *et al.*, 1982) often succeeds in reducing blood pressure and, when given conjointly with potassium, reestablishes a sodium–potassium balance. Although these findings reflect group average effects, there remain many hypertensives who are not salt-sensitive and who will therefore not show the beneficial effects of either antidiuretic medication or salt restriction observed in others (Guyton, 1980). Furthermore, treatment with diuretics or salt restriction may cause marked increases in renin secretion which in turn, through the renin-angiotension system, will negatively affect renal function (DeClue *et al.*, 1978).

Plasma renin activity (PRA) itself tends to vary with age and is elevated only in a relatively small percentage of hypertensives. High PRA is most prevalent among young borderline hypertensives (estimated 30% in Esler, 1977) and is typically associated with relatively low total peripheral resistance (TPR) (Thomas, Ledingham, & Berlin, 1976). As hypertensives get older PRA decreases and TPR increases. An interesting correlate of high PRA is that of a distinct personality feature which is not seen in hypertensives with low PRA levels (Esler *et al.*, 1977; Thailer, Friedman, Harshfield, & Pickering, 1985). These psychological aspects of self-regulation will be discussed in more detail below.

Biopsychological Sequelae of High Blood Pressure

The previous section was entirely devoted to physiological self-regulation of arterial pressure, and little attention was given to potential links between psychological and physiological processes. The available evidence for such a link is somewhat sketchy and speculative. Three main themes seem to prevail: (a) symptom perception processes and how they effect help seeking and compliance with treatment, (b) effects of elevated blood pressure on cognitive abilities in general, and (c) the link between certain personality traits and behavioral skills and elevated arterial pressure.

Symptom perception research has received input from a variety of empirical and theoretical sources: the original "health belief model" (Becker & Maiman, 1975), Leventhal's work on common sense representation of illness danger (Leventhal, Meyer, & Nerenz, 1980; Meyer, Leventhal, & Gutmann, 1985), Pennebaker's extensive analysis of the physical symptom perception process and stages and determinants of perceivability (Pennebaker, 1982), and the "modified health belief model" (Feuerstein & Linden, 1984). This body of research and conceptual analysis converges in noting that high blood pressure is not associated with specific symptoms, there is no pain or significant distress, and there is no reliable self-perception of BP resting levels, or change magnitude, or even direction of change. As a consequence, hypertensives rarely seek treatment on their own; they are not highly motivated to accept and stay in treatment; and even if treatment is initiated most drop out (cf. Meyer *et al.*, 1985). This problem of the inability to perceive change becomes particularly aggravated when the symptom-free (but "ill") hypertensive initiates drug treatment and encounters some of the likely negative side effects of the drug. He or she then tends to feel subjectively and acutely worse than before the treatment, the positive effects of which they do not even perceive. This inconsistency of drug treatment sequelae with common-sense models of illness appears to be a major reason for poor treatment compliance, as Meyer *et al.* (1985) have documented.

The notion of blood pressure elevations affecting cognitive abilities was first put forward by Lacey (1967), who suggested that increases in heart rate or blood pressure led to feedback that inhibited cortical activity. It is quite likely that such cortical inhibition can account for the findings of Wilkie and Eisdorfer (1971), who compared IQ in hypertensives and a matched control group over a 10-year period and found increasing deficits in overall IQ and nonverbal subtests in the hypertensives. These findings were further substantiated by Goldman, Kleinman, Snow, Bidus, and Korol (1974) who, after controlling for age and IQ, also observed that untreated hypertensives made so many errors on a neuropsychology test battery that their scores typically surpassed the criterion levels for brain dysfunction. More recently, it has been reported that after reducing elevated blood pressure with antihypertensive medication, the previously seen deficits on sensory-perceptual, cognitive, and psychomotor tests had reversed when reexamined 15 months later (Miller, Shapiro, King, Gincherean, & Hosutt, 1984). A control group of hypertensives who had not received active treatment remained deficient when compared with normotensive controls. Finally, a fascinating but difficult to interpret study by Dworkin, Filewich, Miller, and Craigmyle (1979) provides further stimulation for research. These researchers increased the blood pressure of laboratory rats with a phenylephrine infusion and noticed that the animals attempted much less frequently to terminate or avoid noxious electrical shocks than was observed in controls who had received blood-pressure ineffective saline infusions. This effect was no longer observed after baroreceptors had been operatively denervated. If it were true for humans as well that blood pressure elevations led to decreased perception of stress symptoms, then one could delineate an operant learning mechanism that would explain why continually elevated blood pressure is not perceived as aversive or may even be perceived as pleasant. Further confirmation of the baroreceptor-cortical inhibition link has been reported by Elbert, Pietrowsky, Kessler, Lutzenberger, and Birbaumer (1985). These researchers replicated Dworkin *et al.*'s findings with a human population in a functionally similar design. Experimental stimulation of the baroreceptors significantly decreased cortical excitability and increased pain sensation threshold in a sample of borderline hypertensives (Elbert *et al.*, 1985).

It is also interesting that the concept of cognitive and behavioral inhibition has an analogue in the literature on personality and hypertension, that is, the repressive-defensive behavior pattern (Linden, 1984; Linden & Feuerstein, 1983; Linden & Frankish, 1984; Morrison, Bellack, & Manuck, 1985; Sapira, Scheib, Moriarty, & Shapiro, 1971). It appears that hypertensives may display deficits in social competence (for example, lack of assertion) and may withhold the expression of particularly negative feelings such as hostility and anger (Sapira *et al.*, 1971; Harburg, Blakelock, & Roeper, 1979). There is much evidence from laboratory-type studies, as well as longitudinal research, that withholding negative affect is dysfunctional. In a series of studies, Hokanson (Hokanson & Edelman, 1966) demonstrated maintained cardiovascular arousal in provoked subjects who were not provided with an appropriate outlet for their hostile feelings, whereas a control group who expressed their feelings showed swift recovery from the provocation. Longitudinally, hostility has been linked with severity of angiographically documented coronary artery disease (Dembroski, MacDougall, Williams, Haney, & Blumenthal, 1985; Williams *et al.*, 1980; MacDougall, Dembroski, Dimsdale, & Hackett, 1985) and general cardiovascular morbidity and mortality (Barefoot,

Dahlstrom, & Williams, 1983; Mathews, Glass, Rosenman, & Bortner, 1977; Shekelle, Gale, Ostfeld, & Paul, 1983).

Although we have been able to cite evidence for a link between repressed hostility and high blood pressure and heart disease in general, it also appears that this personality–behavior pattern applies for a subtype of hypertensives only, individuals with sympathetic hyperreactivity and high renin levels (Esler *et al.*, 1977; Morrison *et al.*, 1985; Thailer *et al.*, 1985).

One very important question relative to these personality and behavior links with hypertension, however, remains unresolved: Does repressed hostility cause hypertension? The limited evidence cited above for cortical inhibition as a correlate of elevated blood pressure makes certain personality–behavior patterns appear more like consequences of EH than like a cause. Evidence for the predictive power of hostility as a factor in heart disease, however, suggests the opposite.

Implications of Biological and Psychobiological Findings for the Behavioral Treatment of Hypertension

From a literature review of behavioral methods of reducing high blood pressure it can be seen that such methods can make a significant contribution and in the case of borderline hypertensives may be an entirely sufficient intervention. When integrating the available knowledge regarding the etiology of essential hypertension with the stated objectives of various behavioral treatments, that is, attempts to reduce sympathetic overarousal, it appears that in principle these methods represent appropriate treatments. However, the intension of this review was not only to investigate whether methods are globally appropriate or inappropriate but also to lead to a critical discussion of how we can improve treatment methods, given the present level of understanding of the biological mechanisms in action. Therefore, the questions that remain to be discussed in this final section of the chapter deal with issues of specificity. In particular, this section is to provide answers to the following questions:

1. Is there one treatment that can be at least of some use for all types of hypertension?
2. Will it be necessary to apply, and are there available, differential forms of treatment for each subtype of hypertension (high versus low renin, high cardiac output versus high peripheral resistance, borderline or low EH versus established chronic EH?

3. Is it recommendable for salt-sensitive versus salt-resistant EH to use different behavioral methods in order to maximize treatment efficacy?
4. Can behavioral methods not only reduce blood pressure *per se* but also facilitate the reversal of damage caused by high blood pressure (e.g., damage in the vessel walls, lesions)?
5. Are there behavioral methods that may facilitate treatment success by augmenting adherence to treatment through interventions of a behavioral nature which will maximize the efficacy of drug treatment programs?

Some of these questions can be answered with fairly well educated guesses; others clearly require extensive future research. Specifically, it is fairly evident, on the basis of the research discussed above, that any treatment attempt that targets and succeeds in reducing sympathetic overarousal will be most effective in dealing with individuals for whom high pressure is primarily a function of high cardiac output. Heightened cardiac output is most often seen in individuals at high risk (parental hypertension) and/or with labile or borderline hypertension. Whether treatments directed at sympathetic overarousal can have any beneficial impact on individuals with chronic hypertension, low cardiac output, no demonstrable sympathetic hyperactivity, but high peripheral resistance is unknown at this time. However, given that at least some of the effects of hypertension are known to be reversible when blood pressure has been reduced, it may ultimately be possible that any reduction in pressure may in turn bring about concurrent systemic changes that help maintain pressure at lower levels. A specific suggestion for investigating this issue can be made based on Light *et al.*'s (1983) study. Subjects were defined as high risk, given that they had at least one hypertensive parent and/or were high versus low reactors. Possible combinations of this factor pattern could be tested further by treating subjects in these four possible cells with relaxation training and investigating in a prepost test design whether reduced sympathetic tone would also improve kidney functioning of individuals at risk during experimental stress. If it could be demonstrated that treatment that reduces sympathetic tone also improves kidney function, at least two interesting and valuable points could be made. First, the finding of reduced sympathetic tone following relaxation would support the notion of sympathetic influences on kidney function *per se*, although this would remain inferential. Second, if reducing sympathetic tone through behavioral means improves kidney function, this treatment result will be particularly useful since improved kidney function on its own contributes to the maintenance of pressure at a lower level by effectively lowering the set point of the servocontrol mechanism. Hence, reduction of sympathetic overarousal could be considered a useful method in resetting the criterion level for blood pressure in the servocontroller, thereby permitting access to this internal control system.

Furthermore, some recent advances in behavioral methods have gone beyond the sole objective of reducing already existing sympathetic overarousal by means of "pacifying" techniques such as relaxation. Specifically, studies involving the prevention of excessive SNS activity through training of active behavioral coping, that is, behavioral assertion or cognitive reappraisal, may be greatly facilitative in modifying the repressed hostility and anger patterns that have been identified in cross-sectional and prospective studies as being a characteristic pattern of emotional response for individuals with high blood pressure as well as individuals with the coronary-prone or Type A behavior pattern (Dembroski *et al.*, 1985; Dimsdale *et al.*, 1979; MacDougall *et al.*, 1985; Shekelle *et al.*, 1983; Williams, Barefoot, & Shekelle, 1985; Williams *et al.*, 1980). The support for the utility of this approach is still very limited in that only two studies have involved complex stress management packages that include behavioral assertion and/or cognitive reappraisal training (Jorgensen *et al.*, 1981; Charlesworth *et al.*, 1984). However, the limited findings that are available were derived from well-designed studies with control groups and follow-up data, as well as reasonably large samples sizes. The main effect sizes of these treatments compare favorably with treatments that are based purely on pacifying training such as relaxation.

The research as presented above provides only limited evidence of the reversibility of hypertension and its sequellae, which on their own may further contribute to the maintenance of hypertension. It is noteworthy, though, that even in drug treatment studies many subjects can be taken off the drug after a few months of treatment and will be able to maintain their blood pressure at lower levels (Maland, Lutz, & Castle, 1983). Similarly, the data available for long-term effects of relaxation training have indicated that blood pressure will remain low over periods of up to 3 years following the end of treatment, thereby suggesting that the pressure-reducing treatments may also have had impact on other systems, which in turn may serve to maintain blood pressure at these reduced levels. One could speculate that these treatments have succeeded in lowering the set point of the servocontrol system.

We have not been able to derive from the present findings any evidence that behavioral treatments, as typically provided, will differentially affect individuals who have the salt-sensitive versus salt-resistant types of hypertension. It is possible that salt-sensitive hypertensives may be satisfactorily treated by a reduced or totally eliminated intake of salt.

There is also good empirical evidence suggesting that salt restriction or use of diuretic medication will bring about this change. Whether behavioral methods could serve as further agents to facilitate or accelerate this success is presently unknown. Equally, we do not know whether subjects who are not of the salt-sensitive type would respond more positively to behavioral treatment methods than do salt-sensitive hypertensives. Again, there is reason to suggest combining both approaches since neither one of them appears to be associated with significant negative side effects or high cost, although compliance may be a problem.

Lastly, on the basis of some recent evidence regarding commonsense models of illness, which individuals apply in a dysfunctional manner to their own hypertension, it is quite likely that treatment suggestions are not adhered to by patients because the course of treatment and the effect of the drugs on improvement of the condition may not concur with their commonsense representation of their illness (Meyer *et al.*, 1985). Facilitation of adherence that may bridge these misrepresentations has been demonstrated by Glasgow *et al.* (1982), who recognized that subjects were not able to directly perceive treatment success and hypothesized that therefore they would not be likely to follow the prescribed treatment regimen (i.e., relaxation). In order to overcome this handicap, all subjects were taught to take their own blood pressure, were given a blood pressure monitor to take home, and registered their own pressure daily. In this manner, subjects had consistent and unequivocal feedback about changes in their resting pressure levels, thus permitting them to attribute their blood pressure changes to changes in their behavior. This method appears promising and deserves replication as it has been demonstrated to be effective. It is also highly consistent with the observations of both Leventhal's group (Meyer *et al.*, 1985) and Pennebaker (1982).

In essence, it appears that behavioral methods, as presently available, are clearly appropriate treatments for essential hypertension, but this review suggests that we know very little about specificity such that particular treatments may be applied with maximal efficacy to particular subtypes of physiologically or psychologically defined hypertensives. Those with the most elevated resting pressure levels seem also to show the largest reductions in pressure when behaviorally treated (Jacob, Kraemer, & Agras, 1977). On the other hand, it has not yet been established whether pressure reduction through behavioral means will decrease mortality and cardiac morbidity as has been documented for the case of drug treatment in the Veterans Administration's cooperative studies (1970, 1972). Therefore the withholding of drug treatment from hypertensives in the moderate and high blood pressure ranges (in favor of behavioral treatment modes) would currently be considered irresponsible by many physicians. Despite the seeming potential of behavioral modes of treatment, they are not generally considered primary choices because of the inherent ethical implications. If, however, drug treatments consistently fail to control the blood pressure of a given patient, behavioral modes promise a low-cost, low-risk alternative. Evidence is available that behavioral modes have particular utility with the borderline hypertensive as drug treatment is generally not indicated for this subgroup. However, for all other known subtypes of hypertension (high versus low renin, salt-resistant versus salt-sensitive, and so on), we have no evidence as yet to differentiate treatment effectiveness. It appears highly worthwhile to study these effects for specific subtypes. The recently devised, more complex stress management packages, which include methods aimed at sympathetic tone reduction as well as improved cognitive and behavioral coping skills, appear promising because they may tap both the biological and psychological components of essential hypertension. Again, more well-controlled outcome studies are called for, because those already available hold promise. The evidence that the kidney does indeed play an important role in the etiology and maintenance of essential hypertension would suggest a need for further study; specifically, the effects of behavioral treatment on kidney functioning in hypertensives has not yet been assessed. It could be that the presently available methods through reduction of sympathetic hyperarousal will also have some positive, although indirect effect on the most important component of the blood pressure control system, the kidney blood-volume servocontroller.

Overall, it appears that research that has emerged during the past 20 years has moved in a promising direction and reviews such as this one may contribute to maximizing the potential of behavioral treatments for treating specific subtypes and stages within the essential hypertension paradigm.

References

Agras, W. S. (1983). Relaxation therapy in hypertension. *Hospital Practice, 19*, 129–137.

Alderman, M. H., & Madhavan, S. (1981). Management of the hypertensive patient: A continuing dilemma. *Hypertension, 3*, 192–197.

Ambrosioni, E., Costa, F. V., Borghi, C., Montebugmoli, L., Giordani, M. F. & Magnani, B. (1982). Effects of moderate salt restriction on intralymphocytic sodium and pressor response to stress in borderline hypertension. *Hypertension, 4*, 789–794.

Barefoot, J. C., Dahlstrom, W. G., & Williams, R. B. (1983). Hostility, CHD incidence, and total mortality: A 25-year follow-up study of 255 physicians. *Psychosomatic Medicine, 45*, 59–63.

Becker, M. H., & Maiman, L. A. (1975). Sociobehavioral determinants of compliance with health and medical care recommendations. *Medical Care, 13*, 10–24.

Benson, H. (1975). *The relaxation response*. New York: William Morrow.

Charlesworth, E. A., Williams, B. J., & Baer, P. E. (1984). Stress management at the worksite for hypertension: Compliance, cost–benefit, health care and hypertension-related variables. *Psychosomatic Medicine, 46*, 387–397.

Chobanian, A. V., Gavras, H., Gavras, I., Bresnahan, M., Sullivan, P., & Melby, J. C. (1978). Studies on the activity of the sympathetic nervous system in essential hypertension. *Journal of Human Stress, 4*, 22–28.

Conway, J. (1984). Hemodynamic aspects of essential hypertension in humans. *Physiological Reviews, 64*, 617–660.

DeClue, J. W., Guyton, A. C., Cowley, A. W., Jr., Coleman, T. G., Norman, R. A., Jr., & McCaa, R. E. (1978). Suppressor angiotension infusion, renal sodium handling, and salt-induced hypertension in the dog. *Circulation Research, 43*, 503–512.

Dembroski, T. M., MacDougall, J. M., Williams, R. B., Haney, I. L., & Blumenthal, J. A. (1985). Components of type A, hostility and anger in relationship to angiographic findings. *Psychosomatic Medicine, 47*, 219–233.

Dimsdale, J. E., Hackett, T. P., Hutter, A. M., Block, P. C., Catanzaro, D. M., & White, P. J. (1979). Type A behavior and angiographic findings. *Journal of Psychosomatic Research, 23*, 273–276.

Dustan, H. P. (1982). Physiologic regulation of arterial pressure: An overview. *Hypertension 4* (Suppl. 3), 62–67.

Dworkin, B. R., Filewich, R. J., Miller, N. E., & Craigmyle, N. (1979). Baroreceptor activation reduces reactivity to noxious stimulation: Implications for hypertension. *Science, 205*, 1299–1301.

Elbert, T., Pietrowsky, R., Kessler, M., Lutzenberger, W., & Birbaumer, N. (1985). Stimulation of baroreceptors decreases cortical excitability and increases pain sensation threshold in borderline hypertensives (Abstract). *Psychophysiology, 22*, 588.

Esler. M., Julius, S., Zweifler, A., Randall, O., Harburg, E., Gardner, H, & DeQuatio, V. (1977). Mild high-venin essential hypertension. *New England Journal of Medicine, 296*, 405–412.

Falkner, B., Onesti, G., Angelakos, E. T., Fernandes, M., & Langman, L. (1979). Cardiovascular response to mental stress in normal adolescents with hypertensive parents. *Hypertension, 1*, 23–30.

Feuerstein, M., & Linden, W. (1984). Psychobiological aspects of health and disease. In H. E. Adams & P. Sutker (Eds.), *Comprehensive handbook of psychopathology* (pp. 809–839). New York: Plenum Press.

Folkow, B. (1975). Vascular changes in hypertension and recent animal studies. In G. Berglund, L. Hansson, & Werkö, E. (Eds.), *Pathophysiology and management of arterial hypertension*. Göteborg: Lindgren & Soener.

Folkow, B. (1982). Physiological aspects of primary hypertension. *Physiological Reviews, 62*, 347–504.

Fredrikson, M., & Engel, B. F. (1985). Cardiovascular and electrodermal adjustments during a vigilance task in patients with borderline and established hypertention. *Journal of Psychosomatic Research, 29*, 235–246.

Fredrikson, M., Dimberg, U., Frisk-Holmberg M., & Stroem, G. (1985). Arterial blood pressure and general sympathetic activation in essential hypertension during stimulation. *Acta Medica Scandinavica, 217*, 309–317.

Frohlich, E. D., Tarazi, R. C., Ulrych, M., Dustan, H. P., & Page, I. H. (1967). Tilt test for investigating a neural component in hypertension: Its correlation with clinical characteristics. *Circulation, 36*, 387–393.

Frohlich, E. D., Tarazi, R. C., & Dustan, H. P. (1969). Hyperdynamic beta-adrenergic circulatory state: Increased beta receptor response. *Archives of Internal Medicine, 123,* 1–7.

Frumkin, K., Nathan, R. J., Prout, M. F., & Cohen, M. C. (1978). Nonpharmacologic control of essential hypertension in man: A critical review of the experimental literature. *Psychosomatic Medicine, 40,* 294–320.

Fujita, T., Noda, H., & Ando, K. (1984). Sodium susceptibility and potassium effects in young patients with borderline hypertension. *Circulation, 69,* 468–476.

Giese, J. (1976). The renin angiotension system and the pathogenesis of vascular disease in malignant hypertension. *Clinical Science and Molecular Medicine, 51* (Suppl. 3), 145.

Glasgow, M. S., Gaarder, K. R., & Engel, B. (1982). Behavioral treatment of high blood pressure. II. Acute and sustained effects of relaxation and systolic blood pressure feedback. *Psychosomatic Medicine, 44,* 155–170.

Goldby, F. S., & Beilin, L. J. (1974). The evolution and healing of arteriolar damage in renal-clip hypertension in the rat: An electron microscope study. *Journal of Pathology, 114,* 139–148.

Goldman, H., Kleinman, K. M., Snow, M. Y., Bidus, D. R., & Korol, B. (1974). Correlation of diastolic blood pressure and signs of cognitive dysfunction in essential hypertension. *Diseases of the Nervous System, 35,* 571–572.

Guyton, A. C. (1980). *Circulatory physiology: III. Arterial blood pressure and hypertension.* Philadelphia: W. G. Saunders.

Guyton, A. C., Cowley, A. W., & Coleman, T. (1972). Interaction between the separate pressure control systems in normal arterial pressure regulation and in hypertension. In J. Genest & E. Koiw (Eds.) *Hypertension.* Berlin: Springer.

Guyton, A. C., Coleman, T. G., Cowley, A. W., Jr., Manning, R. D., Jr., Norman, R. A., Jr., & Ferguson, J. D. (1974). A systems analysis approach to understanding long-range arterial blood pressure control and hypertension. *Circulation Research, 35,* 159–176.

Harburg, E., Blakelock, E. H., Jr., & Roeper, P. J. (1979). Resentful and reflective coping with arbitrary authority and blood pressure. *Psychosomatic Medicine, 41,* 789–202.

Hokanson, J. E., & Edelman, R. (1966). Effects of three social responses on vascular processes. *Journal of Personality and Social Psychology, 3,* 442–447.

Holden, R. A., Ostfeld, A. M., Freeman, D. H., Jr., Hellenbrand, K. D., & D'Atri, D. A. (1983). Dietary salt intake and blood pressure. *Journal of the American Medical Association 250,* 365–369.

Hypertension Detection and Follow-up Program Cooperative Group. (1979). Five-year findings of the Hypertension Detection and Follow-up Program. I. Reduction in mortality of persons with high blood pressure, including mild hypertension. *Journal of the American Medical Association, 242,* 2562–2571.

Hypertension Detection and Follow-up Program Cooperative Group. (1985). Five-year findings of the Hypertension Detection and Follow-up Program. *Hypertension, 7,* 105–112.

Jacob, R. G., Kraemer, H. G., & Agras, W. S. (1977). Relaxation therapy in the treatment of hypertension: A review. *Archives of General Psychiatry, 34,* 1417–1427.

Jorgensen, R. S., Houston, B. K., & Zurawski, R. M. (1981). Anxiety management training in the treatment of essential hypertension. *Behavioral Research and Therapy, 19,* 467–474.

Julius, S., Esler, M. D., & Randall, O. S. (1975). Role of the autonomic nervous system in mild human hypertension. *Clinical Science and Molecular Medicine, 48,* 243–252.

Kaplan, N. M. (1978). *Clinical hypertension.* Baltimore: Williams & Wilkins.

Kasl, S. V. (1978). A social-psychological perspective on successful community control of high blood pressure: A review. *Journal of Behavioral Medicine, 1,* 347–381.

Kawasaki, T., DeLea, L. S., Bartter, I. C., & Smith, H. (1978). The effect of high-sodium and low-sodium intakes on blood pressure and other related variables in human subjects with idiopathic hypertension. *American Journal of Medicine, 64,* 195–198.

Keys, A., Taylor, H. L., Blackburn, H., Brozek, J., Anderson, J. T., & Somonson, E. (1971). Mortality and coronary heart disease among men studied for 23 years. *Archives of Internal Medicine, 128*, 201–214.

Lacey, J. I. (1967). Somatic response patterning and stress: Some revisions of activation theory. In M. H. Apley & R. Trumbull (Eds.), *Psychological stress*. New York: Appleton-Century-Crofts.

Leventhal, H., Meyer, D., & Nerenz, D. (1980). The common-sense representation of illness danger. In S. J. Rachman (Ed.), *Medical psychology* (Vol. 2, pp. 7–30). New York: Pergamon Press.

Libo, L. M., & Arnold, G. E. (1983). Relaxation practice after biofeedback therapy: A long-term follow-up study of utilization and effectiveness. *Biofeedback and Self-Regulation, 8*, 217–227.

Light, K. C., Koepke, J. P., Obrist, P. A., & Willis, P. J., IV. (1983). Psychological stress induces sodium and fluid retention in man at high risk for hypertension. *Science, 220*, 429–431.

Linden, W. (1984). *Psychological perspective of essential hypertension: Etiology, maintenance and treatment*. Basel/New York: S. Karger.

Linden, W., & Feuerstein, M. (1983). Essential hypertension and social coping behavior: Experimental findings. *Journal of Human Stress, 9*, 22–31.

Linden, W., & Frankish, J. (1984). *Cardiovascular reactivity as a function of a repressive psychometric pattern*. Paper presented at the annual meeting of the American Psychological Association, Toronto.

Louis, W. J., Doyle, A. E., & Anavekar, S. (1973). Plasma norepinephrine levels in essential hypertension. *New England Journal of Medicine, 288*, 599–601.

Luborsky, L., Crits-Christoph, P., Brady, J. P., Kron, R. E., Weiss, T., Cohen, M., & Levey, L. (1982). Behavioral versus pharmacological treatments for essential hypertension—A needed comparison. *Psychosomatic Medicine, 44*, 203–213.

MacDougall, J. M., Dembroski, T. M., Dimsdale, J. E., & Hackett, T. P. (1985). Components of Type A, hostility and anger: Further relationships to angiographic findings. *Health Psychology, 4*, 137–152.

Maland, L. J., Lutz, L. J., & Castle, C. H. (1983). Effects of withdrawing diuretic therapy on blood pressure in mild hypertension. *Hypertension, 5*, 539–544.

Mancia, G., Ferrari, A., Gregorini, L., Ludrouk, J., & Zanchetti, A. (1978). Baroreceptor control of heart rate in man. In P. J. Schwartz, A. J. Brown, A. Malliani, & A. Zanchetti (Eds.), *Neural mechanisms in cardiac arrhythmias*. New York: Raven Press.

Manuck, S. B. Kaplan, J. R., & Clarkson, T. B. (1983). Behaviorally induced heart rate reactivity and atherosclerosis in cynomolgus monkeys. *Psychosomatic Medicine, 45*, 95–108.

Matthews, K. A., Glass, D. C., Rosenman, R. H., & Bortner, R. W. (1977). Competitive drive, pattern A, and coronary heart disease: A further analysis of some data from the Western Collaborative Group Study. *Journal of Chronic Diseases, 30*, 489–498.

McCubbin, J. W., Green, J. H., & Page, I. H. (1956). Baroreceptor function in chronic renal hypertension. *Circulation Research, 4*, 205–210.

Meyer, D., Leventhal, H., & Gutmann, M. (1985). Common sense models of illness: The example of hypertension. *Health Psychology, 4*, 115–136.

Miller, R. E., Shapiro, A. P., King, H. E., Gincherean, E. H., & Hosutt, J. A. (1984). Effect of antihypertensive treatment on the behavioral consequences of elevated blood pressure. *Hypertension, 6*, 202–208.

Moehring, J., Moehring, B., Petri, M., Haack, D., & Hackenthal, E. (1975). Studies on the pathogenisis of malignant hypertension in rats. *Kidney International, 8*, 174.

Morrison, R. L., Bellack, A. S., & Manuck, S. B. (1985). Role of social competence in borderline essential hypertension. *Journal of Consulting and Clinical Psychology, 53,* 248–255.

Navar, L. G. (1978). Renal autoregulation: Perspectives from whole kidney and single nephron studies. *American Journal of Physiology,* 234–357.

Pennebaker, J. W. (1982). *The psychology of physical symptoms.* New York: Springer-Verlag.

Sapira, J. D., Scheib, E. T., Moriarty, R., & Shapiro, A. P. (1971). Difference in perception between hypertensive and normotensive populations. *Psychosomatic Medicine, 33,* 239–250.

Schwartz, G. E. (1976). Self-regulation of response patterning: Implications for psychophysiological research and therapy. *Biofeedback and Self-Regulation, 1,* 7–30.

Seer, P. (1979). Psychological control of essential hypertension: Review of the literature and methodological critique. *Psychological Bulletin, 86,* 1015–1043.

Shapiro, A. P., Schwartz, G. E., Ferguson, D. L. E., Redmond, D. P., & Weiss, S. (1977). Behavioral methods in the treatment of hypertension. A review of their clinical status. *Annals of Internal Medicine, 86,* 626–636.

Shekelle, R. B., Gale, M., Ostfeld, A. M., & Paul, D. (1983). Hostility, risk of coronary heart disease, and mortality. *Psychosomatic Medicine, 45,* 109–114.

Shimada, K., Kitazumi, T., Sadakane, N., Ogura, H., & Ozawa, T. (1985). Age-related changes of baroreflex function, plasma norepinephrine, and blood pressure. *Hypertension, 7,* 113–117.

Sleight, P., Robinson, J. L., Brooks, D. E., & Rees, P. M. (1975). Carotid baroreceptor resetting in the hypertensive dog. *Clinical Science and Molecular Medicine Supplementary, 2,* 261s–263s.

Smithwick, R. H., & Robertson, G. W. (1973). Survival rates following splanchnicectomy for essential and malignant hypertension. In G. Onesti, K. E. Kim, & J. H. Moyer (Eds.), *Hypertension: Mechanisms and management* (pp. 847–865). New York: Grune & Stratton.

Southam, M. A., Agras, W. S., Taylor, C. B., & Kraemer, H. C. (1982). Relaxation training: Blood pressure lowering during the working day. *Archives of General Psychiatry, 39,* 715–717.

Swales, J. (1980). Dietary salt and hypertension. *Lancet, 1,* 1177–1179.

Thailer, S. A., Friedman, R., Harshfield, G. A., & Pickering, T. G. (1985). Psychological differences between high, normal, and low renin hypertension. *Psychosomatic Medicine, 47,* 294–297.

Thomas, G. W., Ledingham, J. G., & Beilin, L. J. (1976). Renin responses to intravenous Irusemide in essential hypertension. *Clinical Science and Molecular Medicine, 50,* 19 p.

Veterans Administration Cooperative Study Group on Antihypertensive Agents. (1970). Effects of treatment on morbidity in hypertension. Part 2. *Journal of the American Medical Association, 213,* 1143–1152.

Veterans Administration Cooperative Study Group on Antihypertensive Agents. (1972). Effects of treatment on morbidity in hypertension. Part 3. *Circulation, 45,* 991–1004.

Walker, J. R., & Guyton, A. C. (1967). Influence of blood oxygen saturation on pressure-flow curve of dog hindleg. *American Journal of Physiology, 212,* 506–509.

Weinstein, M. L., & Stason, W. B. (1976). *Hypertension: A policy perspective.* Cambridge, MA: Harvard University Press.

Wilber, J. A., & Barrow, J. C. (1972). Hypertension: A community problem. *American Journal of Medicine, 52,* 653–663.

Wilkie, F., & Eisdorfer, C. (1971). Intelligence and blood pressure in the aged. *Science, 172,* 959–962.

Williams, R. B., Haney, T. L., Lee, K. A., Wong, Y., Blumenthal, J. A., & Whalen, R. E. (1980). Type A behavior, hostility, and coronary atherosclerosis. *Psychosomatic Medicine, 42,* 539–549.

Williams, R. B., Barefoot, J. C., & Shekelle, R. B. (1985). The health consequenes of hostility. In M. A. Chesney, S. E. Goldston, & R. H. Rosenman (Eds.), *Anger, hostility and behavioral medicine*. New York: Hemisphere/McGraw-Hill.

Wilson, N. V., & Meyer, B. M. (1981). Early prediction of hypertension using exercise blood pressure. *Preventive Medicine, 10*, 62–68.

Wood, D. L., Sheps, S. G., Elveback, L. R., & Schirger, A. (1984). Cold pressor test as a predictor of hypertension. *Hypertension, 6*, 301–306.

CHAPTER 8

Psychophysiological Disorders of the Gastrointestinal Tract

Harry S. Shabsin and William E. Whitehead

The gastrointestinal tract is composed of the anatomical structures involved in the transportation and digestion of food, the absorption of nutrients into the blood stream, and the removal of nonabsorbable products from the body (Hassett, 1978; Wolf & Welsh, 1972). Functionally, these structures can be divided into four main components: the esophagus, the stomach, and the small and large intestines. Additionally, the smooth muscle secretory glands composed of the liver, the pancreas, and the gallbladder aid in digestion by providing bile, cholesterol, and other enzymes that enhance the breakdown and absorption of nutrients.

The anatomical structure of the gastrointestinal tract is similar throughout its length. In general, it is composed of an outer layer of longitudinally oriented smooth muscle and an inner circular smooth muscle layer (Barnard & Illman, 1981; Vander, Sherman & Luciano, 1975). These two bands overlay a smaller third muscle layer, the muscularis mucosa, composed of both circular and longitudinal muscle sheaths. Beneath this lie the submucosal and mucosal linings of the lumen which contain exocrine gland cells secreting protective fluids and digestive enzymes, and epithelial cells involved in the absorption of nutrients into the bloodstream. The submucosal layer also contains large amounts of connective tissue. It is the contractions of the outer longitudinal and

Harry S. Shabsin and William E. Whitehead • Division of Digestive Diseases, Francis Scott Key Medical Center, and Johns Hopkins University School of Medicine, Baltimore, Maryland 21224.

circular layers that produce the propulsive or peristaltic movements of the gastrointestinal tract.

The gastrointestinal tract has long been known to be more reactive to external stimuli of psychological significance than most other systems of the body. In a remarkable series of observations Beaumont (1833) first described changes in gastric secretions and mucosal appearance to various events such as food, nondigestable irritants, alcohol, overindulgence, and exercise. Beaumont, an army surgeon, arranged to make direct observations through a gastric fistula in a patient, Alix St. Martin, after an abdominal wound caused by an accidental shotgun blast refused to close completely. This resulted in a natural valve, composed of slightly inverted portions of the inner coats of the stomach, which Beaumont was able to push aside in order to view the inside of the stomach. On several occasions Beaumont observed mucosal changes associated with anger or irritation in his patient and thus provide the earliest direct evidence for emotional influence on the gastrointestinal tract. Since then a number of other investigators, most notably Pavlov (1910) and Cannon (1929), have demonstrated psychological influences on digestive activity. In their well-known patient Tom, Wolf and Wolff (1947) found hyperfunction of the stomach associated with aggression, anger, and restlessness and hypofunction associated with fright, depression, and lethargy. These authors also provocatively reported that these changes occurred during times of unconscious conflict and emotion in their subject.

Several excellent reviews have recently been published describing the relationship between emotional events and gastrointestinal disorders (Drossman, 1983; Weiner, 1977; Whitehead & Bosmajian, 1982; Whitehead & Schuster, 1984). Rather than repeat this process, this chapter will focus on two specific illnesses, the irritable bowel syndrome and esophageal spasms, in an effort to detail the relationship between psychological states, physiological activity, and gastrointestinal disorders.

Irritable Bowel Syndrome (IBS)

The irritable bowel syndrome (IBS), also commonly referred to as spastic colon, mucous colitis, or functional bowel disease, includes a host of symptoms. Among these, the most often reported are abdominal pain, constipation, diarrhea, abdominal distention, gas, and the presence of mucous, in the absence of any detectable organic disease (Schuster, 1984; Smits, 1974; Thompson, 1979). This disorder appears to be more prevalent in women than in men and has a higher incidence in developed countries, possibly because of differences in dietary fiber intake. It is often associated with psychological symptoms (Drossman, Powell, & Sessions, 1977) and is the most common cause for gastrointestinal distress. Irritable bowel syndrome may account for as many as 50%–70% of all gastroenterological complaints (Kirsner & Palmer, 1958), although it appears that only about half as many individuals suffer from it on a chronic basis (Texter & Butler, 1975). In a study of 2,000 patients referred to a gastroenterology clinic by general practitioners, Harvey, Salih, and Read (1983) diagnosed 47.5% with functional disorders of the gastrointestinal tract. Of these, the majority were experiencing abdominal pain with altered bowel habits (50.6%), painless diarrhea (12%), dyspepsia (8.7%), or painless constipation (4.4%). An additional 8.3% were diagnosed as having abdominal symptoms secondary to anxiety or depression, with the remainder falling into miscellaneous categories. In a smaller study employing 50 patients, Waller (1971) reported that 76% of the IBS patients examined presented with abdominal pain associated with altered bowel habits.

Irritable bowel syndrome is a difficult disorder to diagnose because its symptoms are characteristic of a number of organic diseases that may affect the gastrointestinal tract. This had led to recent attempts to develop classification schemata for differentiating the syndrome from other diseases on the basis of symptom questionnaires, either alone or in combination with a medical evaluation. Studying patients primarily with abdominal pain, constipation, or diarrhea, Manning, Thompson, Heaton, and Morris (1978) and Kruis *et al.* (1984) were able to identify symptoms that significantly differentiated IBS patients from those with organic disease. Manning *et al.* found looser stools with the onset of pain to be the best discriminator, followed by more frequent bowel movements with the onset of pain, pain eased after bowel movements, and visible distention. The majority of IBS patients (91%) reported two or more of these syptoms whereas only 30% of those with other diseases reported more than two of these symptoms. Manning *et al.* also reported feelings of incomplete emptying and the passage of mucous by rectum to occur more often in irritable bowel syndrome. However, these differences were not statistically significant when compared to individuals without IBS.

Kruis *et al.* (1984) found alternating bowel movements of constipation and diarrhea or a combination of abdominal pain, flatulence, and irregularities of bowel movement to occur significantly more often in IBS than other gastrointestinal disorders. When used in combination with scores obtained from physical examination, these researchers were able to discriminate IBS from other disorders with a 99% specificity, although they were able to obtain only a moderate rate of sensitivity. The use of this scale has been criticized, however, because the absence of physical signs is weighted more heavily than the presence of symptoms in obtaining a diagnosis (Drossman, 1983).

The inclusion of non physical findings as part of the diagnostic criteria for IBS may also be useful as this disorder is often initially misdiagnose (Waller & Misiewicz, 1969). Although the incidence of organic disease in patients diagnosed with IBS is reported as being only 3%–6% (Kruis *et al.*, 1984; McHardy, Browne, McHardy, Welch, & Ward, 1962), as many as 30% of patients eventually diagnosed as having IBS present with abdomianl scars (Chaudhary & Truelove, 1962; Waller, 1971). It would ther fore appear that efforts to improve the discriminability of measures employed in obtaining a diagnosis are still warranted. Although, as will be discussed below, psychological factors appear to be an important component in IBS. no studeies have as yet included psychological testing as part of the diagnostic criteria.

Psychological Considerations

Functional bowel disorders have been associated with complaints indicative of psychological distress or difficult life situations (Ford, Eastwood, & Eastwood, 1982). McKegney (1977) suggests that dependent and compulsive personality types are often seen with gastrointestinal disorders, and Mendeloff, Monk, Siegel, and Lilienfeld (1970) found a higher incidence of life stresses related to childhood, marital, or employment difficulties in individuals with irritable bowel syndrome. The importance of stressful life events similar to those described by Mendoloff *et al.* in the etiology or exacerbation of IBS has also been shown by others. Hislop (1971) reported that stressful events preceded the onset of abdominal symptoms in 50% of 67 IBS patients he studied; Lisa, Alpers, and Woodruff (1973) found psychological illness to proced IBS in two-thirds of their patients. Chaudry and Truelove (1962) found the presence of psychological factors to result in a poorer prognosis for the IBS patient. They reported that 76% of their patients who experienced life chages that reduced stressful events became symptom-free in comparison with only 22% of those whose life situation did not change.

Anxiety

The two psychological profiles most often diagnosed as accompanying the irritable bowel syndrome are anxiety disorders and general neuroticism. Using the Eysenck Personality Inventory and the Anxiety Scale of the Institute for Personality and Ability Testing Questionnaire, Esler, and Goulston (1973) found an IBS group to be significanstly more anxious and neurotic than a general medical group. However, this difference was statistically significant only for patients whose primary complaint was diarrhea. Patients with predominantly abdominal pain did not differ from controls. Also using the Eysenck Personalality Inventory, along with the Middlexes Hospital Questionnarire, Palmer and his associates (Palmer, Crisp, Stomehill & Walker, 1974) compared 41 IBS patients with a matched group of 25 outpatients suffering from psychoneurotic disorders and with normal values for the Eysenck Personality Inventory obtained from the literature. IBS patients were found to differ significantlty from the two control groups. Although scoring as more neurotic than the normal group on the Eysenck profile, the IBS group was found to be less neurotic than the outpatient group on both psychological measures. No distinction was made between different types of IBS patietns in this study.

In a well-designed study using the Crown–Crisp Experimental Index, Ryan, Kelly, and Fielding (1983) reported significantly higher levels of free-floating and somatic anxiety in an IBS group compared with a group of matched controls. Hislop (1971) also reported anxiety in 69% of his IBS patients versus only 22% for sex- and age-matched controls, although his criteria for diagnosing psychopathology were not clearly stated. A number of other studies (e.g., Dotevall, Svedlund, & Sjodin, 1982; Whitehead, Engle, & Schuster, 1980) have also reported increased levels of anxiety in IBS patients.

Hysteria

Hysteria, the development of physical symptoms in response to stress or psychological conflict (Graham, 1973), is also often reported as being associated with bowel disorders. However, research findings have not been consistent on its occurrence. Both Palmer *et al.* (1974) and Ryan *et al.* (1983) found hysteria to be the only neurotic indicator on which IBS patients scored lower than normals, whereas others have reported it to be the primary disorder in IBS. Using research diagnostic criteria (Feighner *et al.*, 1972), Liss *et al.* (1973) reported that hysteria (followed closely by anxiety) was the most common psychological finding in IBS. Young, Alpers, Norland, and Woodruff (1976), using the same assessment procedure as Liss *et al.*, also reported hysteria to be among the most common finding in IBS patients, although they found depression rather than anxiety to account for a large part of the remaining psychological disorders specifically diagnosed. Further evidence for the role of hysteria in IBS comes from West (1970), who found mucous colitis patients to score higher on the hysteria scale of the MMPI than patients with ulcerative colitis, upper gastrointestinal disorders, hypertension, or skin disorders. In addition, patients with hysteria may be at greater risk for developing IBS. Young *et al.* (1976) reported that in all of their patients diagnosed with hysteria the disorder preceded the occurrence of abdominal pain, whereas in only one of their patients diagnosed with depression was this the case.

Depression

Depression and its associated symptoms, fatigue, decreased mental abilities, sleep disturbances, or saddened affect, is also often mentioned as a psychological disturbance associated with IBS. However, reports of the occurrence of depression and its prevalence in IBS vary widely, ranging from as little as 8% to as much as 77% (Dotevall *et al.*, 1982; Liss *et al.*, 1973). Even in controlled studies comparing IBS groups to normals (e.g., Whitehead *et al.*, 1980; Ryan *et al.*, 1983), IBS patients are not consistently found to differ significantly from normals on measures of depression, although they generally tend to score higher in depressive indices than controls. Although different methods and procedures undoubtedly account for some of these differences, other factors such as increased somatic concern or hypochondriasis may also be involved. For instance, Whitehead, Winget, Fedoravicius, Wooley, and Blackwell (1982) found a random sample of individuals with IBS symptoms to be significantly more likely to have multiple somatic complaints than a normal population, to visit their physicians more often for minor complaints, and to rate their colds and flus more serious than others.

Illness Behavior

Findings similar to those of Whitehead *et al.* (1982) were also reported by Sandler, Drossman, Nathan, and McKee (1984). These studies, along with others by Thompson and Heaton (1980) and Drossman, Sandler, McKee, and Lovitz (1982), indicate that approximately 15% of the general population experiences IBS symptoms but that only 38%–50% seek medical help. This has led to hypotheses that those who seek medical attention are expressing illness behavior as a manifestation of a learned behavior (Whitehead, Fedoravicius, Blackwell, and Wooley, 1979). Latimer *et al.* (1979) suggest that IBS patients differ from other groups in their preoccupation with their bowel symptoms and in their health-seeking behavior. In the only study that looked at psychological measures in individuals with IBS who did and did not visit their doctor for their symptoms, Greenbaum, Abitz, VanEgeren, Mayle, and Greenbaum (1984) found the MMPI to discriminate between these two groups and a control group. IBS subjects not seeking medical care scored significantly lower than those seeking medical care and significantly higher than normals on measures of hypochondriasis, as well as depression and hysteria. It appears that psychological characteristics are important not only in the formation of IBS symptoms but also in the determination of who will seek medical help for these symptoms.

Abdominal Pain

Support for the concept of increased sensitivity to bowel activity in the irritable bowel syndrome is also provided by studies of abdominal pain during colonic distention. Although Latimer *et al.* (1981) in a second study were unable to distinguish IBS patients from controls by the amount of pain they reported during ballon distention of the colon, others have shown IBS groups to be more sensitive along these dimensions. Using a sigmoidoscope for positioning, Ritchie (1973) inflated a balloon in the sigmoid colon of 67 IBS patients and in a control group with no known gastrointestinal disease and no previous abdomianal symptoms. Employing similar balloon diameters and gut wall resistance for both groups, Ritchie found that an inflation level of 60 ml caused reports of pain in 55% of the IBS subjects versus only 6% for controls. It required 120 ml of balloon distention to produce comparable reports of pain from normals. In addition, 52% of the IBS group reported pain at less than the maximun level of colonic distention whereas only 6% of controls did so. Using a similar procedure, Whitehead *et al.* (1979) compared pain ratings in normal subjects and IBS subjects to rectosigmoid distention. They found that more IBS subjects than normals reported pain at all levels of balloon inflation.

Placebo Response

The use of placebo in the treatment of the IBS has also produced results implicating psychological factors in the heightened response to symptoms shown by many IBS patients. Beecher (1965) has shown that up to 35% of individuals experiencing pain respond to placebo with reports of reductions in their symptoms and has suggested that cognitions about pain may affect its perception. Although the experimental situation or the subject's expectations may certainly be a factor in placebo responses (Levitt, 1975), Stroebel (1972) has suggested that there is a direct correlation between the amount of pain relief obtained with placebo and the level of anxiety or stress an individual is experiencing. If anxiety disorders or stress are responsible in some fashion for the complaints presented by those seeking medical help for IBS, Stroebel's hypothesis suggest that one should expect to see these individuals responding favorably to a trial of placebo medication. In general, controlled trials have found that many IBS patients respond as well to placebo as to active medication.

Heefner, Wilder, and Wilson (1978) compared the response of 44 IBS patients to the tricyclic antidepressant desipramine and to placebo. They found that placebo improved abdominal pain, bowel, movemnets, and measures of interference with daily life in 59% or more of thier subjects. These changes were not significantly different from improvements on these measures shown by the drug group, except interference in daily life, although the drug group did show more improvement on these measures than the control group. Interestingly, a higher percentage of patients rated their depression as better on placebo than on antidepressant, although these differences were again not significant. This might suggest that the amount of antidepreseant used in this study was not within an effective therapeutic range.

Lancaster-Smith, Prout, Pinto, Anderson, and Schiff (1982) also compared placebo to the drug Motipress, a combination antidepressant-anxiolytic, in a double-blind, randomized study of IBS patients. They used both physician and patient ratings of diarrhea, constipation, abdominal pain, and feelings of distention to rate patient improvement. At the end of 12 weeks of treatment there were no differences between placebo and drug groups on any of these symptoms except for patient ratings of abdominal pain. In general, both groups showed similar improvement by the end of the study and the authors suggested that the presence of psychoneurotic symptoms has an adverse effect on the short-term medical management of the irritable bowel syndrome.

Placebo has also been reported to be comparable to loperamide, doperidone, trimipramine, and wheat bran in its ability to significantly reduce many of the symptoms associated with IBS (Cann, Read, & Holdsworth, 1983, 1984; Cann, Read, Holdsworth, & Barends, 1984; Myren, Groth, Larssen, & Larsen, 1982). On the whole, the percentage of individuals showing improvement from placebo appears comparable to that achieved with the most effective form of medical management, which involves a combination of antidepressant-anxiolytic, smooth muscle relaxant, and bulking agent (Ritchie & Truelove, 1980).

A study conducted by Svedlund and his associates (Svedlund, Sjodin, Ottosson, & Dotevall, 1983) gives added weight to the involvement of psychological factors with the irritable bowel syndrome. In a well-designed investigation, these researchers divided 101 IBS patients into two matched groups and followed them at 3 and 15 months. Both groups received medical management consisting of bulk forming agents and, when appropriate, anticholinergic agents, antacids, and minor tranquilizers. The control group received only medical management while the experimental group also received ten 1-hour psychotherapy sessions spread over the first three months of the study. At both follow-up periods the group receiving psychotherapy showed significantly more improvement in IBS symptoms than the group receiving only medical management.

Physiological Factors

In order to better understand how stressful environmental events interact with psychological profiles to produce the abdominal symptoms associated with the irritable bowel syndrome, it is necessary to look at physiological as well as psychological functioning. Studies of gastrointestinal functioning will allow for a better appreciation of IBS as either (a) primarily a hysterical manifestation of psychological distress, (b) a short-term physiological alteration in bowel function brought on by stress, or (c) a more permanent alteration in gastrointestinal functioning which predisposes individuals to react physiologically to stress or other environmental events in a fashion that results in the symptoms associated with IBS. The two areas of gut functioning that have received the most attention from researchers interested in this aspect of IBS are colonic motility (the contractions of the large intestine) and the myoelectric activity of the colon associated with such contractions. Because of the difficulty in gaining access to the gastrointestinal tract *in vivo,* most of the studies in humans have involved the sigmoid and rectosigmoid portions of the colon.

Motility

The earliest, and from today's perspective perhaps some of the most interesting, studies of colonic reaction to stress were conducted by Almy and his associates (Almy, 1951; Almy & Tulin, 1947) using medical students without any known abdominal disorders as well as patients reporting IBS symptoms. Almy used both physical and psychological stressors while observing the lower colon endoscopically. Physical stress included submerging an individual's hand or arm into ice water for up to

9 minutes or tightening a headband to produce an artificial headache. Psychological stress involved discussing emotional issues with a subject or the use of hoax to produce a stressful event. For instance, with the collaboration of his co-workers, Almy led one of his subjects to believe that he had found a colonic carcinoma upon insertion of the endoscope and then had the subject sign a release to perform a biopsy. Almy found that these kinds of stressors produced changes in colonic motility in both normals and IBS patients. These changes were reversed upon termination of the stressful situation. However, such reversals took longer in IBS patients than in normals. In addition, in the subjects undergoing painful stressors, Almy reported that colonic changes did not occur with the onset of pain but only after subjects began to have difficulty coping with the pain, indicating self-reproach for agreeing to participate in the study or resentment toward the experimenters for placing them in such a perilous situation. The subjects' attitude also seemed to affect the type of motility change observed. Those subjects expressing hostility, defensiveness, or attempts to cope with the procedure showed increased motility whereas subjects expressing helplessness, defeat, or a subdued manner showed decreases in motility. A similar relationship between emotional expression and motility was also reported by Wolf and Wolff (1947), and Lechin, Van der Dijs, Gomez, Lechin, and Arocha (1983) reported decreased intestinal tone to be associated with increased somatization, fatigue, hypochondriasis, and obsessive compulsiveness, and increased intestinal tone to be associated with increases in guilt, anxiety, agitation, and depersonalization. Wangel and Deller (1965) found motility in normal controls and IBS patients to be affected by stressful interview, although only IBS patients with diarrhea showed a significant change.

Many of the symptoms associated with IBS, such as diarrhea or abdominal pain, have been attributed to disorders in colonic motility (Connell, 1974). For instance, as Burns (1980) points out, diarrhea in IBS is often accompanied by decreases in sigmoid activity whereas constipation is most often associated with increases in motility. This has led a number of researchers to look for physiological differences in motility between IBS patients and various control groups. Discrepancies in various indices of motility between normals and IBS patients have been found during rest (Dinoso, Goldstein, & Rosner 1983; Latimer *et al.*, 1981), after a meal (Sullivan, Cohen, & Snape, 1978), and in response to the presence of gastrointestinal hormones (Snape, Carlson, Matarazzo, & Cohen, 1977). Differences in motility have also been found between diarrhea-prone IBS patients and those with constipation (Taylor, Darby, & Hammond, 1978; Waller, 1971, Wangel & Deller, 1965; Whitehead *et al.*, 1980). These studies, along with others such as that by Harvey and Read (1973), who found IBS patients with postprandial pain to respond with greater contractile activity to cholecystokinin than those patients without meal-related pain, indicate the importance of physiological activity of the colon in the etiology as well as the exacerbation of IBS symptoms.

Slow-Wave Myoelectric Activity

Contractions of the colon are thought to be controlled and coordinated by intrinsic myoelectric activity most likely originating in the cirular smooth muscles of the gut (Christensen, 1975; Durdle, Kingma, Bowes, & Chambers, 1983). In humans, slow-wave myoelectic activity is often observed to occur at frequencies of approximately 6 and 3 cycles per minute (cpm). This kind of activity has been called the basic electrical rhythm or the electrical control activity of the colon. Studies with normal subjects indicate that 6 cpm activity is the more prevalent of the two frequencies (Snape, Carlson, & Cohen, 1977; Taylor, Duthie, Smallwood, Brown, & Linkens, 1974). It may also be possible that there are actually two frequency bands of approximately 2–5 cpm and 6–10 cpm rather than two specific frequencies; several investigators have reported dominant slow-wave frequencies that fall within these two ranges (Altaparmakov & Wienbeck, 1984; Hyland, Darby, Hammond, & Taylor, 1980; Meshkinpour, Hoehler, Bernick, & Buerger, 1981).

Myoelectric investigations with IBS patients have revealed abnormalities in the slow waves of this group and provide additional evidence for a physiological basis for IBS. Although not all studies have shown differences in slow myoelectric activity between normals and IBS patients (e.g., Latimer *et al.*, 1981), a number of investigators have found IBS patients to display a significantly greater proportion of 3 cpm myoelectric activity than normals, both at rest and in response to gastrointestinal hormones (Taylor, Darby & Hammond, 1978; Snape, Carlson, Matarazzo, & Cohen, 1977; Hyland *et al.*, 1980).

As alterations in bowel function might affect myoelectric activity, it is possible that the changes observed in the slow waves of IBS patients are a result of their symptoms rather than being specific to this disorder. Several studies by Taylor and his colleagues (Taylor, Darby, Hammond, & Basu, 1978; Hyland *et al.*, 1980), however, indicate that this is not the case. These investigators compared IBS patients to patients with similar symptoms resulting from organically diagnosed disorders. They found that IBS patients displayed significantly greater amounts of 3 cpm activity than other patients. In Hyland's study, patients with diarrhea arising from diverticular disease did not differ greatly from normals in myoelectric activity, and both IBS patients with diarrhea and patients with diverticular disease were treated with bran for 1 month. Interestingly, treatment did not significantly alter the differences found between these groups prior to the dietary supplement. It is possible that any slow-wave myoelectric contributions to diarrhea-prone IBS symptoms are not amenable to this kind of treatment.

Differences between patients with chronic nonorganic constipation and normals have also been reported. Frieri, Parisi, Corazziari, and Caprilli (1983) found constipated patients to have a significantly higher frequency in the lower slow-wave range than normals. Although much remains to be learned about the relationship between slow waves in the colon and IBS, an increase of 3 cpm myoelectric activity appears to be related to the manifestation of symptoms in this disorder.

Myoelectrical Spike Activity

A second kind of myoelectric activity presently under investigation in both normal subjects and IBS patients involves the occurrence of fast electrical activity in the colon. Recordings of this type of activity typically appear as 5–10 msec monophasic spike potentials occurring as single events or as bursts of electrical activity lasting for periods of up to 30 seconds. Spike bursts may be composed of electrical activity occurring at frequencies as high as 40 Hz. Bursts of spike activity are most often categorized by their duration, which is commonly observed to occur in two temporal frequency bands with mean times ranging between 2 and 4 seconds and between 12 and 20 seconds. These two bands of activity have been called, by various investigators, short and long spike bursts (Bueno, Fioramonti, Ruckebusch, Frexinos, & Coulom, 1980), rhythmic and sporadic spike bursts (Schang & Devroede, 1983), and discrete (DERA) and continuous (CERA) electrical response activity (Sarna, Latimer, Campbell, & Waterfall, 1982).

Rhythmic and sporadic spike activity has been reported to occur with a frequency of 10–40 HZ and 1–20 Hz respectively by Schang and Devroede (1983), and Sarna *et al.* (1982) reported DERA and CERA activity to occur with a frequency between .9 and 10 Hz. A third kind of fast electrical activity that has a frequency range of 25 to 40 cpm has also been reported in normals by Sarna *et al.* (1982) and termed the contractile electrical complex. Spike potentials not associated with spike bursts have also been reported to occur with a frequency of less than 1 per minute to more then 6 per minute (Snape, Carlson, & Cohen, 1976; Altaparmakov & Wienbeck, 1984).

Like slower myoelectric activity, spikes and spike bursts have been related to contractile activity of the colon, and differences have been found between normals and IBS patients. Snape *et al.* (1976) reported that IBS patients have a higher resting incidence of spike potentials in both the rectum and rectosigmoid areas. However, the total number of spikes reported was small and the differences between normals and IBS patients was not significant, even though the IBS group had over twice the number of spikes in the rectosigmoid colon when compared to normals.

Bueno, Fioramonti, Frexinos, and Ruckebusch (1980) also found IBS patients to differ significantly from normals in the number of colonic long and short spike bursts which occurred during resting conditions. In IBS patients, increases in short spike bursts were correlated with constipation and abdominal pain and decreases in short and long spike bursts were correlated with diarrhea. On the other hand, Altaparmakov and Wienbeck (1984) found that loperamide, an antidiarrheal agent, significantly lowered spike activity in normals. Reports of reduced amounts of fast myoelectrical activity during the occurrence of diarrhea and following the administration of medication for the relief of diarrhea points out the need for further research in order to gain a better understanding of the relationship between this sort of myoelectric activity and IBS. However, it appears that alterations in the faster electrical rhythms of the colon are an indication of IBS and may be related to the onset of symptoms in this disorder.

Changes in the pattern of fast electrical activity have also been reported following food ingestion. Such changes are most likely the result of the release of gastrointestinal hormones in response to eating, as similar alterations have been produced by the administration of gastrointestinal hormones such as pentagastrin and cholecystokinin alone (Snape, Carlson, & Cohen, 1977). IBS symptoms have been related to changes in fast myoelectrical activity following a meal by several investigators.

Sullivan *et al.* (1978) found IBS patients to have more prolonged periods of spiking activity following a meal when compared to normals. They attributed this to abnormalities in neural control mechanisms since this temporal increase was reduced by anticholinergic medication. However, the significance of these differences for IBS is hard to interpret at present since Schang and Devroede (1983) found that increases in propigating spike activity following a meal had a time course in normals that was similar to the time course shown by the IBS group in the study by Sullivan *et al.* These discrepancies may reflect differences in the caloric content of the meals used in these two studies as well as other procedural differences.

The absence of aborally propagated long spike bursts has also been reported to be related to postprandial pain by Bueno *et al.* (1980). However, this pattern occurred in only 3 of 35 IBS patients studied. Although it does appear that fast electrical activity of the colon is affected by eating, how such changes after a meal are specifically related to the production of the symptoms seen in IBS needs further clarification.

Disorders of the Esophagus

The esophagus is composed of an inner circular and an outer longitudinal muscle layer and obtains its primary efferent innervation through the common vagal nerve (Code & Schlegel, 1968). Its upper end is bounded by the pharyngoesophageal sphincter and is composed of striated muscle fibers, its lower portion is composed of smooth muscle fibers and is separated from the stomach by the gastroesophageal sphincter. In humans, the esophagus is approximately 21–23 cm in length and functions solely in the movement of material from the mouth to the stomach. Transportation is accomplished by peristalsis involving the distal migration of bands of contracting circular muscle fibers. Motility is initiated primarily by the act of swallowing and secondarily by distention of the esophagus. Once begun, contractions proceed involuntarily in a caudal direction at about 2–4 cm per second, normally terminating in the lower esophageal sphincter. This reflex activity is controlled by the fifth, seventh, ninth, tenth, and eleventh cranial nerves which innervate both the upper and lower portions of the esophagus (Schuster, 1979). Like the colon, the esophagus has often been described as being responsive to emotional events.

Esophageal Spasms

One of the most frequently described motility disorders of the esophagus is diffuse esophageal spasm (DES). This disorder is characterized by repetitive, nonpropulsive, tertiary contractions of the esophagus which occur either spontaneously or following normal contractions initiated by swallowing (Castell, 1982). Unlike normally initiated peristaltic contractions, these contractions appear to be primarily spike-independent (Ouyang, Reynolds, & Cohen, 1983). They may occur in either an oral or a caudal direction and are often accompanied by sensations of pain or difficulty in swallowing.

Using the esophageal transit time of a barium cocktail as a dependent measure, Wolf and Almy (1949) found that spasms of the esophagus could be produced in both normals and patients complaining of dysphagia by a variety of emotionally and physically stressful situations. In an interesting case report, Faulkner (1940) found that he was able to either relieve or produce severe esophageal spasms by simply altering the amount of anxiety one of his patients was experiencing. The patient was a nervous young man experiencing emotional stress related to his economic and home situation at the time. Stacher, Steinringer, Blau, and Landgraf (1979) found that nonpropulsive esophageal contractions could be produced as part of the defense response to loud acoustic stimuli. Rubin, Nagler, Spiro, and Pilot (1962) reported similar increases in nonpropulsive contractions in three of five subjects when they were engaged in a discussion of emotionally charged issues. The amount of nonpropulsive activity was significantly greater during these times than when the subjects were discussing more neutral events.

Psychological disorders have also been implicated in the etiology of esophageal dysfunction. In one of the better studies of its kind, Clouse and Lustman (1983) reported a significant relationship between certain psychiatric illnesses and esophageal contraction abnormalities. Using manometric studies, 50 patients were blindly classified as having contraction abnormalities, other manometric abnormalities (aperistalsis or decreased contractile amplitudes), or no abnormalities. These results were then compared to psychiatric diagnoses (DSM–III criteria) made blindly on the basis of structured interviews. In subjects classified as having contraction abnormalities, 84% also had a psychiatric diagnosis, whereas only 31% without abnormalities and 33% with noncontractile abnormalities were so classified. Most of the psyschiatric diagnoses in this study were accounted for by depression, anxiety, and somatization disorders.

Globus Hystericus

Globus hystericus, the feeling of a lump in the throat, has also often been attributed to psychological disturbances. Although physical disorders such as hiatal hernia, increased cricopharyngeal pressures, reflux esophagitus, or cervical spinal anomalies have been suggested as the cause of globus hystericus (Malcomson, 1966; Watson & Sullivan, 1974), it appears that these disorders do not sufficiently account for the symptms of globus in many patients (Caldarelli, Andrews, & Derbyshire, 1970; Mair, Schroder, Modalsli, & Maurer, 1974). Globus is reported more often in women than in men and occurs primarily between meals. It also appears to be a fairly common phenomenon in the general population. Thompson and Heaton (1982) reported that 34.5% of men and 52.5% of women from a sample of 147 healthy volunteers described feelings of globus. Almost all (95.5%) reported these feelings during times of strong emotion, and many volunteered that the feelings abated with crying.

Glaser and Engel (1977), using a psychoanalytic theoretical model, attributed the symptms of globus to repressed crying related to loss or grief. They cite the relief of symptoms that occurs along with the emotional release in crying as evidence for their theory. On the other end of the psychological spectrum, Schatzki (1964) attributed the sensations of globus to the voluntary behavioral act of repeated swallowing which may occur during times of tension. This results in a reduction of saliva and the accompanying sensation of a lump in the throat, which may become worse as a person focuses on the sensation or increases swallowing in an attempt to get rid of the feeling.

Interestingly, the term *globus hystericus* is a misnomer in that hysteria does not appear to be a common psychiatric factor in globus (Lehtinen & Puhakka, 1976) or other esophageal disorders. In general, when a psychiatric diagnosis is obtained, these patients are found to be more neurotic than others and are usually characterized as having disorders involving anxiety, obsessiveness, or depression. The similarity between this psychological profile and that of individuals with IBS has already been pointed out by others (Clouse & Lustman, 1983; Watson, Sullivan, Corke, Rush, 1978) and gives added weight to a functional explanation for those cases of globus in which a specific medical determination cannot be made. Increased support for a similar psychological etiology in IBS and the esophageal disorders mentioned above is also provided by Watson *et al.* (1978), who found significantly more patients with IBS (51%) than controls (30%) reporting the symptoms found in globus hystericus. It is tempting to speculate that certain disorders of the esophagus are actually a variant of the irritable bowel syndrome and should be treated as a psychosomatic rather than a physiological problem (Thompson, 1979). Additional research in this area should prove valuable in testing such a hypothesis.

Psychological and Behavioral Treatment Approaches for IBS and Esophageal Disorders

With the exception of Svedlund *et al.* (1983), few studies have systematically investigated the effect of psychotherapy on the symptoms associated with IBS or esophageal disorders. Almost all reports in this area suffer from lack of adequate control groups, and most are single case studies. In spite of these difficulties, there appear to be enough consistent findings to suggest that individuals suffering from certain gastrointestinal disorders can benefit from psychotherapeutic procedures. These reports, however, should be considered preliminary, and their importance is more in directing future research than in proving the efficacy of various psychotherapeutic techniques. On the other hand, for the clinician attempting to treat gastrointestinal complaints psychologically, they may provide valuable insights into planning therapeutic strategies.

Few studies have reported on the use of psychodynamic or nondirective psychotherapy for the treatment of IBS. Hislop (1980) described a series of 52 IBS patients whom he provided with brief psychodynamically oriented therapy designed to explore emotional states and to help in the expression of repressed emotions. Recent life events were also explored and reassurance was provided. For the majority of patients, therapy was made available in the form of three or fewer 1-hour sessions spaced 2 to 4 weeks apart. Following treatment, 46% of the patients described their symptoms as absent or improved using self-report questionaires, but no statistical analysis was performed. These results must be accepted with caution, however, as others (Waller & Misiewicz, 1969) have indicated that follow-up contact alone seems to help patients with IBS. In addition, placebo alone has been shown to provide relief from IBS symptoms in over 50% of patients (e.g., Heefner *et al.*, 1978). One must also question how much psychodynamically oriented therapy can be accomplished in 3 hours or less. In general, it appears that this type of therapy may not be as effective as more behaviorally oriented psychotherapeutic techniques such as cognitive restructuring or anxiety reduction and desensitization (Cohen & Reed, 1968; Harrell & Beiman, 1978; Hedberg, 1973).

Good treatment results have been reported in studies employing behavioral methods, particularily those procedures aimed at providing improved coping skills. As already mentioned, Svedlund *et al.* (1983) found significantly greater long-term improvement in IBS symptoms in an IBS group receiving medical treatment plus psychotherapy than in a group of IBS controls receiving only medical treatment. Svedlund and his associates used a variety of techniques, including behavior modification, problem solving, and stress mangement, to help patients modify maladaptive behavior and find solutions to problems. Therapy was focused on ways of coping with stress and emotional problems, and both physical and mental symptoms were used to assess improvements during the study. Physical symptoms consisted of ratings of somatic complaints, abdominal pain, and bowel dysfunction. Mental symptoms were based on scores obtained for total mental symptoms, an asthenic-depressive syndrome, and an anxiety syndrome. Assessments took place prior to the subjects being assigned to groups and at 3-month and 15-month follow-up points.

Both groups studied by Svedlund *et al.* (1983) showed improvement in somatic and mental scores after 3 months of treatment. The experimental group showed significantly greater improvement, however, on total somatization and abdominal pain than the controls at first follow-up, and all three somatic measures were significantly improved over controls at 15 months. In addition, patients receiving psychotherapy continued to show improvement between 3 and 15 months, whereas those receiving only medication regressed toward the initial severity of their symptoms at the 15-month follow-up. No changes in psychological symptoms occurred after 3 months, and the differences in psychological symptoms between groups was not significant at either the 3-month or 15-month follow-up.

When compared with other studies that have shown a poor prognosis for long-term treatment of IBS patients with medication alone (e.g., Waller & Misiewicz, 1969), the Svedlund *et al.* (1983) study suggests that psychotherapy is an effective procedure for use in the treatment of irritable bowel syndrome. It will, one hopes, be influential for researchers and clinicians alike in increasing the availablilty of psychotherapy for IBS patients. In addition, it should encourage more controlled studies to help validate other methods of providing beneficial forms of psychotherapy for treating IBS. For instance, psychotherapy utilizing cognitive and behavioral methods to change attributional styles has been found to be effective in treating the symptoms of IBS in a single case report (Youell & McCullough, 1975), and paradoxical treatment involving aversive behavior therapy has also been reported successful in a single case report (Legalos, 1977).

One of the more useful therapeutic procedures for treating psychophysiological disorders of the gastrointestinal tract appears to be relaxation training. Jacobson (1927) was the first to employ relaxation procedures in the treatment of gastrointestinal disorders and reported several cases of mucous colitis (IBS) and esophageal spasm treated successfully with progressive relaxation. In a more recent study, Phillips (1983) reported progressive relaxation with and without imagery to be more successful than no treatment for a waiting-list control group in relieving pain and discomfort arising from a variety of gastrointestinal disorders, including IBS. Hypnotically induced relaxation has also been reported to reduce symptoms associated with functional gastrointestinal disorders (Dolezalova, Cerny; & Jirak, 1978).

Several clinical studies have combined a number of different psychological procedures in treating IBS. In a single-case study, Mitchell (1978) reported successfully treating spastic colitis using a combination of symptom monitoring, muscle relaxation training, and cognitive restructuring procedures. Neff, Blanchard, and Andrasik (1983) reported successfully reducing abdominal symptoms in two of four IBS patients using a combination of progressive muscle relaxation, thermal biofeedback, and cognitive coping strategies. Utilizing a more comprehensive system of pain management, Khatami and Rush (1978) reported successfully eliminating IBS symptoms in a 32-year-old patient who was so disabled by his symptoms that he had been unable to continue working prior to treatment. Treatment consisted of medical monitoring, EMG biofeedback, and daily practice of relaxation exercises. Psychotherapy was also conducted based on the work of Ellis (1962). This portion of treatment was directed at changing irrational cognitions involving the patient's symptoms as well as other events in his life. In addition, a third component based on the work of Fordyce (1976) was also employed and involved the identification and elimination of behaviors in others that might be reinforcing the continuation of the patient's symptoms. The Khatami and Rush study is noteworthy for its application of behavioral principles for the reduction of illness behavior (e.g., Mechanic, 1983) in a gastrointestinal disorder. Although the maintenance of symptoms through reinforcement has been investigated in other types of disorders, very few studies have reported on this mechanism for gastrointestinal disorders.

Motility disorders of the gastrointestinal tract have also been treated using biofeedback. Latimer (1981) reported on a single case of esophageal spasm treated successfully with frontal EMG feedback and progressive relaxation. Latimer's patient was able to reduce her total perceived spasm time from an initial 10 hours a week to less than 1 hour per week by the end of a 15-week treatment period. Latimer also employed a double swallowing technique that proved helpful for this patient. These gains were maintained at a 6-month follow-up after treatment was terminated. Haynes (1976) reported similar findings using frontalis EMG biofeedback and home relaxation practice in a young woman suffering form esophageal spasms. In a group study employing a waiting-list control population, Giles (1978) found relaxation training using biofeedback to be an effective procedure for treating symptoms arising from functional gastrointestinal disorders. However, the best results were obtained using a combination of biofeedback and psychotherapy.

In a single-case design, O'Connell and Russ (1979) obtained decreases in abdominal pain in an IBS patient with frontalis EMG training. Self-reports of pain reduction were significantly correlated with reductions in EMG activity. These authors also tried biofeedback based on bowel sounds but were unable to find any systematic relationship between changes in bowel sounds and the patient's reports of pain. However, Furman (1973) has reported biofeedback based on bowel sounds to be helpful in treating IBS sympstoms.

Two additional studies employing biofeedback based on the motility of the esophagus and the colon deserve mention. Bueno-Miranda, Cerulli, and Schuster (1976) used biofeedback to alter spastic motility patterns in IBS patients. Feedback was based on pressure recorded from balloons in the rectal and rectosigmoid portions of the colon. The threshold level of distention at which colonic spasms occurred was successfully increased by an average of 82% over baseline in 14 of 21 patients. These patients also showed a decrease in the amplitude, duration, and frequency of spasms. In a separate study, Schuster, Nikoomanesh, and Wells (1973) used biofeedback to teach normal subjects and patients experiencing esophageal reflux to increase the contractile activity of their lower esophageal sphincters. Refluxers, however, were not so sucessful as normals in the amount of increase in lower esophageal sphincter pressure they could produce. These two studies are the only ones known that have used feedback based directly on the motor activity of the gastrointestinal tract in patients with esophageal disorders or IBS. Unfortunately, neither of these studies reported the effects of feedback on gastrointestinal symptoms. However, they do point out the feasibility of designing studies to assess, the usefulness of operant procedures based directly on the activity of the gastrointestinal tract in the treatment of certain types of motility disorders.

Summary

Motility and myoelectric studies of the colon suggest that a biological definition of IBS based on the physiological activity of the gut may be possible. The development of such a diagnostic scoring method would be helpful in distinguishing IBS patients from patients with other gastrointestinal illnesses but similar symptoms. Because IBS is essentially a diagnosis of exclusion, a physiological marker for this disorder would improve confidence in the diagnosis of IBS as well as facilitate the treatment process. However, even though it appears that normals and IBS patients differ in the amount of contractile and myoelectric fast and slow activity of the colon, no systematic studies have as yet attempted to blindly classify subjects on the basis of these criteria.

Differences found in colonic and esophageal functioning between patients and normals also suggest the use of biofeedback as an operant conditioning procedure to investigate the relationship between physiological activity and symptoms arising from psychophysiological disorders of the gastrointestinal tract. As patients experiencing these kinds of disorders have been found to exhibit motor and myoelectrical abnormalities, biofeedback based directly on the physiology of the gastrointestinal tract provides a method for assessing symptoms as dependent variables in relation to voluntary or learned manipulations of colonic and esophageal activity. Bueno-Miranda *et al.* (1976) have already shown the feasibility of such a procedure for IBS, but no attempts have been made toward operant conditioning of the physiological activity of the colon, either as an investigative technique or as a possible therapeutic procedure. The use of biofeedback based on the motor activity of the esophagus is an additional area in which research might prove fruitful. Schuster *et al.* (1973) have shown that biofeedback of this nature is also possible, but, again, no follow-up work has been performed to assess its usefulness in either investigating or treating psychophysiological disorders of the esophagus.

The paucity of research on the effects of operantly conditioning physiological activity of the gastrointestinal tract may be accounted for by several factors. First, the procedure for measuring physiological activity of the gastrointestinal tract is a difficult one requiring a specialized probe containing electrical and pressure sensors. This probe must either be inserted into the colon or swallowed by the patient. In addition, a fair amount of equipment, in the form of electrical transducers and amplifiers, is required in order to process the biological signals in a fashion suitable for analysis. At present, commercial equipment designed specifically for this sort of research is not available. Therefore it is necessary to design a system or develop one from existing equipment in order to test any hypothesis involving the relationship between physiological activity and symptoms in gastrointestinal disorders.

Secondly, although there is little risk involved in the use of direct gastrointestinal recording procedures, they are an invasive technique and require provisions for dealing with any unexpected outcomes. This would tend to limit their use to settings in which medical assistance could be made available if needed. In addition, the methods used in these procedures require some patient preparation time and could probably not be done in less than 1.5 to 2.0 hours. These time constraints, in combination with specialized equipment needs, make this kind of research a costly procedure at present. Nevertheless, studies investigating physiological activity of the colon or esophagus as dependent variables should be undertaken to evaluate their relationship to symptoms in certain types of gastrointestinal disorders. Justification for such studies would certainly appear to be warranted on the basis of the current literature in this area.

In terms of psychological disturbances, for many patients there seems little doubt that psychological conditions are associated with the symptoms of irritable bowel, esophageal spasm, or globus hystericus. The most prevalent of these conditions are anxiety, somatization, and illness behavior. Although depression has been described as a major component of psychosomatic illnesses (Blumer, 1982), it is not clear how much contributes to the appearance of symptoms in IBS or the esophageal disorders discussed above. What is more apparent is that symptoms are brought on or exacerbated during periods of stress. Treatment, therefore, must deal not only with the psychological traits of an individual but also with environmental and behavioral events, as stressful situations appear to be related to symptoms in many individuals with IBS or functional esophageal disorders.

Treatment studies by Svedlund *et al.* (1983), Khatami and Rush (1978), Giles (1978), Latimer (1981), and Jacobson (1927) indicate the importance of using a combination of approaches in the management of psychophysiological disorders of the gastrointesitnal tract. A psychotherapeutic treatment program aimed at individuals with such disorders should provide as many of the following components as necessary in order to help the patient:

- Medical evaluation to rule out organic disorders
- Psychological evaluation including behavioral and cognitive assessments
- A treatment program capable of providing some combination of:
  - Psychotherapy
  - Behavior management
  - Family therapy
  - Stress management
  - Biofeedback and relaxation training

The above therapeutic strategies can easily be carried out on an outpatient basis and should be made available to the patient. At present, psychological and behavioral management programs in conjunction with medical screening appear to provide the best approach to treating the patient with psychophysiological disorders of the gastrointestinal tract.

References

Almy, T. P. (1951). Experimental studies on the irritable colon. *American Journal of Medicine, 9,* 60–67.

Almy, T. P., & Tulin, M. (1947). Alterations in colonic function in man under stress: Experimental production of changes simulating the "irritable colon." *Gastroenterology, 8,* 616–626.

Altaparmakov, I., & Wienbeck, M. (1984). Local inhibition of myoelectrical activity of human colon by loperamide. *Digestive Diseases and Sciences, 29,* 232–238.

Barnard, C., & Illman, J. (Eds.) (1981). *The body machine* (pp. 124–127). New York: Crown.

Beecher, H. K. (1965). Quantification of the subjective pain experience. In P. Hoch & J. Zubin (Eds.), *Psychopathology of perception.* New York: Grune & Stratton.

Beaumont, W. (1833). *Experiments and observations on the gastric juice and the physiology of digestion*. Plattsburgh, NY: F.P. Allen.

Blumer, D. (1982). Chronic pain as a depressive disorder. *Journal of Nervous and Mental Diseases, 170*, 381–406.

Bueno., L., Fioramonti. J., Frexinos, J., & Ruckebush, Y. (1980). Colonic myoelectric activity in diarrhea and constipation. *Hepato-Gastroenterology, 27*, 381–389.

Bueno. L., Fioramonti. J., Ruckebusch, Y., Frexinos, J., & Coulom, P. (1980). Evaluation of colonic myoelectrical activity in health and functional disorders. *Gut, 21*, 480–485.

Bueno-Miranda, F., Cerulli, M., & Schuster, M. M. (1976). Operant conditioning of colonic motility in irritable bowel syndrome (IBS). *Gastroenterology, 70*, 867.

Burns, T. (1980). Colonic motility in the irritable bowel syndrome. *Archives of Internal Medicine, 40*, 247–251.

Caldarelli, D. D., Andrews, A. H., & Derbyshire, A. J. (1970). Esophageal motility studies in globus sensation. *Annals of Otolaryngology*, 1970, *79*, 1098–100.

Cannon, W. B. (1929). *Bodily changes in pain, hunger, fear, and rage* (2nd ed.). New York; Appleton-Century-Crofts.

Cann, P. A., Read, N. W. & Holdsworth, C. D. (1983). Oral domperidone: Double blind comparison with placebo in irritable bowel syndrome. *Gut, 24*, 135–140.

Cann, P. A., Read, N. W., Holdsworth, C. D., & Barends, D. (1984). Role of loperamide and placebo in management of irritable bowel syndrome. *Digestive Diseases and Sciences, 29*, 239–247.

Cann, P. A., Read, N. W., & Holdsworth, C. D. (1984). What is the benefit of coarse wheat bran in patients with irritable bowel syndrome? *Gut, 25*, 168–173.

Castell, D. O. (1982). Pathophysiology and spectrum of clinical syndromes of esophageal motility disorders. *Journal of the Society of Gastrointestinal Assistants, 4*, 17-23.

Chaudhary, N. A., & Truelove, S. C. (1962). The irritable colon syndrome. *Quarterly Journal of Medicine, 31*, 301–322.

Christensen, J. (1975). Myoelectric control of the colon. *Gastroenterology, 70*, 601–609.

Clouse, R. E., & Lustman, P. J. (1983). Psychiatric illness and contraction abnormalities of the esophagus. *New England Journal of Medicine, 42*, 337–342.

Code, C. F., & Schlegel J. F. (1968). Motor action of the esophagus and its sphincters. In C. F. Code (Ed.), *Handbook of physiology. Section 6: Alimentary canal; Vol. 4: Motility*. Washington, DC: American Physiology Society.

Cohen, S. I., & Reed, J. L. (1968). The treatment of "nervous diarrhoea" and other conditioned autonomic disorders by desensitization. *British Journal of Psychiatry, 114*, 1275–1280.

Connell, A. M. (1974). Clinical aspects of motility. *Medical Clinics of North America, 58*, 1201–1216.

Dinoso, V., Goldstein, J., & Rosner, B. (1983). Basal motor activity of the distal colon: A reappraisal. *Gastroenterology, 85*, 637–642.

Dolezalova. V., Cerny, M., & Jirak, R. (1978). Relaxation and EMG activity in neurotics and patients with psychosomatic gastrointestinal disorders. *Activa Nervosa, 1* (Suppl.), 20, 35–36.

Dotevall. G., Svedlund, J., & Sjodin, I. (1982). Symptoms in irritable bowel syndrome. *Scandinavian Journal of Gastroenterology, 79* (Suppl.), 16–19.

Drossman, D. A. (1983). The physician and the patient: Review of the psychosocial gastrointestinal literature with an integrated approach to the patient. In M. H. Sleisenger & J. S. Fordtran (Eds.), *Gastrointestinal disease: Pathophysiology, diagnosis, and management* (Vol. 1, 3rd ed.). Philadelphia: W. B. Saunders.

Drossman, D. A. (1984). Diagnosis of the irritable bowel syndrome. A simple solution? *Gastroenterology, 87*, 224–225.

Drossman, D. A., Powell, D. W., & Sessions, J. T. (1977). The irritable bowel syndrome. *Gastroenterology, 73,* 811–822.

Drossman, D. A., Sandler, R. S., McKee, D. C. & Lovitz, A. J. (1982). Bowel patterns among subjects not seeking health care. *Gastroenterology, 83,* 529–534.

Durdle, N., Kingma, Y., Bowes, K., & Chambers, M. (1983). Origin of slow waves in the canine colon. *Gastroenterology, 84,* 375–382.

Ellis, A. (1962). *Reason and emotion in pswychotherapy.* New York: Lyle Stuart.

Esler, M. D., & Goulston, K. J. (1973). Levels of anxiety in colonic disorders. *New England Journal of Medicine, 288,* 16–20.

Faulkner, W. B. (1940). Severe esophageal spasm. *Psychosomatic Medicine, 2,* 139–140.

Feighner, J., Robins, E., Guze, S., Woodruff, R., Winokus, G. & Munoz, R. (1972). Diagnostic criteria for use in psychiatric research. *Archives of General Psychiatry, 26,* 57–63.

Ford, M. J., Eastwood, J., & Eastwood, M. A. (1982). The irritable bowel syndrone: Soma or psyche? *Psychological Medicine, 12,* 705–707.

Fordyce, W. E. (1976). Behavioral concepts in chronic pain. In P. O. Davidson (Ed.), *The behavioral management of anxiety, depression and pain.* New York: Brunner/Mazel.

Frieri, G., Parisi, F., Corazziari, E., & Caprilli, R. (1983). Colonic electromyography in chronic constipation. *Gastroenterology, 84,* 737–740.

Furman, S. (1973). Intestinal biofeedback in functional diarrhea: A preliminary report. *Journal of Behavior Therapy and Experimental Psychiatry. 4,* 317–321.

Giles, S. L. (1978). Separate and combined effects of biofeedback training and brief individual psychotherapy in the treatment of gastrointestinal disorders. *Dissertation Abstracts International, Part B,* 2495.

Glaser, J. P., & Engel, G. L. (1977). Psychodynamics, pyschophysiology and gastrointestinal symptomatology. In T. P. Almy & J. F. Fielding (Eds.), *Clinics in gastroenterology.* London: W. B. Saunders.

Graham, J. R. (1977). *The MMPI: A practical guide.* New York: Oxford Press.

Greenbaum, D., Abitz, L., VanEgeren, L., Mayle, J., & Greenbaum, R. (1984). Irritable bowel symptom prevalence, rectosigmoid motility and psychometrics in symptomatic subjects not seeing physicians. *Gastroenterology, 84* (5, part 2), 1174.

Hassett, J. (1978). *A primer of psychophysiolgy.* San Francisco: W. H. Freeman.

Harrell, T. H., & Beiman, I. (1978). Cognitive-behavioral treatment of the irritable colon syndrome. *Cognitive Therapy and Research, 2,* 371–375.

Harvey, R., & Read, A. (1973). Effects of cholecystokinin on colonic motility and symptoms in patients with irritable bowel syndrome. *Lancet, 1,* 1–3.

Harvey, R. F., Salih, S. Y., & Read, A. E. (1983). Organic and functional disorders in 2000 gastroenterology outpatients. *Lancet, 1,* 632–634.

Haynes, S. N. (1976). Electromyographic biofeedback treatment of a woman with chronic dysphagia. *Biofeedback and Self-Regulation, 1,* 121–126.

Hedberg, A. G. (1973). The treatment of chronic diarrhea by systematic desensitization: A case report. *Journal of Behavior Therapy and Experimental Psychiatry, 4,* 67–68.

Heefner, J. D., Wilder, R. M. & Wilson, L. D. (1978). Irritable colon and depression. *Psychosomatics, 19,* 540–547.

Hislop, I. G. (1971). Psychological significance of the irritable colon syndrome. *Gut, 12,* 452–457.

Hislop, I. G. (1980). Effect of very brief psychotherapy on the irritable bowel syndrome. *Medical Journal of Australia, 2,* 620–623.

Hyland. J., Darby, C., Hammond, R., & Taylor, I. (1980). Myoelectrical activity of the sigmoid colon in patients with diverticular disease and the irritable colon syndrome suffering from diarrhoea. *Digestion, 20,* 293–299.

Jacobson, E. (1927). Spastic esophagus and mucous colitis. *Archives of Internal Medicine, 39,* 433–455.

Khatami, M., & Rush, J. (1978). A pilot study of the treatment of outpatients with chronic pain: Symptom control, stimulus control, and social system intervention. *Pain, 5,* 163–172.

Kirsner, J. B. & Palmer, W. L. (1958). The irritable colon. *Gastroenterology, 34,* 490–493.

Kruis, W., Thieme, C., Weinzierl, M., Schussler, P., Holl, J., & Paulus, W. (1984). A diagnostic score for the irritable bowel syndrome. *Gastroenterology, 87,* 1–7.

Lancaster-Smith, M. J., Prout, B. J., Pinto, T., Anderson, J., & Schiff, A. A. (1982). Influence of drug treatment on the irritable bowel syndrome and its interaction with psychoneurotic morbidity. *Acta Psychiatrica Scandinavica, 66,* 33–41.

Latimer, P. (1981). Biofeedback and self-regulation in the treatment of diffuse esophageal spasm: A single-case study. *Biofeedback and Self-Regulation, 6,* 181–189.

Latimer, P., Campbell, D., Latimer, M., Sarna, S. Daniel, E., & Waterfall, W. (1979). Irritable bowel syndrome: A test of the colonic hyperalgesia hypothesis. *Journal of Behavioral Medicine, 2,* 285–295.

Latimer. P., Sarna, S., Campbell, D., Latimer, M., Waterfall, W., & Daniel, E. (1981). Colonic motor and myoelectric activity: A comparative study of normal subjects, psychoneurotic patients, and patients with irritable bowel syndrome. *Gastroenterology, 80,* 893–901.

Lechin, R., Van der Dijs, B., Gomez, R., Lechin, E., & Arocha, L. (1983). Distal colonic motility and clinical parameters in depression. *Journal of Affective Disorders, 5,* 19–26.

Legalos, C. N. (1977). Aversive behavior therapy for chronic stomach pain: A case study. *Pain, 4,* 67–72.

Lehtinen, V., & Puhakka, H. (1976). A psychosomatic approach to the globus hystericus syndrome. *Acta Psychiatrica Scandanavica, 53,* 21–28.

Levitt, R. A. (1975). *Psychopharmacology: A biological aproach* (pp.193–194). New York: Wiley.

Liss, J. L., Alpers, D., & Woodruff, R. A. (1973). The irritable colon syndrome and psychiatric illness. *Diseases of the Nervous System, 34,* 151–157.

Mair, W. S., Schroder, K. E., Modalsli, B., & Maurer, H. J. (1974). Aetiological aspects of the globus symptom. *Journal of Laryngology, 88,* 1033–1040.

Malcomson, K. G. (1966). Radiological findings in globus hystericus. *British Journal of Radiology, 39,* 583–586.

Manning. A. P., Thompson, W. G., Heaton, K. W. & Morris, A. F. (1978). Towards positive diagnosis of the irritable bowel. *British Medical Journal, 2,* 653–654.

McHardy, G., Browne, D. C., McHardy, R. J., Welch, G. E., & Ward, S. S. (1962). Psychophysiologic gastrointestinal reactions: Therapeutic observations. *Postgraduate Medicine, 31,* 346–357.

McKegney, P. F. (1977). Psychiatric syndromes associated with gastrointestinal symptoms *Clinics in Gastroenterology, 6,* 675–688.

Mechanic, D. (1983). The experience and expression of distress: The study of illness behavior and medical utilization. In D. Mechanic (Ed.), *Handbook of health, health care, and the health professional.* New York: MacMillan.

Mendeloff, A. I., Monk, M., Siegel, C. I., & Lilienfeld, A. (1970). Illness experience and life stresses in patients with irritable colon syndrome and with ulcerative colitis. *New England Journal of Medicine, 282,* 14–17.

Meshkinpour, H., Hoehler, F., Bernick, D., & Buerger, A. (1981). Electrical control activity in the sigmoid colon: Effect of metoclopramide. *American Journal of Proctology, Gastroenterology, and Colon and Rectal Surgery, 32,* 12–13, 27–28.

Michell, K. (1978). Self-management of spastic colitis. *Journal of Behavior Therapy and Experi-*

mental Psychiatry, 9, 269–272.

Myren, J., Groth, H., Larssen, S. E., & Larsen, S. (1982). The effect of trimipramine in patients with the irritable bowel syndrome. *Scandinavian Journal of Gastroenterology, 17,* 871–875.

Neff, D. F., Blanchard, E. B., & Andrasik, F. (November, 1983). *Behavioral treatment of irritable bowel syndrome.* Paper presented annual meeting of the Association to Advance Behavior Therapy, Washington, DC.

O'Connell, M. F., & Russ, K. L. (February, 1979). *A case report comparing two types of biofeedback in the treatment of irritable bowel syndrome.* Paper presented at the annual meeting of the Biofeedback Society of America, San Diego, CA.

Ouyang, A., Reynolds, J. C., & Cohen, S. (1983). Spike-associated and spike independent esophageal contractions in patients with symptomatic diffuse esophageal spasm. *Gastroenterology, 84,* 907–913.

Palmer, R. L., Crisp, A. H., Stonehill, E., & Waller, S. L. (1974). Psychological characteristics of patients with the irritable bowel syndrome. *Postgraduate Medical Journal, 50,* 416–419.

Pavlov, I. (1910). *The work of the digestive glands.* Translated by W. H. Thompson. London: Griffin.

Phillips, R. H. (November, 1983). *The efficacy of relaxation and imagery procedures in alleviating gastrointestinal discomfort. Preliminary results.* Paper presented at the annual meeting of the Association to Advance Behavior Therapy, Washington, DC

Ritchie, J. (1973). Pain from distension of the pelvic colon by inflating a balloon in the irritable colon syndrome. *Gut, 14,* 125–132.

Ritchie, J. A., & Truelove, S. C. (1980). Comparison of various treatments for irritable bowel syndrome. *British Medical Journal, 281,* 1317–1319.

Ryan, W. A., Kelly, M. G., & Fielding, J. F. (1983). Personality and the irritable bowel syndrome. *Irish Medical Journal, 76,* 140–141.

Rubin, J., Nagler, R., Spiro, H., & Pilot, M. (1962). Measuring the effect of emotions on esophageal motility. *Psychosomatic Medicine, 24,* 170–176.

Sandler, R. S., Drossman, D. A., Nathan, H. P. & McKee, D. C. (1984). Symptom complaints and health care seeking behavior in subjects with bowel dysfunction. *Gastroenterology, 87,* 314–318.

Sarna, S., Latimer, P., Campbell, D., & Waterfall, W. (1982). Electrical and contractile activities of the human rectosigmoid. *Gut, 23,* 698–705.

Schatzki, R. S. (1964). Globus hystericus (globus sensation). *New England Journal of Medicine, 270,* 676.

Schang, J., & Devroede, G. (1983). Fasting and postprandial myoelectrical spiking activity in the human sigmoid colon. *Gastroenterology, 85,* 1048–1053.

Schuster, M. M. (1984). Irritable bowel syndrome: Applications of psychophsiological methods of treatment. In R. Hoelzl & W. E. Whitehead (Eds.), *Psychophysiology of the gastrointestinal tract: Experimental and clinical applications.* New York: Plenum Press.

Schuster, M. M. (1979). Disorders of motility. In P. B. Beeson, W. McDermott, & J. B. Wyngaarden (Eds.), *Cecil Textbook of Medicine* (15th edition). Philadelphia: W. B. Saunders.

Schuster, M. M., Nikoomanesh, P., & Wells, D. (1973). Biofeedback control of lower esophageal sphincter contraction. *Rendiconti di Gastrointerologia, 5,* 14–18.

Smits, B. J. (1974). The irritable bowel syndrome. *Practitioner, 213,* 37–46.

Snape, W., Carlson, G., & Cohen, S. (1976). Colonic myoelectric activity in the irritable bowel syndrome. *Gastroenterology, 70,* 326–33.

Snape, W. Carlson, G., & Cohen, S. (1977). Human colonic myoelectric activity in response to prostigmin and the gastrointestinal hormones. *Digestive Diseases, 22*. 881–887.

Snape, W., Carlson G., Matarazzo, S., & Cohen, S. (1977). Evidence that abnormal myoelectrical activity produces colonic motor dysfunction in the irritable bowel syndrome. *Gastroenterology, 72*, 383–387.

Stacher, G., Steinringer, H., Blau, A., & Landgraf, M. (1979). Acoustically evoked esophageal contraction and defense reaction. *Psychophsiology, 16*, 234–241.

Stroebel, C. F. (1972). Psychophysiological pharmacology. In N. S. Greenfield & R. S. Sternbach (Eds.), *Handbook of psychopysiology*. New York: Holt, Rinehart and Winston.

Sullivan, M., Cohen, S., & Snape, W. (1978). Colonic myoelectrical activity in irritable-bowel syndrome. *New England Journal of Medicine, 298*, 878–883.

Svedlund, J., Sjodin, I., Ottosoon, J., & Dotevall, G. (1983). Controlled study of psychotherapy in irritable bowel syndrome. *Lancet, 2*. 589– 592.

Taylor, I., Duthie, H., Smallwood, R., Brown, B., & Linkens, D. (1974). The effect of stimulation on the myoelectrical activity of the rectosigmoid in man. *Gut, 15*, 599–607.

Taylor, I., Darby, C., & Hammond, P. (1978). Comparison of rectosigmoid myoelectrical activity in the irritable colon syndrome during relapse and remissions. *Gut, 19*, 923–929.

Taylor. I., Darby, C., Hammond, P., & Basu, P. (1978). Is there a myoelectrical abnormality in the irritable colon syndrome? *Gut, 19*, 391–395.

Texter, E. C., & Butler R. C. (1975). The irritable bowel syndrome. *Practical Therapeutics, 11*, 168–170.

Thompson, W. G. (1979). *The irritable gut*. Baltimore: University Park Press.

Thompson, W. G., & Heaton, K. W. (1980). Functional bowel disorders in apparently healthy people. *Gastroenterology, 79*, 283–288.

Thompson, W. G., & Heaton, K. W. (1982). Heartburn and globus in apparently healthy people. *Journal of the Canadian Medical Association, 126*, 46–48.

Vander, A. J., Sherman, J. H., & Luciano, D. S. (1975). *Human physiology: The mechanisms of body function*. New York: McGraw-Hill.

Waller, S. L. (1971). The irritable bowel syndrome: Clinical and pathophysiological features. *Rendiconti di Gastroenterologia, 3*, 80–87.

Waller, S. L., & Misiewicz, J. J. (1969). Prognosis in the irritable bowel syndrome. *Lancet*, 1969, 2, 753–756.

Wangel, A., & Deller, D. (1965). Intestinal motility in man. *Gastroenterolgoy, 48*, 69–84.

Watson, W. C., & Sullivan, S. N. (1974). Hypertonicity of the cricopharyngeal sphincter: A cause of globus sensation. *Lancet, 2*, 676.

Watson, W. C., Sullivan, S. N., Corke, M., & Rush, D. (1978). Globus and headache: Common symptoms of the irritable bowel syndrome. *Journal of the Canadian Medical Association, 118*, 387–388.

Weiner, H. (1977). *Psychobiology and human disease*. New York: Elsevier.

West, K. L. (1970). MMPI correlates of ulcerative colitis. *Journal of Clinical Psychology, 26*, 214–229.

Whitehead, W. E., & Bosmajian, L. (1982). Behavioral medicine approaches to gastrointestinal disorders. *Journal of Consulting and Clinical Psychology, 50*, 972–983.

Whitehead, W. E., & Schuster, M. M. (1985). *Common gastrointestinal disorders: Physiological and behavioral basis for treatment*. New York: Academic Press.

Whitehead, W. E., Fedoravicius, A. S., Blackwell, B., & Wooley, S. (1979). Psychosomatic symptoms as learned responses. In J. R. McNamara (Ed.), *Behavioral approaches in medicine: Application and analysis*. New York: Plenum Press.

Whitehead, W. E., Engle, B., & Schuster, M. M. (1980). Irritable bowel syndrome: Physiological and psychological differences between diarrhea-predominant and constipation-predominant patients. *Digestive Diseases and Sciences, 25,* 404–413.

Whitehead, W. E., Winget, C., Fedoravicius, S. S., Wooley, S., & Blackewell, B. (1982). Learned illness behavior in patients with irritable bowel syndrome and peptic ulcer. *Digestive Diseases and Sciences, 27,* 202–208.

Wolf, S., & Almy, A. P. (1949). Experimental observations of cardiospasm in man. *Gastroenterology, 13,* 401–421.

Wolf, S., & Welsh, J. D. (1972). The gastrointestinal tract as a responsive system. In N.S. Greenfield & R. A. Sternback (Eds.), *Handbook of psychophsiology.* New York: Holt, Rinehart and Winston.

Wolf, S., & Wolff, H. G. (1947). *Human gastric function.* New York: Oxford University Press.

Youell, K. J., & McCullough, J. P. (1975). Behavioral treatment of mucus colitis. *Journal of Consulting and Clinical Psychology, 43,* 740–745.

Young, S. J., Alpers, D. H., Norland, C. C. & Woodruff, R. A. (1976). Psychiatric illness and the irritable bowel syndrome: Practical implications for the primary physician. *Gastroenterology, 70,* 162–166.

CHAPTER 9

Asthma

Thomas L. Creer

No physical disorder is more misunderstood by behavioral scientists than is asthma. Many seem to believe it is a psychological affliction that, like a water faucet, can be turned on and off at will by the patient. This myth survives in the face of reality. Others believe asthma can be cured by psychotherapy. This myth also persists despite a total absence of supporting evidence. Asthma is a complex respiratory condition; not only can a multitude of stimuli precipitate attacks, but an endless number of events, many of which have yet to be delineated, influence the course both of individual attacks and of asthma *per se*. This makes predicting the future direction of a given patient's asthma about as precise as forecasting his behavior. The eloquent models that once promised to permit us to formulate and predict behavior within a simple set of principles have disintegrated in the past two decades. William Estes was recently quoted as saying that what once was regarded with "high optimism" has since been replaced by "strong disillusionment" (Fox, 1983).

Thought regarding the treatment and management of asthma has traveled an equally torturous path. Many remedies have been proposed, usually with little tangible support, as yet another "cure" for the disorder. The passage of time, coupled in some cases with practice or investigation, has proved such claims to be false. There is no cure for asthma; the best that can be expected is that some degree of control can be established over the affliction. Here, as will be argued, self-management can

---

Thomas L. Creer • Department of Psychology, Ohio University, Athens, Ohio 47501. The development and evaluation of the Living with Asthma program was supported in part by contract number 2972 from the Division of Lung Diseases of the National Heart, Lung and Blood Institute.

make a significant contribution. By maximizing the role played by the patient, combined with sound medical treatment, the likelihood that asthma can be controlled is greatly enhanced. The basis for contending that self-management has a major role in the management of asthma will eventually emerge as the major theme of the chapter. Before describing the potential of these procedures, however, the pathophysiological mechanisms that underlie the disorder are described.

Pathophysiology

Current knowledge of asthma serves both to facilitate treatment of the disorder and elucidate constraints that hinder progress in developing a potential cure for the affliction. Clinical features of the disorder have long been reported; descriptions of asthma are found in the writings of Hippocrates, although Aretaeus and Galen in the Christian era presented the first detailed discussion (McFadden & Stevens, 1983). Other notable observers, including Moses Maimonides in the twelfth century (Muntner, 1963) and Sir John Floyer late in the seventeenth century (Sakula, 1984), provided accounts that, although less precise than current descriptions, nevertheless have retained their basic accuracy.

Asthma has long been regarded as a disorder associated with airway abnormality; accordingly, it shares a position with other respiratory disorders including bronchitis, emphysema, bronchiolitis, and chronic obstructive pulmonary disease (COPD). The difference between these disorders is that each category is based on different diagnostic criteria. The diagnosis of chronic bronchitis, for example, is based on etiology, with the most common definition being that the disorder is diagnosed when there is cough or sputum production on most days for at least 3 months of the year (American Thoracic Society, 1962). Emphysema and bronchiolitis are diagnoses based upon anatomical findings. Emphysema is described as an abnormal enlargement of the air spaces distal to the terminal bronchioles, accompanied by destructive changes of the alveoli; bronchiolitis is defined as acute or chronic inflammation of the bronchioles. Both asthma and COPD are based upon clinical findings, but the similarity between the two categories ends here. The latter is a term used to define respiratory diseases of unknown etiology that are characterized by the persistent slowing of airflow during forced expiration. It is a term that should be avoided if more precise diagnoses can be made; on the other hand, COPD is often associated with the presence of the other types of airways abnormality including asthma, bronchitis, bronchiolitis, and, in particular, emphysema (Williams, 1982).

Despite progress made in differentiating asthma from other forms of respiratory disorders, it has proved almost impossible to define. The reasons are twofold (Creer, Harm, & Marion, in press): First, although the definition of asthma in functional terms proposed in 1959 has been-widely accepted, the degree of reversibility required to make a diagnosis of asthma has not been determined (Fletcher & Pride, 1984). It is agreed that some reversibility of airway obstruction must occur if asthma is diagnosed, but the precise degree of reversibility is debatable. As is noted when reversibility in the case of asthma is discussed in greater detail, there are cases wherein little reversibility, if any, is detectable. Second, it has proved impossible to define asthma while excluding all other types of respiratory disorders. A CIBA study team assigned to the task of resolving the question concluded, after considerable deliberation, that their definition would include approximately 25% of patients with chronic bronchitis (Porter & Birch, 1971). As Bernstein (1983) pointed out, differences between chronic bronchitis and asthma in adults are subtle and by no means clear cut. He noted, "Some degree of reversibility is not uncommon in chronic bronchitis and asthma is frequently complicated by episodes of bronchitis" (p. 913).

Difficulties encountered in defining asthma are apparent in presenting three definitions. According to an excellent article by Perlman (1984):

> Asthma is a disorder of the tracheobronchial tree in which there is recurrent, at least partially reversible generalized obstruction to the airflow. It is commonly manifested by cough and expiratory distress and classically by respiratory wheezing. Overt wheezing does not have to occur, however, and the major manifestation may be cough. (p. 459)

In his definition, Perlman notes two important characteristics of the disorder, the *intermittent* and *reversible* nature of the airway obstruction. The remainder of his definition concentrates on clinical signs of asthma. This definition be compared with that of Williams (1982):

> Asthma is defined as reversible airway obstruction. It is characterized by hyperirritability of the airway. Substances that have no effect when inhaled by normal people cause bronchoconstriction in patients with asthma. The principal feature of the condition is extreme variability, both from patient to patient and from time to time in the same patient. It ranges from a mild wheeze with respiratory infection in children, which may disappear in later life, to severe, continuous, and even fatal obstruction of the airways. (p. 23)

Williams's definition also describes the reversibility component of asthma; in particular, however, he emphasizes the *variable* nature of the disorder. Williams also points out that bronchoconstriction is frequently induced by inhaled substances, a topic discussed in more detail in a later section.

The final definition is the most widely cited description of asthma—the definition proposed by a subcommittee of the American Thoracic Society (1962):

> Asthma is a disease characterized by an increased responsiveness of the trachea and bronchi to various stimuli and manifested by a widespread narrowing of the airways that changes in severity either spontaneously or as a result of therapy. (p. 763)

This description suffers from several weaknesses, including its lack of specificity and the questionable contention that asthma is correctly classified as a disease. However, it emphasizes one characteristic of asthma—that the responsiveness of the trachea and bronchi can spontaneously change in severity—that was omitted in the other definitions.

The above descriptions point out the diversity that exists in attempting to define asthma. There are three characteristics of the disorder covered by the definitions, however, that merit special consideration: the intermittent, variable, and reversible nature of asthma. Each characteristic will be described separately.

Intermittence

The attacks of asthma suffered by most patients occur on an intermittent basis. The exact frequency of asthmatic episodes varies from patient to patient and, for any given patient, from time to time. Thus, a patient may experience a burst of attacks over a brief period of time but then may remain free of the disorder for a duration extending over weeks, months, or, in some cases, years. Just how long a period may elapse between attacks was described by Creer (1979). He recounted the comments of an elderly gentleman who complained that he had recently suffered his first asthma attack "since Roosevelt was President." Further conversations with the man revealed that the patient was not referring to Franklin but to his cousin, Theodore! This was undoubtedly an exceptional case, but it does illustrate how long a period may pass without a patient's experiencing any difficulty from asthma.

The frequency of attacks experienced by a patient over time is a function of the stimuli that trigger his or her attacks. Some patients, particularly youngsters, suffer asthma only during certain seasons; airborne allergens, present in the patient's environment, are the chief culprit for this change in the rate of attacks. A patient may suffer an occasional attack during other periods of the year because of an event such as a viral infection: overall, however, attacks are endemic to a given season. In their authoritative review of asthma in children, Siegel, Katz, and Rachelefsky (1983) reported that, regardless of where the youngster resides, asthma attacks generally occur more often and are more severe in the fall of the year. Although the reasons for this finding are unclear, suggested explanations include the increased frequency of viral infections, temperature and humidity changes, increased air pollution, and greater exposure to house dust.

Other patients are less fortunate: they have what is described as perennial asthma and experience attacks during all seasons of the year. There must be some reversibility of the condition, but many patients with perennial asthma experience almost daily symptoms of asthma from a sensation of tightness in the chest to mild wheezing. Although adults can experience seasonal asthma, many are apt to be classified as having perennial asthma.

The primary reason why patients experience perennial asthma is heightened airway responsiveness. As described by Pearlman (1984):

> The lower airways behave as if they were hyperirritable, overresponsive to various chemical mediators of physiologic and inflammatory processes and to a large number of unrelated stimuli, many of which have the capacity to activate or release these substances. (p. 460)

In comparison to those with seasonal asthma, patients with perennial asthma are more responsive to an array of attack triggers to be described, for example, viral infections, allergens, exercise, cold air, chemicals, and environmental factors. Thus, although exposure to the same stimuli will either fail to trigger an attack in a patient with seasonal asthma or will precipitate an occasional mild asthmatic episode, it may trigger what seems an endless series of attacks in the patient with perennial asthma.

Renne and Creer (1985) described three types of problems generated because of the intermittent nature of asthma, and all are relevant to the design and implementation of self-management programs for the disorder. The first problem concerns the inability to recruit a homogeneous population with respect to asthma. Miklich and co-workers (1977) made every conceivable effort to match asthmatic children on such variables as age, sex, and type of asthma. To achieve the latter aim, they recruited only youngsters diagnosed as experiencing perennial asthma. However, although the aim was achieved as well as in any other investigation that has considered this variable, the study demonstrated the inherent fallibility in trying to match patients on this dimension. For example, although all children suffered attacks throughout the year, some experienced more episodes during particular seasons. Perhaps one youngster was more sensitive to pollens present during autumn; a second child, on the other hand, might have experienced more attacks induced by cold winter air. Changes in the pattern of asthma experienced in individual patients resulted in a host of related problems, including alterations in the medication regimen prescribed for a given youngster. These changes and the responses to them, in turn, interfered with the outcome of the investigation conducted by Miklich and his colleagues, a large-scale project, involving both behavioral and medical scientists, that investigated the use of systematic desensitization by reciprocal inhibition as an adjunct treatment for childhood asthma. The study has ben cited (Alexander, 1981; Kinsman, Dirks, Jones, & Dahlem, 1980) as the most definitive test of systematic desensitization for the treatment of the disorder. The study indeed merits this recognition; more significantly, however, it reflects the complex problems encountered both in conducting treatment research with asthma and in interpreting outcome data gathered in such investigation (Renne & Creer, 1985).

The intermittent nature of asthma also makes it difficult to predict how long data should be collected from patients following introduction of an independent variable (Creer, 1982, 1983a; Creer & Kotses, 1983; Renne & Creer, (1985). The paucity of long-term data regarding asthma prompted Leigh (1953) to suggest that studies be initiated to monitor asthmatic patients for up to 15 years. The suggestion is laudable and, with adults, possible (Creer, Harm, & Marion, in press). With childhood asthma, however, it would present the insurmountable task of separating any changes induced by a treatment variable from maturational changes that naturally occur with these youngsters (Renne & Creer, 1985).

The final sets of problems described by Renne and Creer center on expectations acquired by patients and their families because of the intermittent nature of the disorder. Patients with perennial asthma know they can suffer attacks at any time during the year; therefore, at the first indication that they are wheezing or experiencing dyspnea, they usually initiate treatment. Those with seasonal asthma, however, acquire a different set of expectations toward their attacks. They may attempt to escape from the precipitating stimuli with the hope that their response will be the only action required to establish control over the incipient attack. A number of other expectations acquired by those with either perennial or seasonal asthma, including the likelihood of the patient's complying with medication instruction, are further described by Renne and Creer (1985) and Creer, Harm, and Marion (in press).

Problems specific to the self-management of asthma created by its intermittent nature are discussed by Creer and Winder (1986). These run the gamut from difficulties in recruiting subjects to variability in their perceived ability to use self-management skills to control the disorder.

Finally, there is one basic problem alluded to earlier: no matter how careful one is in recruiting potential subjects for such programs, it is impossible to recruit patients with either pure "perennial or intrinsic" asthma or pure "seasonal or extrinsic" asthma. These are not mutually exclusive categories, a fact that has hampered all asthma research (e.g., Stark & Collins, 1977). A patient with perennial asthma may experience more attacks during a particular season whereas a patient with seasonal asthma may experience more virus-induced attacks during a given year. As noted, the heterogeneity of asthma is characterized by the frequency of attacks varying from patient to patient and, for any given patient, from time to time.

Variability

Williams (1980) has suggested that the reason why asthma, a disorder generally recognized by patients and physicians, has eluded precise definition is because it is extremely variable. Variability refers to fluctuations in the severity both of attacks and of the condition itself. Attacks can range from a mild wheeze with a nonbacterial respiratory infection to fatal occlusion of the airways, predominantly by mucus plugs. Williams continued his description by pointing out that although conventional definitions of variable or reversible airway obstruction are sufficiently broad to embrace all patients afflicted with the condition, it necessarily overlaps with other forms of obstructive pulmonary disease.

Attack severity varies from patient to patient and, within the same patient, from episode to episode. At one end of the continuum, there are asthmatic patients who occasionally suffer mild wheezing. For these individuals, asthma is little more than a nuisance; they may experience some unpleasantness during attacks, but the condition does not ordinarily interfere to any extent with their daily lives (Creer, 1983a; Creer, Harm, & Marion, in press). At the other end of the continuum, however, Jones (1976) described patients who experience asthma characterized more by persistent respiratory debilitation than by discrete attacks (although some reversibility of the condition must occur if the diagnosis of asthma is correctly applied). At this extreme, asthma can become a prepotent consideration in dictating the life-style of patients and their families (Creer, 1983a).

Other problems are generated by the variable nature of asthma. A major problem is that there is no standard way of classifying patients as having mild, moderate, or severe asthma or of categorizing any given attack as mild, moderate, or severe. A number of schemes have been suggested to resolve the latter problem—usually based upon the potency, dosage, and schedule of medication taken by patients to control their asthma—but none has found widespread acceptance (Creer, 1982). A valid and reliable solution to the difficulty was proposed by Renne (1982). From the experience of two decades of research with asthmatic children, he suggested that severity of attacks be scored by using a 5 x 5 matrix anchored by two objective indices: peak expiratory flow rates as they deviate from a patient's predicted norms and the potency, schedule, and dosage level of drugs taken to establish control of an attack. Use of the model allows three levels of attack severity to be calculated: (a) no asthma or very mild asthma, (b) mild or moderate asthma, and (c) moderate or severe asthma. With a group of patients, Renne compared attack severity scores calculated with this method to ratings of asthma severity as determined both by a group of experienced allergists and a multidiscipline team composed of psychologists, nurses, and pulmonary technicians who had all worked with the sample group of patients. A correlation calculated on the combined data, collected over a period of time, was $r = .97$. Hence, the procedure developed by Renne proved highly reliable at categorizing attacks as mild, moderate, or severe. Furthermore, on the basis of the percentage of attacks a given individual experiences that are classified as mild, moderate, or severe, it is possible to agree as to whether the patient's asthma *per se* should be classified as mild, moderate, or severe (Creer & Winder, 1986).

Another problem suggested by Renne and Creer (1985) centers on expectations of asthmatic children and their parents. If you only experience minor discomfort during an attack, you and your family are apt to view asthma as little more than a cold. Rest, drinking warm water, or, at the very most, taking a nonprescribed medication will abort most of the attacks you suffer. In these circumstances your expectations about asthma are little different than those of a person with hay fever. In almost any circumstance the attack will be aborted. If you have more serious perennial asthma, however, you acquire other expectations. There is not only greater reliance upon daily medication to control your asthma, but your day-to-day activities are, to a large extent, dictated by your physical condition. The problem described by Renne and Creer (1985) occurs when there is an unexpected change in a patient's asthma. Although, as Williams (1982) suggested, a patient may suffer a very severe attack only once or twice during a lifetime, how you perceive that episode will be important not only in establishing control over that attack but also both in shaping future expectations you and your family have about the disorder and in deciding what responses to make during attacks. For example, Creer (1974) described how panic exhibited by some asthmatic children was acquired because the youngster had observed their parents showing panic during the children's attacks. Although the parents may only have panicked during a particular attack, the youngsters later modeled this parental behavior when they experienced attacks. On the other hand, many patients, particularly adults, overuse nebulized medications (see, e.g., Creer, 1979). This is a serious problem because with overuse patients gradually require more and more of a particular medication to produce bronchodilation and the remission of their symptoms. Again, many patients have explained their behavior by reporting that they once suffered a severe attack and did not wish to experience anything like it in the future; paradoxically, however, their behavior defeats sound medical treatment with respect to the prudent use of asthma medications (Chai & Newcomb, 1973).

A final problem presented by the variability of asthma arises in conducting clinical research on asthma. The difficulties are well described by Clark (1977):

> The benchmark of asthma is its variability and this in itself makes any assessment of treatment most difficult. Trials are usually undertaken in patients who are in a stable state to minimize this problem, but this state is uncharacteristic of the majority of patients who will be requiring the treatment under test and ignores long-term fluctuations in severity. Variability may itself lead to difficulties in assessing the response to treatment particularly when symptoms are present at night. A combination of diary cards and regular measurements of the peak expiratory flow rate has simplified the problem caused by short-term variability but has not excluded them. The problem of assessing variability are compounded by the fact that any measurement of airways obstruction may not reflect all the variable changes in lung function. (p. 225)

The problems would have to be satisfactorily resolved in any study of an intervention program with asthma, including the assessment of a self-management problem.

Reversibility

The airway obstruction that characterizes asthma attacks reverses either spontaneously or with adequte treatment. The reversible increase in the resistance to airflow is the *sine qua non* of asthma (McFadden, 1980); it differentiates the condition from other types of respiratory disorders, emphysema, for instance, in which there is no reversibility of the physical impairment.

The reversibility component of asthma presents a number of major problems to medical and behavioral scientists (Creer & Winder, 1986; Renne & Creer, 1985). As described earlier, asthma is, at best, a relative condition. Thus, although the attacks of many patients completely remit, there are patients in whom the degree of remission is far less clear. For example, a study by Loren and his colleagues (1978) found that many asthmatic patients had reduced airflow which was irreversible with intensive treatment, including the administration of corticosteroids. This casts a shadow over the criterion of reversibility to define and diagnose asthma; if there are patients who, despite fulfilling all other criteria demanded for the diagnosis of asthma, fail to show reversibility of their symptoms, are they correctly diagnosed as having asthma? Only future research, plus considerable refinement of the diagnostic criteria now employed, will eventually answer this question.

Another major problem is that the spontaneous remission of asthma adds a degree of uncertainty regarding the outcome of any treatment procedure (Renne & Creer, 1985; Creer, Harm, & Marion, in press). Simply put, how do we know if the treatment applied resulted in any observable changes? The aim is to answer the question under tightly controlled conditions in which a functional analysis can be established between the application of the treatment procedure and the remission of the asthmatic symptoms. However, even in the laboratory there is still uncertainty, because, in Clark's (1977) words, "the response to treatment appears to be influenced by factors independent of the treatment given" (p. 225). The matter of spontaneous remission becomes even more complex when one is considering the attacks that occur in the daily lives of patients. As Creer (1979) suggested, there are a number of studies in the literature wherein spontaneous remission cannot be ruled out as a possible, perhaps probable, explanation for the treatment outcome observed with asthmatic patients. It is a variable that defies control even in the best designed study.

The fact that a number of separate events occur at the same time provides a probable explanation for some aspects of asthma. Barnes (1984) suggested that nocturnal asthma may be explained by a coincidental occurrence of several rhythms:

> A fall in circulating adrenaline, the delayed effects of steroid withdrawal, and increased vagal cholinergic tone. These factors lead to small changes in the tone of the airways in normal people but to bronchoconstriction in asthmatics because of exaggeration by hyperreactivity and possibly by increased release of mediators. (p. 1398)

Little wonder Barnes concludes that the treatment of nocturnal asthma may be "surprisingly difficult."

The simultaneous occurrence of events has also led to a number of bogus treatments for asthma. The practice can best be called superstitious behavior (Skinner, 1948) in that the patient, physician, or behavioral scientist associates events that occur concurrently with the spontaneous remission of asthma with the latter process. Even though the events are independent of one another, their accidental pairing results in a perceived causal link between the stimulus or stimuli and the amelioration of the condition (Creer, Harm, & Marion, in press). Such folk remedies as patients' balancing pennies on their foreheads, smelling the aromas of certain woods, or carrying around small dogs, usually chihuahuas, were initiated because the patients believed that such activities resulted in the diminution of their asthma. These are worthless treatments and, in the case of carrying around a small dog, may actually exacerbate attacks if animal dander is a precipitant of a patient's asthma. Physicians, too, have promulgated treatments that are just as bogus. Included here would be autogenous urine immunization, a practice condemned by the American Academy of Allergy (1981), and dry cupping, whereby dry cups are applied to the asthmatic patient's back or chest supposedly to reduce airway obstruction by suction. An article by Dearlove, Verguel, Birkin, and Latham (1981) criticized the practice of dry cupping by describing the harmful effects induced by the treatment, including bleeding patients to death.

If medicine has generated worthless treatments for asthma, behavioral scientists are equally guilty of doing so. As Purcell and Weiss (1970) noted:

> It is probably safe to state that at one time or another almost every variety of therapeutic technique, including psychoanalysis, group psychotherapy, environmental manipulation, behavior therapy, hypnosis, and even ECT [electroconvulsive therapy], has been applied in the treatment of bronchial asthma. With the single exception of ECT, claims of success have been filed in all instances. (p. 613)

If Purcell and Weiss were to write their chapter today, they would doubtlessly add other approaches, including Z-therapy and various types of family therapy, to their list.

It is unfortunately true, as proclaimed by Purcell and Weiss, that claims of success were based on studies that failed to satisfy one or more of the basic criteria for adequate treatment studies. A list of such criteria are depicted in Table 1; it reflects a composite of suggestions offered by Purcell and Weiss (1970), Creer (1979, 1982), and Renne and Creer (1985). The list includes the basic standards that should be followed in conducting clinical research by both medical and behavioral investigators.

The possibility of psychological or behavioral techniques having an effect on asthma *per se* is diminished further by considering one other factor: The study by Miklich and his co-workers (1977), described earlier, adhered to the criteria described in Table 1. However, they concluded that even in a well-designed psychological-behavioral intervention study

Table 1. Criteria for conducting intervention research with asthma

1. Confirm the diagnosis of asthma
2. Apply unbiased sample selection procedures
3. Select subjects from similar populations with respect to severity and classification of the disorder, for example, perennial or seasonal asthma
4. Select nonsmoking subjects
5. Recruit matched control groups not treated with an intervention procedure
6. Apply standard treatment procedures
7. Control concurrent independent variables, such as the administration of and compliance with medication instructions
8. Apply acceptable criteria for the evaluation of treatment effects
9. Gather sufficiently extensive follow-up data to rule out normal variability of asthmatic symptoms
10. Recruit large enough samples of subjects to permit appropriate statistical evaluation
11. Apply appropriate statistical procedure

wherein statistically significant outcome data were obtained, the findings paled in clinical significance when compared to outcome data gathered by application of most medical treatments. For example, having a patient drink a cup of coffee—a substance that is similar in chemical composition to theophylline—probably produces greater bronchodilation than any relaxation strategy taken by the patient.

Psychological Factors

At the outset, it was noted that many behavioral scientists believe asthmatic patients can, at will, turn attacks off and on. This assumption is based upon the role played by emotional factors and suggestion in triggering attacks. Each of these topics will be considered.

Emotional Factors

In order to confirm the diagnosis, a patient suspected of suffering from asthma is tested by what is rapidly becoming a standardized procedure. First, he is exposed to minute amounts of stimuli thought to precipitate his attacks. Asthma can be triggered by a variety of stimuli including irritants, exercise, cold air, infections, allergens, aspirin and related substances, and emotional reactions (Reed & Townley, 1978). Usually, the procedure employed entails pricking the patient's skin with a needle containing a minute quantity of the stimulus (a process referred to as a skin test) or by his inhaling a small quantity of the stimulus (a process referred to as a bronchial challenge). The second step in the latter procedure is to measure what occurs when the patient is exposed to such a challenge. This is determined by assessing any changes that may occur in the patient's pulmonary functioning; usually, it involves determining whether there are any changes in measures obtained by having the patient exhale into a spirometer. If there is a 15%–20% reduction, depending upon the criterion established by a given clinician or investigator, in the patient's forced expiratory volume in one second (the FEV_1) that patient may be rightfully diagnosed as having asthma.

Considerable progress has been made both in standardizing stimuli presented to patients and in assessing any changes that may occur because of such exposure (Creer, 1982; Creer, Harm, & Marion, in press). However, in the case of emotional reactions that may trigger asthma there has been more confusion than enlightenment. We know such responses do trigger asthma, but that is almost the extent of our knowledge. There are a number of reasons why this is the case. First, it has proved difficult to standardize any stimulus for inducing an emotional reaction from a patient. What causes emotional reactions is not only idiosyncratic to any given patient but is heavily dependent upon the context in which the provoking stimulus occurs. Usually, the procedure used relies heavily upon hypnotic suggestion or the use of imagery; as is widely known, however, there are wide individual differences in responses obtained with application of either of these techniques. Second, it is difficult to assess the response that does occur. For example, laughing heartily is a reaction that regularly triggers attacks in a number of patients. How would one operationally define laughing, let alone the stimulus used to provoke it, in order to measure the response? Thus far, the question has defied an answer. Third, the nature of the relationship of emotional reactions to asthma is complex and not as yet worked out (McFadden, 1984). Plausible psychological pathways through which emotional events could trigger attacks include hyperventilation, hypocapnea, vagal bronchoconstriction, changes in adrenal or cortical function, and endocrine activity (Reed & Townley, 1978). The difficulty of elucidating the exact pathways in respiration was noted by Cherniack and Cherniack (1983). They pointed out, for example, that it is impossible to provide a complete description of the neural mechanisms involved in human respiration as experiments necessary to obtain the pertinent information cannot be carried out. Finally, the relationship of emotions to asthma has been badly misinterpreted by behavioral scientists. The most prominant mistake was the description of crying and asthma provided by French and Alexander (1941). What they attempted to do has been characterized by Renne and Creer (1985) as anent to Cinderella's stepsisters' attempting to jam their feet into the glass slipper: French and Alexander tried to pry the cause–effect relationship of crying and asthma into a psychoanalytic framework. Although their observations were correct—many asthmatic children do attempt to avoid crying or, if they cry, do so in a stifled manner—their interpretation was only one of a series that have haunted asthmatic dhildren and their families since 1941. What French and Alexander claimed was that the suppressed crying by the children represented a repressed cry for their mothers. No evidence has ever been collected to support this view (Creer, 1978, 1979, 1982), but it has persisted even in the view of conflicting evidence. The best reason why some children avoid crying or cry in an awkward manner was provided by the youngsters themselves. They described to Purcell (1963) how they tried to avoid unnecessary attacks of asthma by engaging in such behavior. This explanation, although accurate because crying does seem to induce asthma through increased vagal activity (Nadel, 1976), has seemingly proved too logical for those who are proponents of psychoanalysis.

Creer (1979) marshalled evidence suggesting that what was important was not emotions *per se* but what the patient did when he or she was emotional. In some cases, asthma may be emotionally induced as a function of specific behaviors such as crying, laughing, yelling, or coughing. Each of these behaviors is capable of serving as an irritant to increase vagal activity. In other cases, however, the emotional response may consist of a number of specific responses. Examples of such patterns would be responding that might be labeled as anger, excitement, or fear; the effect on asthma may be, in these cases, similar to what occurs in exercise-induced asthma. Thus, concluded Creer, the basic argument is that "behavioral components of emotional responding trigger asthma either through mechanical means, probably through stimulation of the vagus nerve, or through exercise" (p. 158). Rees (1984) has extended this argument by suggesting that emotional outbursts may be related to the reaciton of the hyperactive airways to deep inspiration or to the inhalation of cold, dry air. The latter is also regarded by many experts (e.g., McFadden, 1984) as the outcome of exercise and therefore the cause of exercise-induced asthma. Considerably more research must be conducted, however, before there is finally clarification of the role that emotional reactions play in triggering attacks.

Suggestion

In 1886, MacKenzie described bronchospasm occurring in a patient allergic to roses when she was presented with an artificial rose. This study provided the basic impetus for what has since been referred to as investigations of the role of suggestion in triggering attacks. The prototype of such studies was an investigation by Luparello, Lyons, Bleecker, and McFadden (1968). After obtaining baseline measures of airway resistance, asthmatic subjects were told they would be inhaling progressively larger concentrations of an allergen or irritant that could induce bronchospasm. In reality, however, the substance they inhaled was a nebulized saline solution. The suggestion made by the experimenters, coupled with the inhalation of the supposed allergen or irritant, resulted in a significant mean increase in airway resistance for the group. Of the 19 of 40 subjects who responded, 12 developed what Luparello and his coworkers described as full-blown asthma attacks. Control subjects—patients with normal respiratory patterns and patients with restrictive and nonasthmatic lung diseases—did not show changes in airway resistance to suggestion and the inhalation of the bogus irritants or allergens.

Luparello and his colleagues conducted a series of studies on the role of suggestion in precipitating asthma attacks (Luparello, Leist, Lourie, & Sweet, 1970; McFadden, Luparello, Lyons, & Bleecker, 1969; Spector, Luparello, Kopetzky, Souhrada, & Kinsman, 1976); in general, the work supported the initial findings reported by Luparello *et al.* (1968). Other investigators (e.g., Horton, Suda, Kinsman, Souhrada, & Spector, 1978; Philipp, Wilde, & Day, 1972; Strupp *el al.*, 1974) also reported findings supportive of the suggestion hypothesis.

Not everyone was successful in demonstrating that suggestion alters pulmonary functions in asthmatic patients, however. Weiss, Martin, and Riley (1970) investigated the effect of suggestion on the pulmonary physiology of asthmatic children. The youngsters were informed that they were inhaling increasingly larger concentrations of a potential allergen when they actually were presented with saline. Of the 16 subjects, only one responded with decreased flow rates and wheezing to suggestion; the same child, however, displayed the same response in a control session involving saline and no suggestion.

Weiss and his colleagues hypothesized that their findings might have been due to the fact that they used a less sensitive measure of respiratory changes, for instance, peak expiratory flow rates obtained with a peak flow meter rather than the more sensitive measures obtained with a spirometer. Creer (1978), however, noted that methodological differences between the study and previous investigations precluded the possibility of reliable comparisons. The study by Weiss and his coworkers (1970) was also conducted with youngsters at a residential facility for asthma. The context alone—the children were very sophisticated at exposure to challenges such as those presented in the study and were somewhat blasé about attending to instructions—could also have resulted in different findings.

More recently, Lewis, Lewis, and Tattersfield (1984) investigated the effects of suggestion with both normal and asthmatic subjects. Again, substances presented were purposely mislabeled. Thus, it was suggested that the initial five saline solutions contained a bronchoconstrictor and the final five contained a bronchodilator, or vice versa, and that the initial four isoproterenol solutions were inert, whereas the last was a bronchodilator. Nine asthmatic subjects, but one of the normal group, showed bronchoconstriction after the saline inhalation. This was dose-dependent and disappeared when inhaled solutions of 37 degrees centigrade and 100% relative humidity were presented. Lewis and his colleagues demonstrated that suggestion did not affect the airway response to saline or isoproterenol in either group, although it influenced the subjective impression of airway caliber as recorded on a visual analogue scale. They concluded that bronchoconstriction after saline inhalation, previously attributed to suggestion, was actually caused by airway cooling. And, as they demonstrated, this was quickly abolished by presenting the solution at a higher temperature and at full humidity. This study, carefully designed and executed, supports previous work by Weiss and his colleagues; consequently, there are many questions about the role of suggestion and asthma that can be answered through further investigation.

As to the question of whether or not patients can, at their own volition, turn their asthma on and off, the above discussion indicates that, in some cases, a patient may induce an attack by crying, laughing, or displaying some sort of emotional reaction. Mistaken identification of a stimulus as a precipitant may also induce an attack although, as noted, it also requires the proper context. Therefore the answer to the question is partially affirmative; the patient can, in some instances, induce an attack if he or she so desires. However, the observation made by French and Alexander (1941) is still valid: most asthmatic children whose attacks are triggered by such responding attempt not to cry, or, if they do cry, they try to prevent the behavior from causing asthma. By attempting to prevent unnecessary attacks by practicing avoidance behavior, they are demonstrating that they have some knowledge about what triggers their attacks and how they might be controlled. They are, in other words, practicing a self-management skill.

The Self-Management of Asthma

Unlike the case with other physical disorders, there is a strong recent history of attempts to develop and implement self-management programs for asthma, particularly childhood asthma (Creer & Winder, 1986). Not only have a number of programs been generated during the past decade, but the efforts of various groups of investigators have been presented and are available through a conference summary published by the National Institute of Allergy and Infectious Diseases (1981). In addition, several papers describing significant issues in self-management of the disorder, written by experts in their areas, and responses to the papers by individuals with experience in creating and implementing programs were published in a supplemental issue of the *Journal of Allergy and Clinical Immunology* (Green, Goldstein, & Parker, 1983). These sources provide additional background reading for the interested reader.

A paper by Thoreson and Kirmil-Gray (1983), written for the latter journal, reviewed 11 programs developed and applied for the self-management of childhood asthma. They concluded that two programs, the National Asthma Center program and the Family Asthma Project, "deserve recognition for their comprehensive application of the psychology of self-managed change to asthma" (pp. 605–606). These two programs will therefore serve as the basis of discussion. The program developed at the National Asthma Center, hereafter referred to as Living with Asthma, has been thoroughly presented and described by Creer, Backial, Ullman, and Leung (1986); data from the program have been presented by Creer and Leung (1981), Creer and Kotses (1983), Creer and Winder (1986), and, in particular, by Creer *et al.* (1984). The Family Asthma Project was developed and implemented by Michelle Hindi-Alexander and Gerd Cropp. The program was originally described in 1981 (Cropp & Hindi-Alexander, 1981; Hindi-Alexander & Cropp, 1981); more recently, Hindi-Alexander and Cropp (1984) presented a thorough discussion of the data they had gathered with the program.

Rationale

The rationales of the Living with Asthma program and the Family Asthma Project were similar. Creer *et al.* (1984) pointed out that self-management provides the person with skills to assume responsibility for controlling his affliction. He can, in short, become the central component of a health care system geared toward providing him with improved health and well-being. Health no longer becomes the sole province of someone else; it is determined, to some degree, by the patient. To achieve such an aim, Hindi-Alexander and Cropp (1984) noted that it is necessary to increase both the participant's knowledge of asthma, including its treatment, and self-management of coping skills.

Self-Management Training

In concluding their review, Thoresen and Kirmil-Gray (1983) compared the two programs; in doing so, they provided a synopsis of each project:

> The National Asthma Center project [Living with Asthma] is notable for its careful teaching of cognitive and analytic skills, including behavioral analysis, problem solving, and self-monitoring. In addition, the close link between assessment, procedures and treatment techniques is commendable. Several of the measures used to assess change probably served as interventions by helping children and parents become more aware of behavior patterns and providing information that could be used in treatment. For example, daily assessment of pulmonary functioning by use of peak flow meters provided important physiologic information that children and parents used to help decide when and how to intervene and whether their interventions were effective. The National Asthma Center program was also somewhat longer than other programs (eight 80-minute sessions), which allowed skills to be taught in more depth. Skill use was promoted by regular homework assignments that required participants to apply their newly learned skills to situations in their own lives. (p. 606)

The Family Asthma Project is described in the following manner:

> The strength of the Family Asthma Project, on the other hand, was its *in vivo* demonstrations to parents and children of the ability to engage in exercise and to control asthmatic symptoms. Performance accomplishments are a very powerful method of teaching new behavior and increasing personal self-efficacy, especially when the behavior engaged in is one which is feared. This program is also notable for its extensive efforts to build community support for the child with asthma, support that should contribute to the generalization and maintenance of self-management skills. (p. 606)

Despite differences between the programs—the use of the peak flow meter in Living with Asthma (LWA) and the building of community support in the Family Asthma Project (FAP)—the programs are characterized more by their similarity than by their dissimilarity. This becomes evident in reviewing the basic training provided by both programs. Each stressed, in various ways, education and self-management training.

Education

Four major topics were presented and repeatedly reviewed with participants: mechanics, treatment, self-management, and application.

Mechanics of breathing. Basic mechanisms of breathing were presented and discussed. Both programs described the role of diagnostic techniques used to confirm asthma; in addition, both emphasized a discussion of possible triggers of asthma attacks. A number of educational modalities were used to teach participants about the respiratory system and changes that occur during attacks. An assumption in both programs was that a basic knowledge of asthma and its treatments was essential as a cornerstone of any self-management program designed and implemented for the disorder.

Treatment of asthma. Various ways that can be introduced to control asthma were thoroughly described and discussed with participants. Again, a number of educational techniques were employed; included were demonstrations and lectures in the FAP and videotapes and written handouts in LWA. This proved a highly animated portion in both programs as participants were interested not only in how different medictions act to control asthma but also in discussing potential side effects of the drugs. By and large, participants proved themselves to be thoroughly familiar with the potential side effects of all prescribed asthma medications.

Self-management skills. The principles and skills of self-management were presented to participants. Specific skills taught in both programs will be enumerated in the next section.

Application of self-management skills to asthma. Time was devoted in both the FAP and LWA programs to teaching participants how to use self-management skills effectively to control asthma. The emphasis here was to teach patients and their families: (a) to prevent attacks by adhering to prescribed medication regimens or avoiding known precipitants of their attacks; (b) to take whatever steps were required, in a sequential manner, to establish control over attacks; and (c) to manage the myriad of consequences that result from asthma. By acquiring and practicing these skills, it was thought that families could learn to cope with asthma and the many problems it generates.

Self-Management Training

There are specific skills that comprise self-management. These skills were taught to participants in both the FAP and LWA. They include self-monitoring, self-recording, information processing, decision making, and self-instruction.

Self-monitoring. This entails participants' learning to observe and monitor any changes that occur in relation to their asthma. Participants learned to compare sensations of asthma, for instance, wheezing, tightness in the chest, against some sort of standard. In the LWA program, participants learned to compare subjective impressions regarding changes in the children's breathing against peak expiratory flow rates obtained daily with a peak flow meter. This allowed the youngsters' respiratory sensations to be compared against an objective criterion. An unexpected finding was that parents also acquired the ability to correlate behaviors or physical changes exhibited by their children with changes in their asthma (Creer, 1983b; Creer & Leung, 1981; Creer, Renne, & Chai, 1982). Many parents explained that the latter alterations provided a more reliable index of the incipient onset of attacks than did the peak flow meter. Participants in the FAP monitored medications taken by asthmatic children. This measure, too, provided a standard against which participants could compare the children's overall physical condition. A requirement of increased medication could, in some cases, alter the perception of participants regarding the severity of attacks. Such alterations in perception could in turn lead to changes in how the asthma was managed.

Self-recording. Both the FAP and LWA project employed asthma diaries that required participants to record specific information regarding a child's asthma. In LWA, for example, four sources of information were obtained: (a) whether a patient suffered an attack during any given 24-hour period, as well as his perception of the severity of the episode; (b) the highest peak flow values obtained in the morning and evening; (c) how compliant the patient was to any medication instructions; and (d) an estimate of any expenses incurred because of asthma. The self-report diaries provided invaluable information to the investigators on both projects. As self-report data represent both the best and worst information that can be gathered with respect to a patient's asthma (Creer & Winder, 1986), efforts were made to improve the reliability and validity of the data. In both projects, this involved frequent contacts with participants; in the LWA project, it also entailed teaching the children to record data about their condition and to use their parents as a reliability check. This approach improved the overall accuracy of the collected information and in turn enhanced the confidence of the investigators with respect to the validity of the data.

Information processing. By monitoring and recording information related to their asthma, participants initiated an operation of processing information about themselves and their asthma. The acronym for activities specifically engaged in by participants is CAPE. This denotes that participants (a) *collected* data about their condition, (b) continually *analyzed* the information they gathered, (c) detected whether there was a potential *problem* that might require some sort of action, and (d) *evaluated* the problem with respect to possible solutions that might reasonably be taken. An example of information processing is provided by symptom discrimination. Although the detection of asthmatic symptoms may be a simple matter—the patient begins to wheeze and experience breathlessness—it can also be highly complex (Creer, 1983b). The gamut of identified problems related to symptom discrimination ranges from a lack of physiological input to the patient, such as a lack of hypoxic drive, to the patient's misinterpreting physiological changes as symptomatic of asthma when they actually are signals for some other physical change. As noted earlier, asthmatic patients are usually asymptomatic; in this state, they adapt to a certain level or standard of breathing. They continue to collect and analyze information, sometimes with little awareness on their part, and perceive that their breathing is normal. When there is deviation in their breathing from the standard they have adapted to, however, they must first detect such a change and, second, evaluate the input to determine whether it represents a respiratory problem of some nature.

Decision-making. This requires the patient to (a) consider the potential solutions to the problem he has detected and evaluated and (b) select the most appropriate solution from among these choices. Here is where education about asthma is so important in the self-management of the disorder. For example, a child with exercise-induced asthma may do nothing even though he begins to wheeze when running at school. He and his parents may not realize that such activity, healthy for most children, can induce an attack in the asthmatic youngster. Asthmatic children who do know that exercise can trigger their attacks may take a different strategy: they realize their activity is producing the wheezing or tightness they are experiencing and decide to try and abort the symptoms by halting the activity.

Self-instruction. This refers to statements made by oneself to prompt, direct, or maintain behavior (O'Leary & Dubey, 1979). Continuing with the illustration above, an asthmatic child who begins to experience wheezing or tightness may realize that such activity is the consequence of exercising; he or she may halt the action to determine whether there is an amelioration of the symptoms.

Self-instruction was built into every phase of both the FAP and LWA. Both programs featured patients' working out with their physicians the exact behaviors the former should perform in the event of an attack. When the patients later did experience an asthmatic episode, they had to instruct themselves as to the steps they should perform at each stage of the attack. By doing so, they included all of the components of self-management—self-monitoring and recording of behavior, information processing, and decision-making—described in this section. The importance of self-instruction in the LWA program was summarized by Creer and Kotses (1983):

> Self-instruction was the key component of our efforts to teach patients to manage their attacks. From the outset they were taught to conceive of asthma management as a chain of responses. Each link in the response chain occurs in the sequence so that the patient performed one response, then a second, and so on until control was established over the episode. By working in conjunction with the physician, a patient and his or her family could develop a coherent script that could be performed by the patient in the event of an attack. Management of asthma is more readily achieved when a patient follows a predetermined sequence of responses; self-instruction in turn becomes the core of the subsequent recall and performance of such a sequence. (p. 1032)

By managing their asthma in such a manner, the patients were also mimicking the way in which experienced physicians treat asthma: initiate a step, evaluate its effect upon the asthma, initiate a second step if necessary, and so on.

Two other aspects of self-instruction were also stressed in both the FAP and LWA: self-induced stimulus change and self-induced response change. These can be described in the following manner:

1. *Self-induced stimulus change.* If a child has knowledge about what stimuli may trigger attacks, he or she can be taught to avoid, if possible, the stimuli. For example, a youngster who has asthma precipitated by animal dander or cigarette smoke may avoid contact with such stimuli or, in the event of contact, escape from such causal factors. The action of the child is referred to as self-induced stimulus change in that he or she has used self-instruction to initiate such an action.

2. *Self-induced response change.* A description of this tactic was provided by Creer and Kotses (1983):

> A child can alter his or her response to avoid either an asthma attack or a worsening of the episode. This is particularly evident with children who suffer exercise-induced asthma. On one hand, they realize that exercise is an ingredient of good health and in most cases an enjoyable activity. On the other hand, they recognize that exercise can induce an attack. To avoid the latter, they must monitor their behavior and avoid crossing the boundary between healthy activity and inducing unnecessary attacks. (p. 1032)

Design

It is traditional in medical research to use clinical trials with patients randomly assigned to a treatment or control condition. Differences between groups demonstrate the power of the treatment procedure (or independent variable). Characteristics of asthma described earlier, however, have not only frequently subverted the process of matching patients before random assignment to groups but have also eluded experimenter control over the course of the study (Rees, 1983; Stark & Collins, 1977). This problem was richly demonstrated in the study by Miklich and his colleagues (1977) described earlier. Despite a well-designed and reasonable protocol, an ample subject population, and a setting that afforded optimal control to be established by the experimenters, it still proved difficult to conduct such a study and obtain clear-cut results. The same can be said of a study recently reported by Lewis, Rachelefsky, Lewis, de la Sota, and Kaplan (1984), who conducted a randomized trial of an asthma management program Asthma Care Training for children. The results clearly point out the futility of using such a design in a self-management program for asthmatic children. Lewis and his colleagues (a) were unable to assign equal numbers of subjects to treatment and control groups; (b) used an inappropriate control group in that they essentially compared self-management training to patient education (instead of to an untreated control group); (c) employed untested dependent measures of questionable reliability and validity; (d) applied statistical procedures in an inappropriate manner; and, (e) perhaps not surprisingly failed to obtain unequivocal differences between their treatment and control conditions. The results of the study reinforce a statement by Clark (1977) who, in participating in a conference on methods in clinical trials for asthma, emphatically stated: "Patients should wherever possible be used as their own controls and comparisons between subjects should be kept to a minimum" (p. 226).

The FAP and LWA both used subjects as their own controls, but in different experiemental designs. The FAP used a pre–post design wherein participants served strictly as their own controls. After the initial assessment period, participants were exposed to self-management training; depending upon the assessment procedure, specific dependent measures were administered: (a) immediately at the conclusion of intervention, (b) at a 3-month follow-up, and (c) at a 12-month follow-up. The design in LWA featured a waiting-list control group procedure. Consecutive families referred to the project were randomly assigned to one of two groups: intervention or control. The battery of dependent measures was administered for the initial time to members of both groups; in addition, a period of time between assignment and initiation of training permitted baseline data to be obtained on all subjects.

When 10 families had been assigned to both the intervention and control groups, self-management training was initiated for members of the former group. Participants assigned to the control group, on the other hand, served as a control during this period. Both groups of participants were evaluated a second time when self-management training was completed for families assigned to the experimental group; participants assigned to the waiting-list control group were then exposed to self-management training. These participants were evaluated for a third time at the end of training; all participants, whether assigned initially to treatment or control groups, were reevaluated 6 months and 1 year following self-management training.

There are a number of advantages to the design used in LWA (Creer *et al.*, 1984). First, it permitted a statistical analysis and comparison of group data collected with the myriad of paper-and-pencil instruments employed in the study. When required, this allowed us to establish the reliability and validity of particular instruments. Second, the waiting-list characteristic of the design bound a family as a control for only 3 months; pilot data gathered before the onset of LWA showed that beyond 3 months the attrition of participants assigned to such a condition sharply increased. Finally, the nature of the design permitted us to assess progress made by individual children and their families. As argued earlier, having subjects serve as their own control is the most effective design to use with asthma; data gathered from participants over a period of time provided us with the most clinically significant information we collected.

Dependent Variables

A gamut of dependent measures were used to assess the FAP and LWA. These include: paper-and-pencil, the Mini-Wright peak flow meter, and economica and school data.

Paper-and-pencil measures. Wherever possible, both projects relied on paper-and-pencil instruments with established reliability and validity. Major paper-and-pencil instruments were designed to assess knowledge of asthma, attitudes toward the disorder, locus of control, and daily information about the patient's asthma. Specific types of measures included:

1. *Initial interviews.* Both the FAP and LWA used questionnaires during an initial interview to gather in-depth information about such factors as history of asthma, names and types of medications, and so forth. It took approximately one hour in each program to gather information from a child and his parents. The instrument used in LWA was the Asthma Problem Behavior Checklist (Creer, Marion, & Creer, 1983), an instrument with demonstrated reliability and validity.

2. *Knowledge quizzes.* Both projects developed quizzes to detrmine whether participants' knowledge of asthma increased as a result of self-management training. Instruments were tailored for a specific program

whether it was the FAP or LWA; reliability and validity were established for each instrument.

3. *Locus of control.* The purpose of a locus of control measure is to assess whether the individual perceives either himself or external factors (for example, others, chance) as basically responsible for his health. The FAP employed two standardized instruments: the Multidimensional Health Locus of Control (MHLC) developed for adults by Walston, Walston, and DeVellis (1978) and the Children's Health Locus of Control (CHLC) developed by Parcel and Meyer (1978). Both have proven validity and reliability. LWA used the I–E Locus of Control Scale (Rotter, 1966) with adults and, although it is not a locus of control instrument, the Piers-Harris Children's Self-Concept Scale (Piers & Harris, 1966). This instrument permitted us to determine whether there were any changes in the attitudes of children toward themselves as a result of their acquiring self-management skills.

4. *Asthma diaries.* The diary used in LWA was described earlier; the diary used in the FAP assessed similar dimensions of asthma, including medications, mórbidity data, and disability level.

5. *Attitude surveys.* The LWA project staff developed and tested two surveys designed to assess participants' attitudes toward asthma, the Adult Attitude Survey and the Children's Attitude Survey (Creer *et al.*, 1984). Both instruments have established reliability and validity; both are widely used with other self-management programs, particularly with the Superstuff materials developed by the American Lung Association (Weiss, 1981).

6. *Report of asthma attack or episode.* This one-page form was designed to be completed following each attack suffered by a participant (Creer, 1980). Information is checked off with respect to: (a) the severity of the attack; (b) whether the patient was compliant with any medication instructions prior to the attack; (c) where and when the episode occurred; (d) types and amounts of medications taken during the attack; and, (e) in an approximate order, the sequence of steps taken by the child and his family to establish control over the asthmatic episode.

7. *Medical cost information.* This was a record used in LWA to assess the financial impact of asthma (Marion, Creer, & Reynolds, 1985; Creer *et al.*, 1984). It permitted us to calculate changes in the costs of asthma that were achieved because of the acquisition and practice of self-management skills.

The Mini-Wright peak flow meter. This simple instrument, used in LWA, consists of a mouthpiece attached to a plastic cylinder. A person blows through the mouthpiece into the cylinder and activates a meter to record the amount of air exhaled in the initial 10 sec of the expiration. The amount of expired air, referred to as the peak expiratory flow rate (PEFR), is reflected on the meter in terms of liters per minute. It provides a convenient way to assess airway resistance; an increase in airway resistance, in general, signals pulmonary obstruction and the increased likelihood of an asthma attack. Peak expiratory flow rates are useful in estimating both the severity and progress of the airway obstruction. Advantages of the peak flow meter are simplicity, economy, portability, and the fact that values obtained with the instrument correlate with data gathered with the spirometer (Wright & McKerrow, 1959).

Economic and school data. LWA gathered data on the costs of asthma in order to determine whether they were affected by the practice of self-management skills; both the FAP and LWA gathered information regarding the impact of self-management on school absenteeism. As will be noted, the latter proved to be an excellent dependent variable in both studies.

Results

The dependent variables employed in the FAP and LWA focused on measuring the morbidity of asthma. It was thought that a demonstration of changes in morbidity indices would, more than any other evidence, reflect the true value of a self-management program designed and implemented for the disorder. In addition, a large number of participants were involved with the programs: 147 and 343 individuals were involved with the FAP and LWA, respectively. Although space limitations prevent a thorough discussion of the findings, what appear as the most salient data from both studies will be presented.

Paper-and-pencil measures. As noted, a number of paper-and-pencil instruments were employed in the studies. The most prominent findings obtained with these measures are as follows:

1. *Knowledge of asthma.* A statistically significant change in knowledge of asthma was noted with subjects in both programs as a result of self-management training. Participants became knowledgeable about asthma, and their knowledge, as suggested earlier, was essential for the overall success of self-management. In LWA, no changes were noted with subjects assigned to the control groups during the 3 months they served in this condition.

2. *Locus of control.* As a result of self-management, statistically significant changes occurred with both locus of control scales administered in the FAP. Participants shifted their view from perceiving that external

factors had control of their health to perceiving that they themselves had responsibility. A similar finding was made in LWA with the I–E Locus of Control Scale after self-management training; in addition, youngsters in LWA reported an improvement in their self-concept as measured on the Piers-Harris Children's Self-Concept Scale. The changes on both of these instruments were statistically significant.

3. *Attitude Surveys.* According to both the adult and child asthma surveys administered in LWA, participants acquired more positive attitudes toward the disorder and their ability to control it; these changes occurred as a result of self-management training and were statistically significant. No changes were noted in the administration of the two surveys with participants while they served as control subjects in the study.

4. *Report of asthma attacks and episodes.* In LWA, 84 families turned in as many as 94 completed reports; the mean number of reports submitted per family was 13.03. A rich vein of information was tapped by this instrument. For example, it was noted that the leading stimuli perceived as triggering attacks included infections, exercise, allergens, and overexertion; furthermore, 60% of the attacks were observed to occur at home, with a lesser percentage occurring when children were playing outside or at school. Only 37% of the participants reported that they were fully compliant with medication instructions before an attack suffered by a given child. This percentage was higher than that reported in more stringent clinical tests by Eney and Goldstein (1976); Sublett, Pollard, Kadlec, and Karibo (1979); and Miller (1982); but it still reflected a considerable degree of noncompliance.

5. *Diary data.* Participant self-report, as recorded in a diary, provided important information collected in both the FAP and LWA. A wealth of data was obtained; in LWA, for example, information was gathered for almost 10,000 days by the participants. Data reported on the instrument were verified in a number of ways: First, as noted, LWA taught children to complete the diary and had parents serve as a reliability check. This greatly enhanced our confidence in the measure. Second, both studies verified data reported in the diary against external checks. This included, for example, information gathered from school, hospitals, or, in the case of asthma costs, from insurance companies. The result was that in both the FAP and LWA the information is unlike much self-report data (Creer & Winder, 1986) in that it is both reliable and valid.

A number of significant findings were reported by the FAP (Hindi-Alexander & Cropp, 1984). These investigators found that a statistically significant increase in total activity experienced by participants occurred as a result of the acquisition and practice of self-management skills; this increase in activity was accompanied in turn by a statistically significant decrease in both health care visits and school absenteeism (more on the latter will be described below). Hindi-Alexander and Cropp also reported a 24% decrease in emergency visits, a 10% decrease in the participants' medication scores (indicating that they required less medication), and a 44% reduction in hospital admissions.

Major findings obtained with the diary used in LWA included improvements in peak expiratory flow rates (to be discussed next) and in both school absenteeism and costs for asthma (also described below). One statistically significant finding was a reduction in the number of asthma attacks suffered by children involved in the project. In the year prior to self-management training, participants reported that they had suffered an average of five attacks per month; this suggests that, on the average, they suffered over one attack per week. In the year following their participation, however, they experienced an average of only one attack per month.

Mini-Wright peak flow meter. Information gathered with the peak flow meter proved invaluable. First, data gathered from individual children during baseline were compared against their predicted peak flow values. The latter scores were calculated according to the height of individuals. It was found that there was a statistically significant difference between the youngsters' flow rates, obtained in both the morning and evening, and their predicted flow rates. During self-management training, at the 6-month follow-up and again at the 12-month follow-up, however, these differences disappeared. In other words, the youngsters' flow rates came to approximate their predicted flow values.

Second, the peak flow data proved useful in predicting attacks of individual children; this has been described by Taplin and Creer (1978) and Harm, Kotses, and Creer (1984). Both studies entered flow rates into conditional probability equations to predict asthma within a 12-hour period. Taplin and Creer (1978) predicted the occurrence of asthma in two children. The base rate, or prior probability for the occurrence of asthma, and a critical PEFR value which most enhanced the predictability of asthma was determined for each child. Two conditional probabilities were calculated for each subject; the first was the probability of asthma in a 12-hour period following a flow value less than or equal to the critical value; the second was the probability of asthma in a 12-hour period following a PEFR greater than the critical value. Taplin and Creer found approximately a 300% increase over the base rate in predicting future attacks of both children.

Harm and her colleagues (1984) extended the procedure and examined its usefulness with a larger group of children, including many who participated in LWA. Twenty-five children recorded flow rates twice daily, along with the date and time of their asthma attacks. Two conditional posterior probabilities—identical to those calculated by Taplin and Creer (1978)—and the ratio of hits to misses was calculated for each child at successively lower flow rates. The average improvement in predictability from the prior to the highest posterior probability was 491%. These studies demonstrate even further the value of adding peak flow meters as a dependent measure in self-management studies for asthma.

School and economic data. As noted earlier, the FAP found that there was almost a 50% decrease in school absenteeism for the asthmatic children who participated in their program. The mean number of days of absence from school was 17.5 in the year prior to children's involvement with LWA; this decreased to 6.4 days in the year after the children received self-management training. This represents a 273% decrease in the number of days of absence from school.

School absenteeism data from LWA can be interpreted in a number of ways: First, the number of days of absence decreased to a point at which it was almost identical to that reported for all children in Colorado where LWA was developed and evaluated (6.4 to 6.3 days, repectively). There was, therefore, no difference in the absence rate between participants in LWA and their nonasthmatic peers. Second, the method by which children's health is classified, according to criteria established by the federal government, is based on the number of days they are absent from school (*Vital and Health Statistics,* 1983). According to these standards, the change in health status of participants changed from poor to good. Finally, it is important to describe savings to school districts because of the reduction in school absenteeism. In the year before participants received self-management training in LWA, school districts would have lost approximately $160 in tax revenue because of an asthmatic child's absence record; this amount was reduced to approximately $58, a decrease of almost 276%, per child in the year following participation in LWA. Similar savings could also have been calculated for each youngster involved with the FAP. Projecting what would occur if similar findings were obtained with each asthmatic child in the United States—assuming that each youngster was taught and practiced self-management skills—the savings would amount to approximately half a billion dollars annually to school districts.

An even greater economic saving was found in LWA with respect to the costs of asthma. A determined and sophisticated effort was made to obtain cost information for participants. The best data collected was that obtained from families who initially paid the costs incurred because of their child's asthma but who were later reimbursed by insurance companies. On the basis of data presented by Creer and colleagues (1984), involvement in LWA resulted in a 66% reduction in the health care costs of these participants. Again, by projecting what this would mean on a national level, the acquistion and practice of self-management skills by asthmatic children could save them and their families a health care bill of approximately $5 billion annually. This amount is almost equal to the annual budget of the National Institutes of Health, including the National Heart, Lung, and Blood Institute, the agency that sponsored LWA. The decrease in health care costs assumes even greater importance if indirect costs are considered. According to Marion *et al.* (1985), these costs represent a larger burden to some families of asthmatic children than do the direct costs of health care services.

Conclusions

The presentation of findings from the FAP and LWA points out that the self-management of asthma is indeed a practical method of controlling the disorder. And, at the same time, it offers a proven way to break the bonds of soaring medical costs that threaten to bankrupt our society.

There are three points that must be considered. First, as Creer and co-workers (1984) emphasize in their presentation of LWA, their findings *must be interpreted within the context of solid medical treatment*. The physicians who referred participants to the project were, to a person, highly skilled and knowledgeable about asthma. They treated and advised patients enrolled in the program in a most effective and enlightened manner; self-management techniques, in turn, augmented the ability of patients to apply this medical instruction and advice so that it proved maximally effective. The synthesis of solid and proven medical treatment to self-management skills by patients cannot be overemphasized in discussing either the FAP or LWA; data from both studies must be considered as a function of blending physician and patient skills. By the same token, Creer and Winder (1986) caution that teaching patients to practice self-management skills can have disastrous effects if the patient is given poor medical advice. An illustration of this potential would be seen if, during self-management training, a patient were taught to comply with potentially harmful medication instructions. Medications commonly prescribed for asthma are potent; furthermore, different studies have indicated that they are frequently overprescribed (e.g., Sublett *et al.*, 1979) or prescribed to be taken in combination with other asthma medications. The latter is particularly fraught with peril as there are suggestions that the combination of two widely prescribed generic asthma medications, theophylline and beta agonists, may have harmful, perhaps fatal, consequences (Lehr & Guideri, 1983; Wilson & Sutherland, 1982). This possibility further accentuates the need for asthma self-management programs for a full integration of behavioral self-management training and the most current medical advances.

The second point concerns the need for refinement of the measures used to assess self-management programs (Creer & Winder, 1986). Excellent data were obtained in both the FAP and LWA , but there is a need to use more sophisticated measures for assessing, among other variables, activity limitations and the costs of asthma. The major contribution of self-management programs will be to alter the morbidity factors produced by the disorder. The technology of self-management is, as argued by Creer and Winder (1986), available; what is needed are better ways to assess the application of these programs. The assessment of self-management programs for asthma currently serves as the major behavioral constraint for the technology; future research will be directed at expanding these boundaries. At the same time, what is achieved with application of self-management to asthma will hinge upon the characteristics of the disorder and progress made by medical scientists in overcoming many of the problems previously discussed. As demonstrated over the years, limitations of knowledge regarding asthma present the major barrier to its understanding and eventual control.

Finally, it is becoming progressively more evident that all of the 10 million asthma patients in the United States require self-management training. A report by Strunk, Wolfson, La Brecque, and Mrazek (1984) described the deaths of 21 asthmatic children, former residents at a treatment facility for the disorder, in the period between 1973 and 1982. What was distressing was that Strunk and his colleagues suggested that these children had died from what they called psychological factors, primarily the lack of self-management skills. Such a finding is inexcusable from two viewpoints. First, self-management skills, although known to be effective, were not taught to these youngsters. At other residential care facilities, there are reports of occasional deaths among former residents. However, as noted by Creer and co-workers (1984), these deaths were always due to physical problems, for instance, cardiac arrest occurring during severe attacks, and never to what Strunk and his co-workers (1984) referred to as psychological factors. Second, there is the unavoidable conclusion that the deaths of many of the youngsters described by the latter investigators might have been avoided had the children been taught self-management skills. With the technology available, deaths from asthma can be reduced; morbidity factors certainly can, as demonstrated in the FAP and LWA, be altered. What is required is the wholehearted commitment by physicians and behavioral scientists to introduction of the self-management technology described in this chapter to achieve such an aim.

References

Alexander, A. B. (1981). Behavioral approaches in the treatment of bronchial asthma. In C. K. Prokop & L. A. Bradley (Eds.), *Medical psychology: Contributions to behavioral medicine* (pp. 373–394). New York: Academic Press.

American Academy of Allergy. (1981). Position statements—Controversial techniques. *Journal of Allergy and Clinical Immunology, 67,* 333–338.

American Thoracic Society Committee on Diagnostic Standards for Nontuberculous Diseases. (1962). Definitions and classifications of chronic bronchitis, asthma, and pulmonary emphysema. *American Review of Respiratory Disease. 85,* 762–768.

Barnes, P. J. (1984). Nocturnal asthma: Mechanisms and treatment. *British Medical Journal, 288,* 1397–1398.

Bernstein, L. I. (1983). Asthma in adults: Diagnosis and treatment. In E. Middleton, Jr., C. E. Reed, & E. F. Ellis (Eds.)., *Allergy: Principles and practice* (pp. 901–934). St. Louis: C. V. Mosby.

Chai, H., & Newcomb, R. W. (1973). Pharmacologic management of childhood asthma. *American Journal of Diseases of Children, 125,* 757–765.

Cherniack, R. M., & Cherniack, L. (1983). *Respiration in health and diseases* (3rd ed.). Philadelphia: W. B. Saunders.

Clark, T. J. H. (1977). Definition of asthma for clinical trials. In J. E. Stark & J. V. Collins (Eds.), Methods in clinical trials in asthma. *British Journal of Diseases of the Chest, 71,* 225–226.

Creer, T. L. (1974). Biofeedback and asthma. *Advances in Asthma and Allergy, 1,* 6–11.

Creer, T. L. (1978). Asthma: Psychologic aspects and management. In E. Middleton, Jr., C. E. Reed, & E. F. Ellis, (Eds.), *Allergy: Principles and practice* (pp. 796–811). St. Louis: C. V. Mosby.

Creer, T. L. (1979). *Asthma therapy: A behavioral health care system for respiratory disorders.* New York: Springer.

Creer, T. L. (1980). Self-management behavioral strategies for asthmatics. *Behavioral Medicine, 7,* 14–24.

Creer, T. L. (1982). Asthma. *Journal of Consulting and Clinical Psychology, 50,* 912–921.

Creer, T. L. (1983a). Respiratory disorders. In T. G. Burish & L. A. Bradley (Eds.), *Coping with chronic diseases: Research and applications* (pp. 316–336). New York: Academic Press.

Creer, T. L. (1983b). Response: Self-management psychology and the treatment of childhood asthma. *Journal of Allergy and Clinical Immunology, 72* (Part 2), 607–610.

Creer, T. L., & Kotses, H. (1983). Asthma: Psychologic aspects and management. In E. Middleton, Jr., C. E. Reed, & E. F. Ellis (Eds.) *Allergy: Principles and practice* (2nd ed., pp. 1015–1036). St. Louis: C. V. Mosby.

Creer, T., & Leung, P. (1981). The development and evaluation of a self-management program for children with asthma. In *Self-management educational programs for childhood asthma: Vol. 2. Manuscripts* (pp. 107–128). Bethesda, MD: National Institute of Allergy and Infectious Diseases.

Creer, T. L., & Winder, J. A. (1986). The self-management of asthma. In K. A. Holroyd & T. L. Creer (Eds.) *Handbook of self-management in health psychology and behavioral medicine.* (pp. 269–303). New York: Academic Press

Creer, T. L., Renne, C. M., & Chai, H. (1982). The application of behavioral techniques to childhood asthma. In D. C. Russo & J. W. Varni (Eds.) *Behavioral pediatrics: Research and practice* (pp. 27–66). New York: Plenum Press.

Creer, T. L., Marion, R. J., & Creer, P. P. (1983). The Asthma Problem Behavior Checklist: Parental perceptions of the behavior of asthmatic children. *Journal of Asthma, 20,* 97–104.

Creer, T. L., Backial, M., Burns, K. L., Leung, P., Marion, R. J., Miklich, D. R., Taplin, P. S., & Ullman, S. (1984). *The self-management of childhood asthma.* Unpublished manuscript, Ohio University, Athens, Ohio.

Creer, T. L., Backiel, M., Ullman, S., & Leung, P. (1986). *Living with asthma.* (NIH Publication No. 84-2364). Bethesda, MD: National Heart, Lung, and Blood Institute.

Creer, T. L., Harm, D. L., & Marion, R. J. (In press). Asthma. In D. K. Routh (Ed.), *Handbook of pediatric psychology.* New York: Guilford.

Cropp, G., & Hindi-Alexander, M. (1981). Program at Children's Hospital in Buffalo. In *Self-management educational programs for childhood asthma: Vol. 2. Manuscripts* (pp. 246–256). Bethesda, MD: National Institute of Allergy and Infectious Diseases.

Dearlove, J., Verguel, A. P., Birkin, N., & Latham, P. (1981). Anachronistic treatment for asthma. *British Medical Journal, 283,* 1684–1685.

Eney, R. D., & Goldstein, E. O. (1976). Compliance of chronic asthmatics with oral administration of theophylline as measured by serum and salivary levels. *Pediatrics, 57,* 513–517.

Fletcher, C. M., & Pride, N. B. (1984). Definitions of emphysema, chronic bronchitis, asthma, and airflow obstruction: 25 years on from the CIBA symposium. *Thorax, 39,* 81–85.

Fox, J. (1983). Debate on learning theory is shifting. *Science, 222,* 1219–1222.

French, T. M., & Alexander, F. (1941). Psychogenic factors in bronchial asthma. *Psychosomatic Medicine Monographs,* No. 4.

Green, L. W., Goldstein, R., & Parker, S. R. (Eds.). (1983). Workshop proceedings on self-management of childhood asthma. *Journal of Allergy and Clinical Immunology, 72* (Part 2), 519–626.

Harm, D. L., Kotses, H., & Creer, T. L. (1985). Improving the ability of peak expiratory flow rates to predict asthma. *Journal of Allergy and Clinical Immunology, 76,* 688–694.

Hindi-Alexander, M., & Cropp, G. J. A. (1981). Community and family programs for children with asthma. *Annals of Allergy, 46,* 143–148.

Hindi-Alexander, M., & Cropp, G. J. A. (1984). Evaluation of a family asthma program. *Journal of Allergy and Clinical Immunology, 74,* 505–510.

Horton, D. J., Suda, W. L., Kinsman, R. A., Souhrada, J., & Spector, S. L. (1978). Bronchoconstriction suggestion in asthma: A role for airways hyperreactivity and emotions. *American Review of Respiratory Diseases, 117,* 1029–1038.

Jones, R. S. (1976). *Asthma in children.* Action, MA: Publishing Sciences Group.

Kinsman, R. A., Dirks, J. F., Jones, N. F., & Dahlem, N. W. (1980). Anxiety reduction in asthma: Four catches to general application. *Psychosomatic Medicine, 42,* 397–405.

Lewis, C. E., Rachelefsky, G., Lewis, M. A., de la Sota, A., & Kaplan, M. (1984). A randomized trial of A.C.T. (Asthma Care Training) for kids. *Pediatrics, 47,* 478–486.

Lewis, R. A., Lewis, M. N., & Tattersfield, A. E. (1984). Asthma induced by suggestion: Is it due to airway cooling? *American Review of Respiratory Diseases, 129,* 691–695.

Lehr, D., & Guideri, G. (1983). More on combined beta-agonists and methylxanthines in asthma. *New England Journal of Medicine, 309,* 1581–1582.

Leigh, D. (1953). Asthma and the psychiatrist: A critical review. *International Archives of Allergy and Applied Immunology, 4,* 227–246.

Loren, M. L., Leung, P. K., Cooley, R. L., Chai, H., Bell, T. D., & Buck, V. M. (1978). Irreversibility of obstructive changes in severe asthma in children. *Chest, 74,* 126–129.

Luparello. T., Lyons, H. A., Bleecker, E. R., & McFadden, E. R., Jr. (1968). Influences of suggestion on airway reactivity in asthmatic subjects. *Psychosomatic Medicine, 30,* 819–825.

Luparello, T., Leist, N., Lourie, C. H., & Sweet, P. (1970). The interaction of psychologic stimuli and pharmacologic agents on airway reactivity in asthmatic subjects. *Psychosomatic Medicine, 32,* 509–513.

MacKenzie, J. N. (1886). The production of "rose asthma" by an artificial rose. *American Journal of Medical Sciences, 91,* 45–57.

Marion, R. J., Creer, T. L., & Reynolds, R. V. C. (1985). Direct and indirect costs associated with the management of childhood asthma. *Annals of Allergy, 54,* 1–4.

McFadden, E. R., Jr. (1980). Asthma: Pathophysiology. *Seminars in Respiratory Medicine, 1,* 297–303.

McFadden, E. R., Jr. (1984). Pathogenesis of asthma. *Journal of Allergy and Clinical Immunology, 73,* 413–424.

McFadden, E. R., Jr., Luparello, T., Lyons, H. A., & Bleecker, E. (1969). The mechanism of action of suggestion in the induction of acute asthma attacks. *Psychosomatic Medicine, 31,* 134–143.

McFadden, E. R., Jr., & Stevens, J. B. (1983). A history of asthma. In E. Middleton, Jr., C. E. Reed, & E. F. Ellis (Eds.), *Allergy: Principles and practice* (2nd ed., pp. 805–809). St. Louis: C. V. Mosby.

Miklich, D. R., Renne, C. M., Creer, T. L., Alexander, A. B., Chai, H., Davis, M. H., Hoffman, A., & Danker-Brown, P. (1977). The clinical utility of behavior therapy as an adjunctive treatment for asthma. *Journal of Allergy and Clinical Immunology, 60,* 285–294.

Miller, K. A. (1982). Theophylline compliance in adolescent patients with chronic asthma. *Journal of Adolescent Health Care, 3,* 177–179.

Muntner, S. (Ed.). (1963). *Moses Maimonides: Treatise on asthma.* Philadelphia: Lippincott.

Nadel, J. A. (1976). Airways: Autonomic regulation and airways responsiveness. In E. B. Weiss & M. S. Segal (Eds.), *Bronchial asthma: Mechanisms and therapeutics* (pp. 155–162). Boston: Little, Brown.

National Institute of Allergy and Infectious Diseases. (1981). *Self-management educational programs for childhood asthma: Vol. 2. Manuscripts.* Bethesda, MD: National Institute of Allergy and Infectious Diseases.

O'Leary, S. G., & Dubey, D. R. (1979). Applications of self-control procedures by children: A review. *Journal of Applied Behavior Analysis, 12,* 449–465.

Parcel, G. S., & Meyer, M. P. (1978). Development of an instrument to measure children's health locus of control. *Health Education Monographs, 6,* 149–159.

Pearlman, D. S. (1984). Bronchial asthma: A perspective from childhood to adulthood. *American Journal of Diseases of Children, 138,* 459–466.

Philipp, R. L., Wilde, G. J. S., & Day, J. H. (1972). Suggestion and relaxation in asthmatics. *Journal of Psychosomatic Research, 16,* 193–204.

Piers, E. V. & Harris, D. B. (1964). Age and other correlates of self-concept in children. *Journal of Educational Psychology, 55,* 91–95.

Porter, R., & Birch, J. (Eds.). (1971). Report of the working group on the definition of asthma. *Identification of asthma.* London: Churchill Livingston.

Purcell, K. (1963). Distinctions between subgroups of asthmatic children: Children's perceptions of events associated with asthma. *Pediatrics, 31,* 486–494.

Purcell, K., & Weiss, J. H. (1970) Asthma. In C. C. Costello (Ed.), *Symptoms of psychopathology* (pp. 597–623). New York: Wiley.

Reed, C. E., & Townley, R. G. (1978). Asthma: Classification and pathogenesis. In E. Middleton, Jr., C. E. Reed, & E. F. Ellis (Eds.), *Allergy: Principles and practice* (pp. 659–677). St. Louis: C. V. Mosby.

Rees, J. (1983). Clincial trials in asthma. *British Medical Journal, 287,* 376–377.

Rees, J. (1984). ABC's of asthma: Precipitating factors. *British Medical Journal, 288,* 1512–1513.

Renne, C. M. (1982). *Asthma in families: Behavioral analysis and treatment.* (Final report, Grant No. RO1-HL 22021). Bethesda, MD: National Heart, Lung, and Blood Institute.

Renne, C. M., & Creer, T. L. (1985). Asthmatic children and their families. In M. L. Wolraich & D. K. Routh (Eds.), *Advances in developmental and behavioral pediatrics* (pp. 41–81) Greenwich, CT: JAI Press.

Rotter, J. B. (1966). Generalized expectancies for internal versus external control of reinforcement. *Psychological Monographs, 80* (1, Whole No. 609).

Sakula, A. (1984). [Review of] Sir John Floyer's *A Treatise of the Asthma. Thorax, 39,* 248–254.

Siegel, S. C., Katz, R. M., & Rachelefsky, G. S. (1983). Asthma in infancy and childhood. In E. Middleton, Jr., C. E. Reed, & E. F. Ellis (Eds.), *Allergy: Principles and practice* (2nd ed., pp. 863–900). St. Louis: C. V. Mosby.

Skinner, B. F. (1948). Superstition in the pigeon. *Journal of Experimental Psychology, 38,* 168–172.

Spector, S. L., Luparello, T. J., Kopetzky, M. T., Souhrada, J., & Kinsman, R. A. (1976). Response of asthmatics to methacholine and suggestion. *American Review of Respiratory Diseases, 113,* 43–50.

Stark, J. E., & Collins, J. V. (Eds.). (1977). Methods in clinical trials in asthma. *British Journal of Diseases of the Chest, 71,* 225–244.

Strunk, R. C., Wolfson, G. S., LaBrecque, J. F., & Mrazek, D. Predictors of a fatal outcome in childhood asthma (Pt. 2). *Journal of Allergy and Clinical Immunology, 73,* 122.

Strupp, H. H., Levenson, R. W., Manuck, S. B., Snell, J. D., Hinrichsen, J. J., & Boyd, S. (1974). Effects of suggestion on total respiratory resistance in mild asthmatics. *Journal of Psychosomatic Research, 18,* 337–346.

Sublett, J. L., Pollard, S. J., Kadlec, G. J., & Karibo, J. M. (1979). Non-compliance in asthmatic children: A study of theophylline levels in a pediatric emergency room population. *Annals of Allergy, 43,* 95–97.

Taplin, P. S., & Creer, T. L. (1978). A procedure for using peak expiratory flow rate data to increase the predictability of asthma episodes. *Journal of Asthma Research, 16,* 15–19.

Thoreson, C. E., & Kirmil-Gray, K. (1983). Self-management psychology and the treatment of childhood asthma (Pt. 2). *Journal of Allergy and Clinical Immunology, 72,* 596–606.

Vital and Health Statistics. (1983). Disability days: United States, 1980. (Series 10, 43). Washington, DC: U.S. Government Printing Office.

Wallston, K. A., Wallston, B. S., & De Vellis, R. (1978). Development of the multidimensional health locus of control (MHLC) scales. *Health Education Monographs, 6,* 160–170.

Weiss, J. H. (1981). Superstuff. *Self-management educational programs for childhood asthma: Vol. 2. Manuscripts* (pp. 273–293). Bethesda, MD: National Institute of Allergy and Infectious Diseases.

Weiss, J. H., Martin, C., & Riley, J. (1970). Effects of suggestion on respiration in asthmatic children. *Psychosomatic Medicine, 32,* 409–415.

Williams, M. H., Jr. (1980). Clinical features. *Seminars in Respiratory Medicine, 1,* 304–314.

Williams, M. H., Jr. (1982). *Essentials of pulmonary medicine.* Philadelphia: W. B. Saunders.

Wilson, J. D., & Sutherland, D. C. (1982). Combined beta agonists and methylxanthines in asthma. *New England Journal of Medicine, 307,* 1707.

Wright, B. M., & McKerrow, C. B. (1959). Maximum forced expiratory flow rates as a measure of ventilatory capacity. *British Medical Journal, 2,* 1041–1047.

CHAPTER 10

Pain

Ruth V. E. Grunau and Kenneth D. Craig

Pain is a complex experience central to human existence. The burden it places on individuals and society is of enormous cost. Accidental injury, disease, and physical trauma inflicted during acts of aggression are virtually universal events. Of particular importance is chronic pain, which imposes economic, social, and emotional hardships on patients, their families, and society, and is a major source of disability in North America today (Bonica, 1983). Our ability to prevent and treat pain in its many manifestations has been limited by our conceptual models and theories; yet these have been surprisingly transitory.

With the advent of modern medicine and basic medical sciences in the nineteenth century, pain came to be conceptualized almost exclusively as a sensory phenomenon, and the search for neurophysiological afferent and central processing mechanisms was initiated. Strategies for pain management developed which were designed to reduce the perception of pain by interrupting the transmission of "pain messages" from "pain receptors" to a "pain center" in the brain, predominantly through pharmacological and surgical techniques. Affective and cognitive components associated with pain were relegated to a secondary position as a "reaction" to pain (Beecher, 1959; Craig, 1984), whereas physiological and psychophysical analyses of sensory input were studied in detail. From this perspective, cognitive and affective processes were conceptualized as if they were "contaminants" to effective medical management or sources of experimental error that needed to be controlled.

Ruth V. E. Grunau and Kenneth D. Craig • Department of Psychology, University of British Columbia, Vancouver, British Columbia, Canada V6T 1Y7.

This unidimensional sensory focus remained well entrenched until its inadequacies became apparent in the last several decades (Melzack & Wall, 1982). Traditional medical intervention based on this model had proved to be only partially successful, leaving a large proportion of patients with either no improvement or, in some cases, increased pain (Bonica, 1980). Numerous clinical phenomena defied explanation in a rigid sensory-specificity model of pain transmission (Melzack & Wall, 1982). Examples of these include: (a) phantom limb pain in amputees, (b) severe pain in paraplegics in specific areas of the trunk or limbs below the level of a known spinal transection, and (c) the lack of success in certain pain syndromes of attempts to provide permanent relief through surgical lesions of the peripheral and central nervous system.

A major transformation in concepts of pain has taken place during recent decades. Melzack and Wall (1965) developed a model in which pain is conceived as a multidimensional phenomenon comprising major cognitive and affective components as well as sensory processes. Tissue stress or damage was reconstrued as activating neural input of both affective-motivational and sensory aspects. Gate control theory postulated that initial neural input can trigger central control systems which inhibit or facilitate input at various levels of the brain and spinal cord. Central messages reflecting attentional, emotional, and experiential factors can descend from the brain through the spinal cord and influence nociceptive messages from peripheral receptors (Melzack & Wall, 1982). Thus, neurophysiological signals from injured tissues come to be integrated with emotional, arousal, and thought processes. At higher brain levels, complex processes occur wherein nociceptive signals are integrated with beliefs, expectations, and immediate social demands that reflect socialization and cultural processes (Craig, 1983a).

This profound shift in the conceptualization of pain away from the sensory-specific model has been reflected in the definition of pain adopted by the International Association for the Study of Pain (1979), which describes pain as "an unpleasant sensory and emotional experience associated with actual or potential tissue damage, or described in terms of such damage" (p. 250). The broader formulations incorporating psychological and social dimensions have received a great deal of experimental support from physiological studies of gating mechanisms in the spinal cord and central nervous system (Bonica, Lindblom, & Iggo, 1983; Wall & Melzack, 1984). Recent discoveries of the endorphinergic regulation of pain have also contributed potential biological bases for endogenous pain modulation systems (Terman, Shavit, Lewis, Cannon, & Liebeskind, 1984).

With the development of enthusiasm for direct interventions into psychological and social parameters of pain, it would be a mistake not to recognize the identity of these processes with the biological substrates of all behavior. Given that pain is now broadly conceived as intrinsically far more than a sensory phenomenon, the biological and psychological phenomena of attention, memory, decision-making, and other self-regulatory processes have become pertinent to our understanding of pain. These processes are inherently superordinate to the contents of all experience and impose limits upon what we think and feel (Mahoney, 1983; Rosenthal & Zimmerman, 1978). From this perspective, all experience, whether painful or not, is an active construction of the nervous system with the biological constraints dictating how people attend to their environment, the assimilation and organization of experience, and decision-making strategies (Craig, 1984). Comprehensive models of pain will have to attend to these complexities.

Acute versus Chronic Pain

Differences in the etiology, physiopathology, symptoms, diagnosis, and therapy of acute as compared with chronic pain have been recognized as important only recently (Bonica, 1974; Sternbach, 1974). Acute pain now is viewed as arising rapidly due to injury or disease processes and persisting only as long as tissue pathology itself in disorders that resolve through healing processes. Chronic pain is associated with persistent, recurrent, or progressive tissue stress or damage. It may arise from ineffective treatment of acute pain or it may represent the pain persisting beyond the period normal for healing of acute injury or disease. These basic distinctions have also made it clear that the appropriate treatment and palliatives for acute pain are contraindicated for some people with chronic disorders. Risk of chronicity is increased for some people if potent analgesics are prescribed for a protracted period of time, if extensive convalescence and inactivity are recommended, and if there is escape or release from ongoing life rsponsibilities such as work or family routines (Fordyce, 1976; Sternbach, 1984).

In chronic pain, factors conveniently described as psychological have been found to be progressively more important; thus, pain which commences as a nociceptive event may persist longer than necessary as a result of psychological and behavioral factors. Whereas distinctions between acute and chronic pain have functional utility in determining management, most recently the complexities and commonalities of both acute and chronic pain in terms of interdependence of psychological and sensory aspects have been emphasized. Thus, proper management of acute pain related to injury, disease, or surgery requires recognition that it reflects a constellation of sensory, emotional, and cognitive experiences and associated autonomic, psychological, and behavioral responses (Chapman & Bonica, 1983). It is now recognized that psychological influences may frequently have profound effects on acute, nociceptively generated pain as well as on chronic pain and that these play an important role in management (Benedetti & Murphy, 1985).

Furthermore, chronic pain has frequently been dichotomized into either *organic* or *functional* subtypes. Pain that persisted despite medical or surgical intervention and absence of an apparent organic basis was viewed as psychogenic in origin. Most often, functional diagnoses have been the result of excluding plausible organic bases for the pain rather than positive evidence of psychological factors contributing to the disorder. Some underlying emotional dysfunction requiring treatment with psychotherapy or psychoactive medication was presumed. However, chronic pain has been unresponsive not only to traditional medical treatment but also to classical psychotherapeutic or psychiatric treatment as well. The organic versus functional distinction is currently viewed as semantically misleading and irrelevant (Roberts, 1983). Chronic pain sufferers all experience "real" pain; so-called psychogenic pain is organic, namely, a function of the brain. However, it does appear useful to discriminate between prior etiological events versus ongoing mechanisms such as reinforcement contingencies, maladaptive cognitive styles, and abnormal illness behavior in maintaining chronic pain.

Psychological Approaches to Pain Management

A broad range of management techniques have been applied to pain, including operant conditioning, cognitive-behavioral methods, biofeedback, relaxation training, hypnosis, and group therapy. Many chronic pain treatment centers offer multimodal treatment in an interdisciplinary setting and use a variety of these techniques. Although it has been difficult to assess the utility of each approach, this will be attempted, as the object of this volume has been to evaluate the extent to which psychological approaches to behavioral medicine have been successful and to address applications in which they may have been oversold. Methodological problems with research in the clinical efficacy of these procedures is recognized (Fordyce, Roberts, & Sternbach, 1985; Tan, 1982; Turner & Chapman, 1982b) and are not discussed here. Attention was directed in particular to the interplay between explicitly biological and psychological processes. In considering the compatibility of psychological intervention methods with our current understanding of psychological processes, two areas to be reviewed emerged as particularly problematic: biofeedback as a technique for controlling physiological factors in pain, and claims for psychological management of childbirth pain.

Operant Models

In 1968, Fordyce, Fowler, Lehmann, and Delateur described behavioral management techniques based upon operant conditioning principles for treating problems associated with chronic pain. Their model focused on the presence of social reinforcers in the social-occupational-familial environment of the patient which were delivered contingent upon pain behaviors. These included the pain-relieving and mood-elevating effects of analgesics, attention from family, and avoidance of aversive activities such as unpleasant work or home responsibilities. In most instances, pathophysiological processes were ignored in this model in favor of explicitly behavioral processes, whether the patient were free of biological threat, as in the case of "benign" chronic pain, or suffering from progressive, painful disorders. The aim of treatment became to render pain patients as capable of displaying normal well behavior as possible. The primary objective in this approach was not to modify pain experience, although changes in behavior may produce this outcome, and subjective reports of painful distress were of little or no interest (Sternbach, 1984).

Turner and Chapman (1982b) and Fordyce *et al.* (1985) have recently reviewed the behavior modification treatment literature and concluded that the effectiveness of altering social reinforcement contingencies on long-term pain behavior has been demonstrated for carefully selected patients. Studies have reported significant decreases in amount of medication used and increases in activity levels and well behavior with follow-ups between 5 months and 8 years (Anderson, Cole, Gullickson, Hudgens, & Robert, 1977; Cairns, Thomas, Mooney, & Pace, 1976; Fordyce, Fowler, Lehmann, DeLateur, Sand, & Treischmann, 1973; Roberts & Reinhardt, 1980). Roberts (1983) observed that it is known that many pain patients improve significantly simply through withdrawal of all medications. He maintains that pain treatment programs should aim to withdraw rather than reduce or alter medications, and that solely operant techniques are needed, with no other psychological or complimentary adjuncts. This extreme position deserves respect because of the success of the approach, but not all behavior psychologists would agree with this restrictive focus on behavior.

Behavioral methods broadly defined are now used in virtually every legitimate pain treatment program (Fordyce *et al.*, 1985). When one considers that these methods are usually applied to patients who have shown little or no improvement despite traditional medical and surgical interventions, the outcomes reported appear quite favorable.

Cognitive-Behavioral Methods

Cognitive methods attempt to modify thought processes and thereby attenuate pain. The assumption is that expectations and ideas influence what people feel; thus, fears and negative thoughts increase anxiety, depression, and pain. Changes in cognitions and the focus of attention are viewed as capable of potentiating changes in pain experience and behavior (McCaul & Mallot, 1984; Tan, 1982; Turk, Meichenbaum, & Genest, 1983). A variety of techniques have been developed including provision of preparatory information prior to a medical procedure such as surgery, hypnosis, and cognitive coping strategies including distraction and imagery. Stress-inoculation training provides a comprehensive approach from this perspective by providing a conceptual framework for understanding pain experience, instruction, and practice with a variety of coping mechanisms such as relaxation, deep breathing, distraction, imagery strategies, and techniques for improving self-statements (Meichenbaum, 1977).

The broad range of cognitive methods have been applied to both acute and chronic pain; the area has been reviewed recently by McCaul and Mallot (1984), Tan (1982), Turk *et al.* (1983), and Turner and Chapman (1982b).

Turk (1982) reviewed controlled laboratory studies of cognitive coping skills. Typically, a group given instructions to employ a specific strategy had been compared with a no-treatment group or a group instructed in a different strategy. The primary skills taught have focused on imagery techniques and of diversion attention. Turk concluded that the view that any cognitive control strategy would increase coping had received limited support, at least in the laboratory situation. Although there is some evidence that imagery strategies are more effective than methods in which imagery is not employed, results remain inconclusive.

Some interesting findings have emerged in which the utility of certain techniques appears to be a function of individual differences. Thus, cognitive interventions may be differentially effective depending on personality variables such as coping style (Andrew, 1970), perceived locus of control (Strickland, 1978), and physical-danger trait anxiety (Kim, 1978).

A complicating factor in determining efficacy of coping strategies has been that a number of strategies have shown that, typically, individuals generate their own coping strategies spontaneously when faced with pain, so that the no-treatment groups are not "inert" (Tan, 1982). If patients do this effectively on their own, there would be little justification for behavioral psychologists to provide intervention. The limiting factor would appear to be the capacity of patients to use these self-regulatory skills in the face of distressful clinical pain. Fear, anxiety, and interpretational and situational variables would appear to be far more potent in clinical pain than laboratory analogues (Craig, 1984).

The renewed emphasis on cognitive factors provides a reminder that pain must be conceptualized from a multidimensional perspective and measurement strategies must be applied to sensory, affective, and cognitive variables at the level of subjective experience and to behavioral and physiological events at the level of direct observation. Frequently, when positive outcomes have been reported for some treatment, the investigation has been criticized because either no self-report measures of discomfort were obtained or, although objective measures such as length of hospitalization or amount of medication were lower than for the control group, subjective ratings might not be. Some reviewers take this to be an indication that the treatment is ineffective or the results inconclusive (e.g., Tan, 1982), whereas others maintain that effecting changes in subjective ratings is not an aim of their approach, and therefore their results should not be judged on that basis. The issue of adequate dependent measures for assessing pain is important. Most reviewers are now emphasizing a need for multiple outcome measures to be included in all studies.

In summary, cognitive-behavioral treatment methods are viewed as showing potential, but as yet it is not clear which techniques are effective with particular types of pain problems or patients.

Biofeedback

The aim of biofeedback techniques has been to control ostensive peripheral physiological factors responsible for generating pain. The rationale has been that through feedback of electronically monitored and amplified physiological events patients can learn to become aware of and bring under control certain processes underlying pain. On occasion, complementary operant conditioning and relaxation strategies are employed to enhance self-control. Although biofeedback has been applied to a wide range of chronic pain problems, the majority of studies evaluating its effectiveness have examined headaches.

Beyond the general principles, the application of biofeedback has been based on assumptions about the processes mediating each specific form of pain. For example, tension headache has been treated with electromyogram (EMG) biofeedback from the facial and head musculature because sustained muscle contraction has been viewed as responsible. Two methods of biofeedback have been employed with migraine sufferers, based on quite different rationales: (a) cephalic vasomotor responses have been used to train vasoconstriction of the temporal artery on the assumption that migraine headache results from cranial and cerebral vasculature dilation, and (b) finger-tip temperature feedback has been used to achieve hand-warming in the interest of reducing sympathetic activity, on the assumption that excess sympathetic activity causes migraine.

A number of review articles on biofeedback therapy in the past few years (Jessup, 1984; Jessup, Neufeld, & Mersky, 1979; Philips, 1983; Turner & Chapman, 1982a; Zitman, 1983) have challenged the specific effects of biofeedback as a physiological technique. Current reviews acknowledge the efficacy of the clinical application of biofeedback techniques for treatment of headache but conclude that there is little evidence to support beliefs about the specific effects upon which the applications are predicated. If biofeedback techniques were in fact treating underlying physiological causes of pain, there would be demonstrable correlations between physiological changes and symptom changes. Many lines of investigation have been unable to demonstrate correlations of this type. Indeed, the evidence indicates that biofeedback effects may be mainly nonspecific.

For example, EMG feedback recorded from the frontalis muscle to treat tension headaches has been based on the assumption that these headaches are caused by contractions of the face, scalp, and neck muscles. EMG biofeedback training has been demonstrated to be effective compared with no treatment or untrained self-relaxation (e.g., Haynes, Griffin, Mooney, & Parise, 1975). However, it appears that EMG activity at one muscle site does not necessarily generalize automatically to other muscles involved in the pain syndrome (Nuechterlein & Holroyd, 1980).

There is little evidence for a direct relationship between tension in the frontalis muscle and reported headache activity. In fact, varying degrees of association between EMG level and headache have been found (e.g., Epstein, Abel, Collins, Parker, & Cinciripini, 1978; Haynes *et al.*, 1975; Nuechterlein & Holroyd, 1980; Philips & Hunter, 1982). There appears to be strong evidence that EMG biofeedback training is no more effective than relaxation training in decreasing tension headaches (Jessup, 1984; Turner & Chapman, 1982a; Zitman, 1983).

Bidirectional treatment designs that attempt to change the target physiological parameter in opposite directions have demonstrated that at least some biofeedback effects are nonspecific. For example, Andrasik and Holroyd (1980) provided EMG feedback training designed to decrease frontalis muscle tension in one treatment group, to increase frontalis muscle tension in another group, and to stabilize frontalis muscle tension in a third; a no-treatment group also was included. All three treatment groups showed equivalent substantial improvement in tension headaches at 3-month follow-up. They were equally better than the no-treatment group. This was a particularly well-controlled study, as built-in checks demonstrated that the subjects had acquired frontalis muscle control as trained for their treatment group. The physiological assumption on which the rationale for frontalis muscle feedback has been based is that only frontalis EMG decreases should relieve headache. The fact that training *increases* in frontalis tension have been found to be equally effective in biofeedback treatment of muscle contraction headache conclusively demonstrates that the biofeedback effect depends upon more than the putative muscle contractions. Hence the nonspecific expression is used, and the physiological model that had provided the treatment rationale now is deemed to be inadequate. Thus, learned reduction of EMG activity appears to play little specific role in outcomes obtained with biofeedback. Treatment effects appear to be due to other factors not included in the physiological model. A broader formulation of pain incorporating subjective, behavioral, and contextual considerations would have more promise (Philips, 1983).

A further example of two physiologically conflicting procedures that have both been reported as effective concerns techniques designed to treat migraine headaches. Whereas hand warming is specifically aimed at decreasing sympathetic activity, temporal artery constriction requires increased sympathetic activity. Success in ameliorating migraines has been reported for each of these procedures, despite the fact that they are physiologically antagonistic (Jessup, 1984). As both methods appear to be effective for reducing migraines, despite contradictory assumptions behind them, the effects of one or both of these biofeedback techniques must be nonspecific as defined above. Jessup *et al.* (1979) reviewed 28 studies of hand-temperature biofeedback for treatment of migraine headaches and concluded, in summary, that they failed to demonstrate specific benefits. Reductions in migraine symptoms were apparently attributable to nonspecific features of the experience. In contrast, evidence has indicated that cephalic vasomotor response feedback may be more directly effective for migraine (e.g., Bild & Adams, 1980; Friar & Beatty, 1976). Turner and Chapman (1982a) concluded that more controlled group outcome studies were needed to establish whether success with this technique is due to more than nonspecific factors. Undoubtedly, greater attention to the biological, psychological, and social bases for migraine will render the origins of the disorder and the treatment effects less nonspecific.

One important consideration in evaluating biofeedback as a treatment has been that although arguments for the physiological origins of the disorders may prove invalid, biofeedback may serve as an effective form of relaxation training for certain patient subgroups. In addition, Qualls and Sheehan (1981) have suggested that person–treatment interaction studies are needed. Personality and individual difference variables have been suggested as predictors of treatment success (e.g., Zitman, 1983). For example, Corrobles, Cardona, and Santacreu (1981) identified a large group of chronic headache sufferers who were responsive simply to headache recording and a smaller group who were not. For this latter group EMG biofeedback was more beneficial. Presumably, this variance arose from patient differences in perception or expectation of efficacy of the treatment alternatives.

It is noteworthy that research on the effectiveness of biofeedback strategies has had a substantial impact on clinical practice. The application of EEG biofeedback to the treatment of headache is a case in point. Zitman (1983) reviewed evidence indicating that, contrary to earlier expectations, EEG alpha levels were related to ocular motor changes rather than reflecting a specific relaxation state and were not related to pain sensitivity. Thus, alpha EEG biofeedback was not found to be promising in pain management and is rarely used.

Turner and Chapman (1982a) concluded that the potential for widespread applications of biofeedback in management of chronic pain may have been overoptimistic. On the other hand, Jessup (1984) points out that in the long run the most important contribution of biofeedback research has been to emphasize the potency of nonspecific treatments in pain management.

Childbirth

The joint efforts of prepared childbirth trainers in collaboration with obstetricians and anesthetists has resulted in considerable progress toward the common goal of achieving physical safety for the mother and infant and providing psychological fulfillment for the mother. Psychological techniques for pain management during labor have been credited with reduced use of analgesic and anesthetic medication, significant decreases in length of labor, and a lower incidence of obstetric interventions such as forceps deliveries, episiotomies, and cesarian section (for reviews see Beck & Hall, 1978; Genest, 1981; Turk *et al.*, 1983).

However, assumptions behind prepared childbirth training must be examined in order to evaluate and place in perspective the actual value and role of psychological methods for reducing labor pain. Bonica (1980, 1984) has been in the forefront of efforts to bring a multidisciplinary and broad conception of pain to bear on the problem of pain during childbirth.

Many proponents of natural childbirth have maintained that labor is inherently painless and argue that when it does occur it is a reflection of modern cultural and environmental factors (Dick-Read, 1953; Lamaze, 1956). Their position has been that because childbirth is a natural process, it must be painless, and when pain occurs it has been learned through fear and tension. This view is based on the assumptions that: (a) because animals show no evidence of pain during labor, therefore pain in women has been learned, and (b) women in primitive cultures have painless births. Both assumptions are wrong (Melzack, 1984).

A review of parturition in nonhuman primates presents evidence of significant pain and discomfort. Because of structural anatomical differences between four-legged animals and the upright human female, the entire process of birth is far more complex in humans (Beischer & MacKay, 1976). Moreover, studies of innervation of the human uterus, pelvic floor, and perineum show conclusively that during intense contractions and stretching, pain production can be assumed to occur, rather than the reverse (Bonica, 1984; Krantz, 1959). Melzack (1984), in considering studies of primitive cultures, concluded that labor pain was experienced by all women in all cultures and, moreover, it is often extremely severe. Melzack, Taenzer, Feldman, and Kinch (1981) found that average ratings for labor pain were higher than those reported by patients with other forms of chronic and acute pain known to be severe, although there was a wide range in pain scores. Because of a positive association between menstrual and labor pain, it has been suggested that women who suffer severe labor pain may produce excessive prostaglandins, known to trigger uterine contractions (Marx, 1979; Melzack, 1984). Bonica (e.g., 1984) has repeatedly maintained that labor is often extemely painful. Moreover, he has described the physiological by-products of prolonged severe pain, which can be dangerous to women with cardiovascular problems, and to the high-risk fetus during protracted complicated deliveries. Pain of uterine contractions is a powerful ventilatory stimulus, resulting in hyperventilation followed by transient periods of hypoventilation, which may then result in significant repercussions on the fetus in the form of heart rate decelerations. The degree of increase of maternal cardiac output is influenced by pain. Increases in heart rate and systolic blood pressure are tolerated by healthy women but may pose risks for those suffering from heart disease, toxemia, hypertension, or severe anemia.

Of course, one assumption of prepared childbirth advocates is clearly correct, that psychological methods designed to reduce fear and anxiety should theoretically also decrease pain. The literature abounds with articles suggesting ameliorative effects of preparative information, relaxation, distraction, and other techniques during labor (see Genest, 1981). Turk *et al.*, (1983) have discussed the problems inherent in drawing conclusions from these studies, as, of necessity, they are uncontrolled. The most consistent finding reported has been that trained mothers receive less medication than untrained. However, this may be due to motivational factors reflecting self-selection in the groups. In the absence of random assignment to experimental and control groups, which is unavoidable in this clinical setting, clear-cut cause-and-effect statements have been precluded in this area. Factors such as maternal anxiety level, socioeconomic status, and reaction to pregnancy and childbirth, which are known to be related to childbirth experience (Klusman, 1975; Zax, Sameroff, & Farnu, 1975), have not been incorporated into studies of efficacy of prepared childbirth techniques, and a great deal remains to be done.

Melzak (1984) has provided data indicating that although prepared childbirth training has been consistently associated with lower levels of pain, as reported on the McGill Pain Questionnaire, the levels reported still remain high. Thus, trained women report less pain than untrained, but dramatic reductions in pain have not been evident, even though they were provided by a self-selected sample of patients with positive attitudes. Melzack concluded that the fact that current training procedures show statistically significant effects on pain is encouraging and indicates that psychological intervention is valuable. However, the small reduction in pain suggests a need for further development of these procedures.

Concerns have been raised that childbirth preparation classes which suggest that painless labor is possible if techniques are used properly may be doing a disservice to women. By instilling unrealistic expectations of labor, which are then violated by the actual labor experience, they may lead women to feel personally responsible for failure. Need for medication or obstetric procedures thereby implicate women as unsuccessful in their endeavor, which would have been otherwise if she had "done it right." Guilt and feelings of helplessness may ensue (Stewart, 1982). Lumley and Astbury (1980) emphasized the need to provide preparatory childbirth information which will match what actually happens during labor. They found that childbirth classes typically provided unrealistic expectations regarding pain. As the pain model provided in classes presents pain as a form of psychological failure, the women judged their labor pain accordingly in this context. Profound negative attitudes toward themselves, childbirth, and the medical staff were described as the outcome of such "failure."

Melzack (1984) concluded that the emphasis of the prepared childbirth movement on removing pain has been misleading and unfortunate. More accurate recognition of the physiological bases of labor pain and the wide range of individual differences in the course of labor is an essential next step for trainers in childbirth preparation. Only then can psychological techniques be implemented in such a way that they can be responsive to and useful for optimizing actual rather than idealized labor and childbirth experiences. Nevertheless, the movement is in an excellent position to incorporate advances in psychological methods for acute pain management, in training coping strategies for labor pain, and in teaching adaptive responses to anxiety and stress in a manner that is compatible with obstetric management by medical personnel.

Biological Mechanisms in Pain

There would appear to be advantages to examining our current understanding of basic biological systems in pain to identify limits on the potential for behavioral intervention.

The prospects for direct intervention with neural processes modulating pain would seem least likely at the level of the primary afferent receptor. Noxious mechanical, thermal, or chemical stimuli activate injury-sensitive receptors (nociceptors) that are free nerve endings. Nociceptors have no special structure for detecting injury. The traditional view of morphologically specific receptors beneath each sensory spot on the skin assigned to each of the four modalities of touch, heat, cold, and pain has not been supported by physiological studies. However, the assumption that skin receptors have specialized physiological properties remains valid, but not in the modality-specific sense. Rather, receptors may generate different temporal patterns of nerve impulses as a function of threshold to mechanical distortion, threshold to negative and positive temperature change, threshold to chemical change, rate of adaptation to stimulation, size of receptor field, duration after-discharge, and possible interrelationships among these variables (Melzack & Wall, 1982).

Afferent nerve fibers are classified in three main groups: A, B, and C. Class A fibers are myelinated and larger in diameter than those in classes B and C. Approximately 10%–25% of A-delta fibers (which are thinly myelinated) carry noxious impulses, initiated by strong stimuli which are potentially or frankly damaging to tissues. Approximately 20%–50% of class C fibers (slow-conducting and unmyelinated) respond to innocuous stimulation, the remainder to noxious stimuli (Chapman & Bonica, 1983). There are C "polymodal fibers" that respond to pressure, heat, and chemicals. However, any nerve fiber hit hard enough and fast enough will give off an injury discharge (Melzack & Wall, 1982).

It is interesting that the two classes of peripheral receptors cause subjectively different pain. Stimulation of A-delta nociceptive fibers results in well-localized, sharp, distinct pain that is not particularly persistent but is immediately associated with the injury. C-fiber activation is dull, poorly localized, and persistent and arises slowly after injury. Qualitative differences between these two types of pains have been related not only to the peripheral nociceptors but also to spinothalamic pathways and higher centers (Dubner, 1980).

Perl (1976) reported that repeated noxious stimulation lowers the threshold of nociceptors, so eventually *innocuous* stimulation can cause their activation, resulting in pain and hyperalgesia. He found that, unlike most sensory receptors, which habituate with repeated activation, repetitive stimulation of polymodal nociceptors increases activity and decreases firing threshold. This kind of data may have far-reaching implications for understanding some features of chronic pain.

There are many paradoxes yet to be explained (Chapman & Bonica, 1983). For example, one perplexing problem to neurophysiologists is the differences in the nature of the adequate stimulus necessary for nociception between cutaneous, deep, and visceral organs, despite the fact that the same sensory end organs serve the skin and visceral organs. Another puzzle is the existence of clinically significant pain in which nociception from peripheral receptors plays no role. Chapman and Bonica describe classical trigeminal neuralgia, an excruciatingly painful syndrome of repeated paroxysmal unilateral episodes of facial pain. This pain cannot be aroused by injurious stimulation such as pinprick, but rather can be triggered with light touch, such as drawing a cottonball across the skin. Phantom limb pain similarly defies explanation from what is known about peripheral neurophysiology. Amputation at higher levels not only does not cure the pain but can actually make it worse. Improvement has been achieved with electrical or vibratory stimulation of the stump. Chapman and Bonica have emphasized that the complexity of such neurological disorders underscores the importance of the fact that rigid distinctions between organic and psychogenic pain should be abandoned. Findings have been reported recently on mechanisms that may be involved in central nervous system pathobiology causing pain, in the absence of peripheral nociception, referred to as "deafferentation pain" (Zimmerman, 1983).

Endogenous Pain Modulation

The microenvironment of the nociceptor consists of a complex biochemical milieu, as well as smooth muscle, blood capillaries, and efferent sympathetic nerve fibers. These may undergo pathophysiological changes through a wide diversity of possible mechanisms that may influence excitability of the nociceptor (Zimmerman, 1983). Chemical substances have been identified such as H^+ ions, serotonin, bradykinin, and prostaglandins which occur endogenously and excite or sensitize nociceptors. The action of these algesic substances on nociceptors is complex. For example, excitation of muscle nociceptors by bradykinin is greatly increased if serotonin or prostaglandin E^2 is simultaneously present. It has been hypothesized that these and other facilitatory chemical interactions play a role in chronic pain (Zimmerman, 1983). Substance P, released from some sensory nerve endings, has been proposed to be another factor in pain referred to as neurogenic inflammation. Excitation of certain nociceptive fibers results in release of substance P, which causes vasodilation and local edema (Lembeck & Gamse, 1982).

Nociceptive afferents, which have cell bodies located in the spinal ganglia, enter the dorsal horn posteriorly and terminate by making synaptic contact with the cells of the successive layers, or laminae, I, II, III, and V, of the dorsal horn of the spinal cord (Kerr, 1980; Melzack & Dennis, 1978). From the peripheral spinal nerves, nociceptive sensory information is transmitted to dorsal horn cells and then to higher parts of the neuraxis through ascending neural systems. In contrast to the outdated concept of straight-through pain transmission, it is now evident beyond any doubt that there is an extraordinary degree of modulation all along the course of transmission of impulses. Modulation occurs at the first synapse in the dorsal horn and at every level of the neuraxis thereafter. Studies have shown that, contrary to the traditional view of the dorsal horn as a simple relay station, it is actually a highly complex structure containing many varieties of neurons and synaptic arrangements. A great deal of sensory processing takes place at the level of the dorsal horn, achieved through complex interaction of excitatory and inhibitory influences coming from the periphery, adjacent neurons, the brain, and various other parts of the central nervous system (Bonica, 1974).

At the time that Melzack and Wall (1965) proposed the existence of a pain modulating system in their gate control theory, evidence for descending control of pain was limited. Subsequently, systems of descending control have been identified by anatomical, physiological, and pharmacological means (see Willis, 1982). It is not yet known to what extent these different systems cooperate and interact or how they are normally activated.

Focal electrical stimulation of specific discrete brain sites results in behavioral changes to noxious stimuli, namely, suppression of pain-related behavior (Terman *et al.*, 1984). Many of the brain structures from which analgesia and descending inhibition can be induced by focal electrical stimulation are rich in opiate receptors (Zimmerman, 1983).

Discovery of endogenous opioid peptides and description of specific pain-modulating neural networks in the brain stem and spinal cord have resulted in tremendous progress in understanding pain control mechanisms of the central nervous system (Kosterlitz, 1983). It is now clear that the brain produces a variety of morphine-like peptide substances. The main types are enkephalins and endorphins. The binding of enkephalins to specific receptors appears to inhibit release of substance P, which may transmit noxious impulses to higher brain centers. Enkephalins have been viewed as acting mainly at the spinal cord level to inhibit transmission of nociception, but they have also been found at higher points of the central nervous system such as in the hypothalamus, periaqueductal grey, and nucleus raphe magnus.

Beta-endorphin has attracted particular attention for clinical research as its effects are longer lasting than those of the enkephalins and it is believed to act mainly at the periaqueductal grey area, where it appears to initiate activity in a descending inhibitory system (Chapman & Bonica, 1983). Although there have been reports that certain types of chronic pain are associated with low levels of beta-endorphin in cerebrospinal fluid (Terenius, 1984), conclusions so far are tentative. However, this appears to be a promising area of research that may in the long run have important implications for understanding and treatment of acute and chronic pain.

In addition to the endogenous opioid-mediated system activated by longer duration, relatively higher intensity pain stimuli, a less well characterized non-opioid-mediated analgesia system has been identified. This system can be activated by nonpainful stressors and by noxious stimuli of short duration (Devor, 1984; Levine, 1984).

There is currently considerable interest in the effects of physical and psychological stressors on central and peripheral neurochemistry. The importance of the pituitary-adrenal and sympatho-adrenal systems in adaptive response to stress has long been recognized (Selye, 1956). Participation of hormonal systems in stress-induced analgesia appears likely. Relationships between neurochemical and behavioral consequences of nociception and stress also are being identified (Tricklebank & Curzon, 1984).

Although biological and psychological dimensions of pain are conceptualized as only representing different facets of behavior in the active organism, an ontogenetic perspective on pain permits isolation of the relative impact of inherited genetic as opposed to socialization determinants of pain expression (Craig, 1980, 1984; Owen, 1984). It is now unreasonable to conclude that infants are relatively insensitive to pain in the early days and weeks of life. Systematic observation of motoric and cry behavior when neonates are subjected to the heel lance incision for diagnostic blood sampling purposes discloses reaction patterns that are readily identified as expressive of pain (Grunau & Craig, 1987). Even at this stage of life pain does not represent a reflexive, sensory-specific reaction pattern. The pattern of expression varied systematically with the state of behavioral arousal. Thus, for example, infants who were wide awake and inactive were substantially more responsive than those who were alert and active or in different states of sleep. Even neonates display a capacity at this early stage of development for ongoing functional activity to modulate pain reactions. In bioevolutionary terms, it would be adaptive for newborns to be sensitive to pain and responsive to variations in context and to have a highly developed signal system for communicating distress to caretakers.

Reactions to immunization injections also vary systematically between the 1st and 2nd years of life (Craig, McMahon, Morison, & Zaskow, 1984). Children less than a year of age reacted in a manner that was more spontaneous, global, and linked to the actual time of the injection. In contrast, children aged 13 to 24 months were characterized as displaying more anticipatory distress, descriptive language, and voluntary, self-protective movements. Systematic description of the progression of changes in pain expression during normal development, as well as accounts of what constitutes significant deviation from normal development, will be of considerable usefulness to clinicians.

Conclusions

Discovery of the existence of endogenous pain control mechanisms in the central nervous system demanded a reappraisal of concepts of the relationships between so-called psychological and physiological phenomena and of the rationales for pain management that have prevailed. It has become clear that vestiges of mind–body dualism in approaches to clinical pain must be abandoned. For example, concepts of placebo effects as being "in the mind" must be revised in the light of evidence that analgesic effects of placebo may be mediated by release of endogenous opioids (Levine, 1984). For biological beings, all cognitive representation of necessity has some physical analogue.

Most psychological interventions for pain management include relaxation training in some form and have been very successful (Turner & Chapman, 1982a). Elicitation of the relaxation response results in physiological changes thought to reflect an integrated hypothalamic function (Benson, Pomerantz, & Kutz, 1984). Physiological changes of the relaxation response are consistent with decreased sympathetic nervous system activity. The neuromuscular mechanisms whereby relaxation produces analgesia (biochemical or neurophysiological) remain unclear as yet. It has been proposed that relaxation may evoke an endorphinergic mechanism; however, attempts to test this hypothesis have been inconclusive (Benson *et al.*, 1984). Activity in endogenous pain control systems may ultimately account for much of the observed wide individual differences and variability in pain experience, behavior, and clinical response of pain patients (Levine, 1984).

Traditionally, pharmacological pain research has been concerned with developing drugs the "true" action of which is analgesic. This model attributes analgesia solely to drug action, placebo responses or other extraneous psychological variables representing merely "noise" to be eliminated. Chen and Dworkin (1983) recently proposed an alternative model, namely, that pharmacological analgesia can be synergistically enhanced through psychological mechanisms. Thus, treatment effects reflect drug action plus psychological analgesia. Their work on modification of nitrous oxide analgesia through provision of information or suggestion prior to treatment supported this model. In treatment of intractable pain in cancer patients, drug action has been found to be significantly more effective in care units providing psychological support (Mount, 1984). Guided self-hypnosis appears to be a useful adjunct to medical care in pain syndromes with specific organic etiologies such as changing burn dressings over long periods of time, repeated bone marrow aspirations, and cancer pain, particularly with children (Katz *et al.*, 1982).

Suggestions regarding mechanisms for mediation of psychological interventions, that is, the way in which psychological factors may influence the physiology of pain, are emerging from a number of lines of research. Anxiety, tension, depression, and perceived lack of control have been shown to modulate production of stress hormones, neurotransmitters, and autonomic arousal (Turk, *et al.*, 1983).

Currently, the issue is no longer whether psychological treatments of pain are effective; it has long been established that psychological therapies do help pain patients (Sternbach, 1984). Now it is necessary to examine which treatment approaches are more effective than others, and for which patients. Relationships between psychological and physiological or biochemical transmission will be of interest and importance in understanding mechanisms of pain control. Although current emphasis on psychological and environmental influences on chronic pain is overdue, it must be emphasized that there is a very wide diversity of chronic pain syndromes. Widespread acceptance of the suggestion by Black (1980) that the term *chronic pain syndrome* be limited to persistent pain mainly related to operant mechanisms may mislead and confuse some practitioners into considering all chronic pain to arise from psychological or operant factors (Bonica, 1983). Bonica (1984) has recently expressed concern that care must be taken lest grave injustice be done to millions of patients with chronic pain due to arthritis, cancer, visceral pain, and a host of other disorders in which persistent pain is due to pathological processes that cause activation and/or dysfunction of the nociceptive system.

References

Anderson, T. P., Cole, T. M., Gullickson, G., Hudgens, A., & Robert, A. H. (1977). Behavior modifications of chronic pain: A treatment program by a multidisciplinary team. *Clinical Orthopsychiatry, 129*, 96–100.

Andrasik, F., & Holroyd, K. A. (1980). A test of specific and non-specific effects in the biofeedback treatment of tension headache. *Journal of Consulting and Clinical Psychology, 48*, 575–586.

Andrew, J. M. (1970). Recovery from surgery, with and without preparatory instruction, for three coping styles. *Journal of Personality and Social Psychology, 15,* 223–226.

Beck, N. C., & Hall, D. (1978). Natural childbirth: A review and analysis. *Obstetrics and Gynecology, 52,* 371–379.

Beecher, H. K. (1959). *Measurement of subjective responses: Qualitative effects of drugs.* New York: Oxford University Press.

Beischer, N. A., & MacKay, E. V. (1976). *Obstetrics and the newborn.* Philadelphia: Saunders.

Benedetti, C., & Murphy, T. (1985). Non-pharmacological methods of acute pain control. In G. Smith & B. Covino (Eds.), *Acute pain* (pp. 257–269).London: Butterworth.

Benson, H., Pomeranz, B., & Kutz, H. (1984). The relaxation response and pain. In P. D. Wall & R. Melzack (Eds.), *Textbook of pain* (pp. 817–822). Edinburgh: Churchill Livingstone.

Bild, R., & Adams, H. (1980). Modifications of migraine headaches by cephalic blood volume pulse and EMG biofeedback. *Journal of Consulting and Clinical Psychology, 48,* 51–57.

Black, R. G. (1980). The clinical syndrome of chronic pain. In L. K. Y. Ng & J. J. Bonica (Eds.), *Pain, discomfort and humanitarian care.* Amsterdam: Elsevier.

Bonica, J. J. (1974). Neurophysiologic and pathologic aspects of acute and chronic pain. *Archives of Surgery, 112,* 750–761.

Bonica, J. J. (1980). Pain research and therapy: Past and current status and future needs. In L. K. Y. Ng & J. J. Bonica (Eds.), *Pain, discomfort and humanitarian care* (pp. 1–46). New York: Elsevier.

Bonica, J. J. (1983). Pain research and therapy: Achievements of the past and challenges of the future. In J. J. Bonica, U. Lindbolm, & A. Iggo (Eds.), *Advances in pain research and therapy* (Vol. 5, pp. 1–36). New York: Raven Press.

Bonica, J. J. (1984). Pain research and therapy: Recent advances and future needs. In L. Kruger & J. C. Liebskind (Eds.), *Advances in pain research and therapy* (Vol. 6, pp. 1–22). New York: Raven Press.

Bonica, J. J., Lindbolm, U., & Iggo, A. (Eds.). (1983). *Advances in pain research and therapy. Proceedings of the Third World Congress on Pain.* New York: Raven Press.

Carrobles, J. A., Cardona, A., & Santacreu, J. (1981). Shaping and generalization procedures in the EMG-biofeedback treatment of tension headaches. *British Journal of Clinical Psychology, 20,* 49–56.

Cairns, D., Thomas, L., Mooney, V., & Pace, B. J. (1976). A comprehensive treatment approach to chronic low back pain. *Pain, 2,* 301–308.

Chapman, C. R., & Bonica, J. J. (1983). *Acute pain.* Kalamazoo: Upjohn.

Chen, A. C. N., & Dworkin, S. F. (1983). Cognitive synergism of pharmacological analgesia: A new focus for analgesic treatment. In J. J. Bonica, U. Lindblom, & A. Iggo (Eds.), *Advances in pain research and therapy* (Vol. 5, pp. X). New York: Raven Press.

Craig, K. D. (1980). Ontogenetic and cultural influences on the expression of pain in man. In H. W. Kosterlitz & L. Y. Terenius (Eds.), *Pain and society* (pp. 37–52). Weinheim: Verlag Chemie.

Craig, K. (1983). Modeling and social learning factors in chronic pain. In J. J. Bonica, U. Lindblom, & A. Iggo (Eds.), *Advances in pain research and therapy* (Vol. 5, pp. 813–326). New York: Raven Press.

Craig, K. D. (1984). Psychology of pain. *Postgraduate Medical Journal, 60* 835–840.

Craig, K. D., McMahon, R. J., Morison, J. D., & Zaskow, C. (1984). Developmental changes in infant pain expression during immunization injections. *Social Science and Medicine, 19,* 1331–1338.

Devor, M. (1984). Pain and 'state'-induced analgesia: An introduction. In M. D. Tricklebank

& G. Curzon (Eds.), *Stress-induced analgesia* (pp. 1–18). New York: Wiley.

Dick-Read, G. (1944). *Childbirth without fear*. New York: Harper.

Dubner, R. (1980). Peripheral and central mechanisms of pain. In L. K. Y. Ng & J. J. Bonica (Eds.), *Pain, discomfort and humanitarian care* (pp. 61–82). New York: Elsevier.

Epstein, L. H., Abel, G. G., Collins, F., Parker, L., & Cinciripini, P. M. (1978). The relationship between frontalis muscle activity and self-reports of headache pain. *Behavior Research and Therapy, 16*, 153–160.

Fields, H. L., & Basbaum, A. I. (1984). Endogenous pain control mechanisms. In P. D. Wall & R. Melzak (Eds.), *Textbook of pain*. New York: Churchill Livingstone.

Fordyce, W. E. (1976). *Behavioral methods for chronic pain and illness*. St. Louis: C. J. Mosby.

Fordyce, W. E., Fowler, R. S., Lehmann, J. F., & DeLateur, B. J. (1968). Some implications of learning in problems of chronic pain. *Journal of Chronic Diseases, 21*, 179–190.

Fordyce, W. E., Fowler, R. S., Lehmann, J. F., DeLateur, B. J., Sand, P. L., & Treischmann, R. B. (1973). Operant conditioning in the treatment of chronic pain. *Archives of Physical Medicine and Rehabilitation, 54*, 399–409.

Fordyce, W. E., Roberts, A. H., & Sternbach, R. A. (1985). The behavioral management of chronic pain: A response to critics. *Pain, 22*, 113–125.

Friar, L., & Beatty, J. (1976). Migraine: Management by trained control of vasoconstriction. *Journal of Consulting and Clinical Psychology, 44*, 46–53.

Genest, M. (1981). Preparation of childbirth: A selected review of evidence for efficacy. *Journal of Obstetric, Gynecologic and Neonatal Nursing, 10*, 82–85.

Grunau, R. V. E., & Craig, K. D. (1987). *Cry and facial behavior during induced pain in neonates. Pain, 28*, 395–410.

Haynes, S., Griffin, P., Mooney, D., & Parise, M. (1975). Electromyographic biofeedback and relaxation instruction in treatment of muscle contraction headaches. *Behavior Therapy, 6*, 672–678.

Jessup, B. A. (1984). Biofeedback, In P. D. Wall & R. Melzak (Eds.), *Textbook of pain* (pp. 776–786). New York: Churchill Livingstone.

Jessup, B. A., Neufeld, R. W. J., & Mersky, H. (1979). Biofeedback therapy for headache and other pain: An evaluative review. *Pain, 7*, 225–270.

Katz, E. R., Sharp, B., Kellerman, J., Marston, A. R., Hershman, J. J., & Siegel, S. E. (1982). Endorphin immunoreactivity and acute behavioral distress in children with leukemia. *Journal of Nervous and Mental Disease, 170*, 72–77.

International Association for the Study of Pain. (1979). Pain terms: A list with definitions and notes on usage. *Pain, 6*, 249–252.

Kerr, F. W. L. (1980). The structural basis of pain: Circuitry and pathways. In L. K. Y. Ng, & J. J. Bonica (Eds.), *Pain, discomfort and humanitarian care* (pp. 49–60). New York: Elsevier.

Kim. S. (1978). Preparatory information, anxiety, and pain: A contingency model and its nursing implications. *Dissertation Abstracts International, 39*, 2224B–2225B.

Klusman, L. E. (1975). Reduction of pain in childbirth by the alleviation of anxiety during pregnancy. *Journal of Consulting and Clinical Psychology, 43*, 162–165.

Kosterlitz, H. W. (1983). Opiod peptides and pain: An update. In J. J. Bonica *et al.* (Eds.), *Advances in pain research and therapy* (Vol. 5). New York: Raven Press.

Krantz, K. E. (1959). Innervation of the human uterus. *Annals of the New York Academy of Science, 75*, 770–785.

Lamaze, F. (1970). *Painless childbirth: Psychoprophylactic method*. Chicago: Regnery.

Lembeck, F., & Gamse, R. (1982). In R. Porter & M. O'Connor (Eds.), *Substance P in the nervous system*. London: Pitman.

Levine, J. (1984). Pain and analgesia: The outlook for more rational treatment. *Annals of*

Internal Medicine, 100(2), 269–276.

Lumley, J., & Astbury, J. (1980). *Birth rites, birth rights: Childbirth Alternatives for Australian Parents*. Melbourne: Sphere Books.

Mahoney, M. J. (1983). Cognition, consciousness, and processes of personal change. In K. D. Craig & R. J. McMahon (Eds.), *Advances in clinical behavior therapy*. New York: Appleton-Century-Crofts.

Marx, J. L. (1979). Dysmenorrhea: Basic research leads to a rational theory. *Science, 205*, 175–176.

McCaul, K. D., & Mallot, J. M. (1984). Distraction and coping with pain. *Psychological Bulletin, 95*, 516–533.

Meichenbaum, D. H. (1977). *Cognitive-behavior modification: An integrative approach*. New York: Plenum Press.

Melzack, R. (1984). The myth of painless childbirth. *Pain, 19*, 321–337.

Melzack, R., & Dennis, S. G. (1978). Neurophysiological foundations of pain. In R. A. Sternbach (Eds.), *The psychology of pain*. New York: Raven.

Melzack, R., Taenzer, P., Feldman, P., & Kinch, R. A. (1981). Labour is still painful after prepared childbirth training. *Canadian Medical Association Journal, 125*, 357–363.

Melzack, R., & Wall, P. D. (1965). Pain mechanisms: A new theory. *Science, 50*, 971–979.

Melzack, R., & Wall, P. D. (1982). *The challenge of pain*. New York: Penguin.

Mount, B. M. (1984). Psychologist and social aspects of cancer pain. In P. D. Wall & R. Melzack (Eds.), *Textbook of pain* (pp. 460–471). Edinburgh: Churchill Livingstone.

Nuechterlein, K., & Holroyd, J. (1980). Biofeedback in the treatment of tension headache. *Archives of General Psychiatry, 37*, 866–873.

Owen, M. E. (1984). Pain in infancy: Conceptual and methodological issues. *Pain, 20*, 213–230.

Perl, E. R. (1976). Sensitization of nociceptors and its relation to sensation. In J. J. Bonica & D. Albe-Tessard (Eds.), *Advances in pain research and therapy*, (Vol. 1, pp. 17–28). New York: Raven Press.

Philips, C. (1983). In K. D. Craig & R. J. McMahon (Eds.), *Advances in clinical behavior therapy* (pp. 194–210). New York: Brunner/Mazel.

Philips, C., & Hunter, M. (1982). The psychophysiology of tension headache. *Headache, 22*, 173.

Qualls, P. J., & Sheehan, P. W. (1981). Electromyograph biofeedback as a relaxation technique: A critical appraisal and reassessment. *Psychological Bulletin, 90*, 21–42.

Roberts, A. H. (1983). Contingency management methods in the treatment of chronic pain. In J. J. Bonica, U. Lindbolm, & A. Iggo (Eds.), *Advances in pain research and therapy* (Vol. 5, pp. 789–794). New York: Raven Press.

Roberts, A. H., & Reinhardt, L. (1980). The behavioral management of chronic pain: Long-term follow-up with comparison groups. *Pain, 8*, 151–162.

Rosenthal, T. L., & Zimmerman, B. J. (1978). *Social learning and cognition*. New York: Academic Press.

Selye, H. (1956). *The stress of life*. New York: McGraw-Hill.

Sternbach, R. A. (1974). *Pain patients: Traits and treatments*. New York: Academic Press.

Sternbach, R. A. (1984). Acute versus chronic pain. In P. D. Wall & R. Melzak (Eds.), *Textbook of pain* (pp. 173–177). New York: Churchill Livingstone.

Stewart, D. E. (1982). Psychiatric symtoms following attempted natural childbirth. *Canadian Medical Association Journal, 127*, 713–716.

Strickland, B. R. (1978). Internal-external expectancies and health-related behaviors. *Journal of Consulting and Clinical Psychology, 46*, 1192–1211.

Tan, Siang-Yang. (1982). Cognitive and cognitive-behavioral methods for pain control: A selective review. *Pain, 12*, 201–228.

Terenius, L. (1984). The endogenous opioids and other central peptides. In P. D. Wall & R. Melzak (Eds.), *Textbook of pain*. New York: Churchill Livingstone.

Terman, G. W., Shavit, J. W., Lewis, J. W., Cannon, J. T., & Liebeskind, J. C. (1984). Intrinsic mechanisms of pain inhibition: Activation by stress. *Science, 226*, 1270–1277.

Tricklebank, M. D., & Curzon, G. (Eds.). (1984). *Stress-induced analgesia*. New York: Wiley.

Turk, D. C. (1982). Cognitive learning approaches in health care. In D. M. Doleys, R. L. Meredith, & A. R. Ciminero (Eds.), *Behavioral medicine: Assessment and treatment strategies*. New York: Plenum Press.

Turk, D. C., Meichenbaum, D., & Genest, M. (1983). *Pain and behavioral medicine: A cognitive-behavioral perspective*. New York: Guilford Press.

Turner, J. A., & Chapman, C. R. (1982a). Psychological intervention for chronic pain: A critical review. I. Relaxation training and biofeedback. *Pain, 12*, 1–22.

Turner, J. A., & Chapman, C. R. (1982b). Psychological intervention for chronic pain: A critical review. II. Operant conditioning, hypnosis and cognitive-behavioral therapy. *Pain, 12*, 22–46.

Wall, P. D., & Melzak, R. (1984). *The textbook of pain*. New York: Churchill Livingstone.

Willis, W. D. (1982). Control of nociceptive transmission in the spinal cord. In D. Ottoson (Ed.), *Progress in sensory physiology* (Vol. 3, pp. 1–159). Berlin: Springer-Verlag.

Zax, M., Sameroff, A. J., & Farnum, J. E. (1975). Childbirth education, maternal attitudes and delivery. *American Journal of Obstetrics and Gynecology, 123*, 185–190.

Zimmerman, M. (1983). Introduction to neurobiological mechanisms of pain and pain therapy. In T. Yokota & R. Dubner (Eds.) *Current topics in pain research and therapy*. Amsterdam: Excerpta Medica.

Zitman, F. G. (1983). Biofeedback and chronic pain. In J. J. Bonica, U. Lindblom, & A. Iggo (Eds.), *Advances in pain research and therapy* (Vol. 5, pp. 795–808). New York: Raven Press.

Chapter 11

Understanding and Preventing Relapse

Kelly D. Brownell, Edward Lichtenstein, G. Alan Marlatt, and G. Terence Wilson

This chapter examines relapse by integrating knowledge from the disorders of alcoholism, smoking, and obesity in an attempt to emphasize in a prototypical manner the overlap in etiological mechanisms and treatment rationales for disorders with powerful, underlying biological self-regulation components. Commonalities across these areas suggest at least three basic stages of behavior change: motivation and commitment, initial change, and maintenance. A distinction is made between the terms *lapse* and *relapse*, with *lapse* referring to the process (slips or mistakes) that may or may not lead to an outcome (*relapse*). The natural history of relapse is discussed, as are the consequences of relapse for patients and the professionals who treat them. Information on determi-

---

Kelly D. Brownell • Department of Psychiatry, University of Pennsylvania School of Medicine, Philadelphia, Pennsylvania 19104. *Edward Lichtenstein* • Department of Psychology, University of Oregon, and Oregon Research Institute, Eugene, Oregon 97403. *G. Alan Marlatt* • Department of Psychology, University of Washington, Seattle, Washington 98195. *G. Terence Wilson* • Department of Psychology, Rutgers University, New Brunswick, New Jersey 08854. This chapter originally appeared in *American Psychologist*, 1986, *41* (7), 765–783. The work was supported in part by Research Scientist Development Award MH00319 from NIMH and by a grant from the MacArthur Foundation to Kelly D. Brownell, Grant HL29547 to Edward Lichtenstein from MHLBI, Grant AA00259 to G. Terence Wilson from NIAAA, and Grant AA05591 to G. Alan Marlatt from NIAAA.

nants and predictors of relapse is evaluated, with the emphasis on the interaction of individual, environmental, and physiological factors. Methods of preventing relapse are proposed and are targeted to the three stages of change. Specific research needs in these areas are discussed.

The problem of relapse remains an important challenge to dealing with disorders characterized by biological self-regulation, particularly the addictive disorders. This is true for obesity (Brownell, 1982; Rodin, 1981; Stunkard & Penick, 1979; Wilson, 1980), smoking (Lando & McGovern, 1982; Lichtenstein, 1982; Ockene, Hymowitz, Sexton, & Broste, 1982; Pechacek, 1979; Shiffman, 1982), and alcoholism (Marlatt, 1983; Miller & Hester, 1980; Nathan, 1983; Nathan & Goldman, 1979).

The purpose of this chapter is to focus on relapse by integrating the perspectives of four researchers and clinicians who have worked with one or more of the addictive disorders (Brownell, 1982; Lichtenstein, 1982; Marlatt, 1983; Wilson, 1980). We discuss the natural history of relapse, its determinants and effects, and methods for prevention. We hope that our collective experience and different perspectives will aid in developing a model for evaluating and preventing relapse.

Commonalities and Differences in the Addictions

Compelling arguments can be marshaled for both commonalities and differences in the addictive disorders. Many differences exist, both among the disorders and among persons afflicted with the same disorder. For example, genetic contributions to both alcoholism (McClearn, 1981; Schuckitt, 1981) and obesity (Stunkard *et al.*, 1986) suggest separate pathways for their development. There may be key differences in the pharmacology of nicotine and alcohol (Ashton & Stepney, 1982; Best, Wainwright, Mills, & Kirkland, Chapter 4 in this volume; Gilbert, 1979; Myers, 1978; Pomerleau & Pomerleau, 1984), and food abuse fits even less neatly with concepts of physical dependency, withdrawal, and tolerance. Treatment goals also vary, with abstinence the target in some cases and moderation in others.

Individual differences within the addictions are also impressive. Variable treatment responses are an example. There are also striking differences in patterns of use. Some smokers, alcoholics, and overeaters engage in steady substance use, whereas others go on binges. Combinations of physiological, psychological, social, and environmental factors may addict different people to the same substance. Finally, as in previous chapters of this volume, we will attempt to demonstrate how different processes may govern the initiation and maintenance of the disorders.

There is also increasing emphasis on commonalities. One reason is that rates for relapse appear to similar. In 1971, Hunt, Barnett, and Branch found nearly identical patterns of relapse in alcoholics, heroin addicts, and smokers. The picture is the same today (Marlatt & Gordon, 1985). There may also be common determinants of relapse (Cummings, Gordon, & Marlatt, 1980). These factors suggest important commonalities in the addictive disorders. Progress may be aided by viewing these disorders from multiple perspectives (Levison, Gerstein, & Maloff, 1983; Marlatt & Gordon, 1985; Miller, 1980; Nathan, 1980; and as presented throughout this book).

The notion of commonalities gained support from expert panels assembled by two government agencies. The National Institute on Drug Abuse (NIDA) convened a panel of researchers in alcoholism, obesity, smoking, and drug abuse and found both conceptual and practical similarities in the areas (NIDA, 1979). Similar conclusions appeared in a more extensive report by the National Academy of Sciences (Levison *et al.*, 1983). Both reports noted the importance of relapse and suggested the utility of combining perspectives from different forms of addiction.

The question of whether the addictions are more similar than different is difficult to answer. It may be the case, for example, that there are common psychological adaptations to different physiological pressures. Nicotine dependence may be the central issue for a smoker, excessive fat cells for a dieter, and disordered alcohol metabolism for an alcoholic, but there may be common social or psychological provocations for relapse, emotional reactions to initial slips, and problems in reestablishing control. Our hope is to expand the information to be focused on relapse by considering both similarities and differences. In so doing, both conceptual and practical ideas may emerge that would not be suggested by the knowledge available in any one area.

Rates and Definition

Relapse rates for the addictions are assumed to be in the range of 50% to 90% (Hunt *et al.*, 1971; Hunt & Matarazzo, 1973; Marlatt & Gordon, 1980, 1985). This underscores the importance of the problem. However, defining specific rates is difficult. Hidden within these averages is large variability. The rates depend on characteristics of the addiction, individual variables, the success of treatment, and so forth.

The figures generally cited for relapse could overestimate or underestimate actual rates. Because most data are from clinical programs, rates are based on those people who have received formal treatment. These figures could overstate the problem because only difficult cases are seen and because only one attempt at change is studied (Schachter, 1982). Schachter notes also that persons attempting to change on their own may be more successful and may well relapse less frequently. The vast majority of persons who change do so on their own (Ockene, 1984). These data could understate the case because clinical programs are most likely to provide effective treatments. In addition, various criteria are used to define relapse. For example, relapse in alcohol studies could be defined as number of days intoxicated, number of days hospitalized or jailed, number of days of drinking out of control, or the use of any alcohol. This points to the need for standard definitions and for the study of the natural history of relapse.

Lapse and Relapse: Process Versus Outcome

There are two common definitions of relapse, each reflecting a bias regarding its nature and severity (Marlatt & Gordon, 1985). *Webster's New Collegiate Dictionary* of 1983 gives both definitions. The first is "a recurrence of symptoms of a disease after a period of improvement." This refers to an *outcome* and implies a dichotomous view because a person is either ill and has symptoms or is well and does not. The second definition is "the act or instance of backsliding, worsening, or subsiding." This focuses on a *process* and implies something less serious, perhaps a slip or mistake.

The choice of the process or outcome definition has important implications for conceptualizing, preventing, and treating relapse. We suggest that *lapse* may best describe a process, behavior, or event (Marlatt & Gordon, 1985). *Webster's* defines *lapse* as "a slight error or slip...a temporary fall esp. from a higher to a lower state." A lapse is a single event, a reemergence of a previous habit, which may or may not lead to the state of relapse. When a slip or mistake is defined as a lapse, it implies that corrective action can be taken, not that control is lost completely. There is support for this distinction in smokers (Coppotelli & Orleans, 1985; Mermelstein & Lichtenstein, 1983) and in dieters (Dubbert & Wilson, 1984). In these cases, different determinants were found for lapses (slips) and relapses.

The challenge with this approach is defining the point at which one or more lapses become a relapse. One former smoker may lose control with the first transgression, whereas another may smoke one cigarette each month and never lose control. A lapse, therefore, could be defined concretely as use of the substance in the case of smoking and alcoholism or violation of program guidelines for a dieter. The individual's *response* to these lapses determines whether relapse has occurred. This varies from person to person and may be best defined by perceived loss of control. Reliable measures do not yet exist for this assessment. Research in this area is important for the field.

The Nature and Process of Relapse

Surprisingly little is known about relapse in its natural state. Most data are from clinical programs in which different treatments are used with different populations; it is difficult, therefore, to isolate the factors that influence relapse. In addition, few researchers have done careful evaluations of patients when they are most likely to relapse, that is, after treatment has ended. Because periodic follow-ups in groups are the only contacts with patients in most studies, repeated, intensive assessments are needed. There would be great value in learning more about the nature and process of relapse.

The Need for a Natural History

A metaphor that describes traditional thought on relapse is of a person existing perilously close to the edge of a cliff. The slightest disruption can precipitate a fall from which there is no return. A person is always on the brink of relapse, ready to fall at any disturbance. There may be physiological, psychological, or social causes of the disturbances, but the outcome is just as final. The first slip creates momentum so that a complete relapse is certain.

This metaphor may be inadequate. It does not explain why a relapse occurs in the same circumstances that the person managed before. An eating binge may precipitate relapse in a dieter, but such an individual has probably recovered from similar binges in the past. A smoker may relapse after being offered a cigarette, but there are cases wherein this same person refused the cigarette or prevented the lapse from becoming a relapse. Also, the metaphor is based on observations of people who have relapsed, not of those who have not; therefore, successful recovery is seldom seen.

Information on natural history could address the question of whether the probability of relapse increases or decreases with time. If relapse occurs when treatment "wears off," the probability should increase with time. If the metaphor used above is valid, the chance of relapse should increase with time simply because more disturbances could occur. One can speculate, however, that a person learns to cope effectively as time passes and that those who "survive" beyond the initial period are those who will succeed. To the extent to which withdrawal symptoms precipitate relapse, particularly in smoking and alcoholism, the likelihood of relapse should decrease as the body adapts to the absence of the addictive substance.

It is in this context that the concept of a "safe" point arises. This is a point in time before which relapse is likely and beyond which relapse is unlikely. In the work of Hunt *et al.* (1971) on heroin addiction, smoking, and alcoholism, relapse curves stabilized after the first 3 months. It is appealing to conclude that individuals who abstain for three months are likely to succeed thereafter, but more recent evidence does not support a specific safe point (Lichtenstein & Rodrigues, 1977; Wilson & Brownell, 1980). Defining such a point would have important conceptual and practical implications, and more study on this topic could pay high dividends. Interpreting relapse curves may be the first step.

Relapse curves are one kind of survival curve. The figures must therefore be interpreted with several facts in mind (Elandt-Johnson & Johnson, 1980; Marlatt & Gordon, 1985; Sutton, 1979). Group averages do not represent individuals. Marlatt, Goldstein, and Gordon (1984) found that abstinence rates for smokers after quitting on the basis of a New Year's resolution were 21% both 4 and 12 months later, implying that relapse rates stabilize and show a safe point at 4 months. However, different individuals formed the 21% on these two occasions; some moved from abstinence to relapse, whereas equal numbers moved in the opposite direction. Second, the cumulative nature of the curves implies that a person who relapses will continue to do so; survival curves are negatively accelerating by their nature. Schachter (1982) noted that cure for many persons follows several relapses. Third, the probability of survival for the entire group increases with time because the persons at highest risk are most likely to leave the sample. Life-table analyses have been designed to deal with these issues (Elandt–Johnson & Johnson, 1980). Therefore, it may be possible in future research to develop a time line for the relapse process and to determine whether there are indeed safe points.

Some information does exist on the natural history of the addictions. Vaillant's (1983) report on the long-term progress of 110 alcohol abusers, 71 of whom were alcohol-dependent, shows the complexity of the issue. Vaillant's book and an article by Vaillant and Milofsky (1982) showed the importance of cultural and ethnic factors in alcoholism. Many personal and environmental factors influenced the propensity to drink excessively. It was clear from these data that a lapse does not necessarily become a relapse and that this transition has many determinants.

Schachter (1982) interviewed 161 persons from the Psychology Department at Columbia University and from a resort community. In their retrospective accounts, they reported much higher rates of success at dieting and smoking cessation than suggested by the literature. Almost all successes were achieved without professional aid. Although Schachter's methods have been questioned (Jeffery & Wing, 1983; Prochaska, 1983), he made several important points. He noted that cure rates are based on clinical samples and that self-quitters may differ from therapy-assisted quitters, a notion supported by DiClemente and Prochaska (1982). Second, he found that many of the successful quitters had made numerous attempts to change before finally succeeding.

Marlatt and Gordon (1980, 1985) have examined the natural history of the relapse itself. Beginning with a high-risk situation, their cognitive-behavioral model addresses the coping process (Figure 1). The absence of

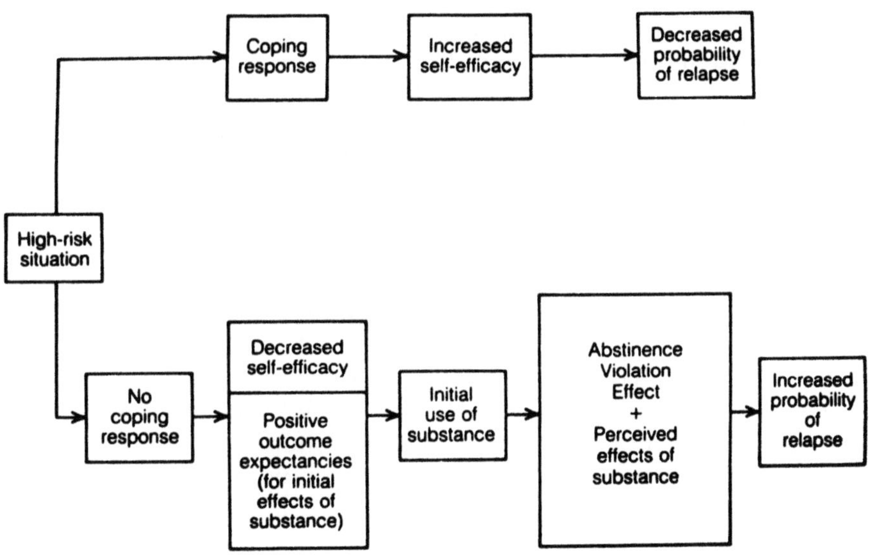

Figure 1. A cognitive-behavioral model of the relapse process beginning with the exposure to a high-risk situation. From *Relapse prevention: Maintenance strategies in addictive behavior change* (p. 38) by G. A. Marlatt and J. R. Gordon, 1985, New York: Guilford Press. Copyright 1985 by Guilford Press. Reprinted by permission.

a coping response leads to decreased self-efficacy (Bandura, 1977a,b), then to use of the substance, and then to the cognitive phenomenon they call the "abstinence violation effect." This phenomenon involves the loss of control that follows violation of self-imposed rules. The end result of this process is increased probability of relapse. Recent data from an analysis of relapse episodes in smokers showed a significant difference in attributions for slips between subjects who slipped (smoked at least one cigarette) and regained abstinence and those who relapsed (Goldstein, Gordon, & Marlatt, 1984). Persons who relapsed made more internal, characterological attributions for the slip. This model is useful in conceptualizing the relapse process from the point at which the person is in a high-risk situation.

Marlatt and Gordon's (1985) model allows for multiple determinants of high-risk situations but emphasizes cognitive processes thereafter. Other factors of a physiological or environmental nature may also be important. For example, the use of nicotine or alcohol after a period of abstinence may create a physiological demand for additional use. An environmental example is that of a smoker whose lapse occurs in a social setting in which others are smoking. The resulting cues may provoke further use. Grunberg and colleagues have found powerful effects of nicotine on the regulation of body weight and food preferences in both humans and animals (Grunberg, 1982; Grunberg & Bowen, 1985; Grunberg, Bowen, Maycock, & Nespor, 1985; Grunberg, Bowen, & Morse, 1984). Stopping smoking can create physiological pressure to change food intake and gain weight. This in turn has psychological and environmental consequences that can precipitate relapse. Therefore, it is important to consider the interaction of individual, environmental, and physiological factors in all stages of the change process.

There is much to be learned about the natural history of relapse. More descriptive information is needed on lapses and their associations with relapse. This research is not easy because the work must be prospective and because qualitative and quantitative work must be combined. As an example, Lichtenstein (1984) followed treated smokers at intervals of 1, 2, 3, 6, and 12 months intervals with telephone calls. Relapses were preceded by slips for 41 subjects; 19 subjects reported slips but did not relapse. More information of this nature would be useful.

Stages of Change

Several attempts have been made to divide the change process into stages (DiClemente & Prochaska, 1982: Horn, 1976; Marlatt & Gordon,

1985; Prochaska, 1979; Prochaska & DiClemente, 1982, 1983, 1984; Rosen & Shipley, 1983). There appears to be a convergence of opinion that at least three fundamental stages exist.

Horn (1976) first proposed four stages of change in smoking cessation; (a) contemplating change, (b) deciding to change, (c) short-term change, and (d) long-term change. This is similar to the three-stage models suggested by DiClemente and Prochaska (1982), Rosen and Shipley (1983), and Marlatt and Gordon (1985), which involve the decision and commitment to change, initial change, and maintenance of change.

Prochaska and DiClemente have done the most thorough work in this area by evaluating stage models of smoking cessation and therapy in general. Prochaska (1979) reviewed 300 therapy outcome studies and proposed five stages, three of which involved "verbal processes" and two "behavioral processes." DiClemente and Prochaska (1982) used this model to compare smokers who quit on their own to those who used commercial programs. They proposed the three stages mentioned above and described six verbal and four behavioral processes within the stages. In their recent work, Prochaska and DiClemente (1983, 1984) suggested five stages: (a) precontemplation, (b) contemplation, (c) action, (d) maintenance, and (e) relapse.

More work is needed to test the utility of the various stage models. They are similar in many respects. Each has at least one stage wherein motivation and commitment are central, followed by initial change and then the maintenance of change; therefore we will use these three fundamental stages to organize the description of relapse prevention later in this chapter. Whichever stage model prevails, we feel that relapse must be considered in light of the stages that precede it. This will draw attention to the early determinants of relapse and the importance of the many factors that influence long-term success.

A stage model may also be helpful for relapse itself. A model might include the time prior to a lapse, the lapse itself, and the period in which the person does or does not relapse. The work of Lichtenstein, Antonuccio, and Rainwater (1977), Cummings *et al.* (1980), and Shiffman (1982, 1984) suggests the utility of such an approach.

An important conceptual advance has been the emphasis of Prochaska and DiClemente (1982, 1984) on a circular rather than a linear model of change. Linear models have stages that occur in a specific sequence, with relapse occurring at the last stage. A circular model shows relapse leading back to an earlier stage from which an individual may make another attempt to change. Relapse can be viewed in a less negative light from this perspective, as an individual may acquire information or skills that may be helpful later. This is consistent with Schachter's (1982) notion that success for most individuals comes after several relapses. Taking this to the extreme, one could suggest that relapse is a *necessary* step on the path to success. We do not support this extreme, but we do feel that relapse may provide valuable experience and that persons who relapse should be instructed accordingly.

The Consequences of Relapse

Relapse could provoke a variety of responses in the individual. It is generally assumed that these responses are negative, but this may not be true in all cases. This is an important issue because these responses may determine the likelihood of success in subsequent attempts to change.

It would appear at first glance that relapse has negative emotional effects. Disappointment, frustration, and self-condemnation are apparent in people who relapse. Family and friends are unhappy and sometimes angry. However, learning may occur before or during the relapse, and therefore some benefit may accrue. One study tracked depression in subjects who lost weight and then regained it (Brownell & Stunkard, 1981). Depression scores dropped as weight declined but returned halfway to baseline as half of the weight was regained. Although these subjects were not successful maintainers, the net change in mood was still positive.

There may also be physiological effects of relapse. When a person stops smoking, the body begins the healing process, and risk for premature death declines (U.S. Department of Health and Human Services, 1983). Because there is a dose–response relationship between smoking and disease, bouts of abstinence may incur some benefit and the smoker who relapses may be better off medically than one who never quit. This is highly speculative, but it does show that this issue deserves more attention.

The picture may be different in the matter of weight loss; relapse may have detrimental metabolic and health effects. A recent study found that repeated cycles of weight loss and regain in animals was associated with increased metabolic efficiency (Brownell, Greenwood, Shrager, & Stellar, 1986). As a result, the animals lost weight at half the rate when they were put on a diet a second time even though intake was the same on both diets. When allowed to eat freely, the animals regained at three times the rate on the second diet than on the first diet. Dieting and relapse made subsequent dieting more difficult. Epidemiology studies with humans show positive effects of weight loss on blood pressure, cholesterol, glucose tolerance, and so forth (Simopolous & Van Itallie, 1984). However, when an equal amount of weight is regained, the negative effects on blood pressure and cholesterol may be greater than the positive effects when the weight is lost (Ashley & Kannel, 1974).

Relapse: Failure or Incremental Learning?

We wonder whether repeated attempts to change followed by relapse increase or decrease the chance for later success. There is evidence that persons who have dieted many times have a poor prognosis (Jeffery *et al.*, 1984; Jeffery, Snell, & Forster, 1984), although Dubbert and Wilson (1984) did not find this result. A relapse could be a failure that strengthens the person's view that the problem is beyond his or her best efforts. However, relapse may have positive consequences if the experience somehow prepares the individual for later success. This more optimistic view is consistent with Schachter's (1982) suggestion that multiple attempts occur before many people succeed. A person who relapses may be acquiring information about his or her weaknesses and may learn ways to prevent lapses in the future.

This view of incremental learning could be useful to both professionals and patients. If relapse can be a constructive experience, experimentation with programmed relapse might be warranted (Marlatt & Gordon, 1985). This approach involves planning and executing a relapse that would not occur otherwise, to teach patients to recover with self-management techniques. This approach will be discussed in more detail below.

A point that has received little attention is the effect of patients who relapse have on the professionals who treat them. Following patients through the emotional roller coaster of success and relapse is discouraging and can make professionals pessimistic with new patients. Whether this pessimism is justified depends on perspective. It is a failure viewed in the short term, but some long-term effect may occur. Most patients will make other attempts, and some will succeed.

Determinants and Predictors of Lapse and Relapse

We make several assumptions here. The first is that there are similarities in relapse across the addictive disorders (Marlatt & Gordon, 1985). Our second assumption is that different processes govern initial change and maintenance (Bandura, 1977a). This assumption has been substantiated by research on alcoholism (Cronkite & Moos, 1980; Marlatt & Gordon, 1985), smoking (Lichtenstein, 1982; Pomerleau, Adkins, & Pertschuk, 1978; Shiffman, 1982, 1984), and obesity (Brownell, 1982; Dubbert & Wilson, 1984; Wilson, 1978). The third assumption is that the risk for relapse is determined by an interaction of individual, situational, and physiological factors.

The initial attempts to classify relapse situations were made by Marlatt (1978), Marlatt and Gordon (1980), and Cummings *et al.* (1980). The Cummings *et al.* analysis evaluated 311 initial relapse episodes in drinking, smoking, compulsive gambling, excessive eating, and heroin addiction. Several determinants emerged, which can be broadly grouped into individual (intrapersonal) and situational (environmental) categories. These two categories are supported by work on smoking (Mermelstein & Lichtenstein, 1983; Shiffman, 1982, 1984) and obesity (Dubbert & Wilson, 1984). We feel it is important to add physiological variables, as their critical role is becoming more clear (Best *et al.*, in press; Brownell, 1982; Lichtenstein, 1982; Myers, 1978; Nathan & Wiens, 1983; Pomerleau & Pomerleau, 1984).

Individual and Intrapersonal Factors

Negative Emotional States

Stress, depression, anxiety, and other emotional states are related to relapse. Cummings *et al.* (1980) found that negative emotional states accounted for 30% of all relapses. Shiffman (1982, 1984) evaluated reports of relapse in 264 ex-smokers who called a telephone hotline service (Stay Quit Line). Subjects were interviewed soon after the relapse, so reports were recent even if based only on self-report. Most of the subjects (71%) had negative affects preceding the relapse, with the most common mood state being anxiety, followed by anger or frustration, and depression (Shiffman, 1982). Ossip-Klein, Shapiro, and Stiggins (1984) have also used a telephone hotline to study relapse in smokers. Mermelstein, Cohen, and Lichtenstein (1983) found 43% of relapses to occur under stress. Pomerleau *et al.* (1978) reported that those who smoke to reduce negative affect are at increased risk for relapse. A careful study of smokers by Abrams *et al.* (1986) supported these notions by using physiological behavioral, and self-report data.

In a study with smokers, Mermelstein aned Lichtenstein (1983) studied by lapses (slips) and relapses. Lapses were more commonly associated with situational factors, whereas relapses occurred during negative emotional states or stressful events. When the data from these studies with different addictive behaviors are combined, it is clear that negative emotional states greatly increase the chance of relapse. More specifically, negative moods may increase the chance that a lapse will become a relapse.

Inadequate Motivation

It is surprising that so little work has been done on motivation and commitment. It would appear that all persons who set out to change are motivated, particularly those who enter professional programs. However, there are degrees of motivation, and it is common for a person to begin the change process in a burst of enthusiasm without appreciation for the long-term effort involved. In other cases, motivation may be more external than internal, when social pressure forces a symbolic if not real attempt to change.

There are three relevant aspects of the motivation issue. The first is the need to evaluate motivation so that high-risk subjects can be detected. To our knowledge, this has not been done in the addictions area. Second, screening for motivation is important if treatment should be directed at those with a chance for success. Third, methods may be available for increasing motivation, to improve a person's "readiness" for change (Marlatt & Gordon, 1985; Prochaska & DiClemente, 1984). The second and third points have implications for treatment, as we will discuss.

Response to Treatment

There is some evidence that initial responses to treatment predict later success. Weight loss in the first weeks of treatment has been related to success (Foreyt *et al.*, 1982; Graham, Taylor, Hovell, & Siegel, 1983; Jeffery, Wing, & Stunkard, 1978). Pomerleau *et al.* (1978) found that early compliance (self-monitoring) was related to positive outcome in smokers, and Glasgow, Shafer, and O'Neill (1981) found that self-reported compliance was related to success in self-quitters. Inability to stop smoking on the assigned target date (usually midway in treatment) is a poor prognostic sign (Lichtenstein, 1982).

One of us (K.D.B.) has observed informally a paradoxical relationship between early program adherence and outcome in persons on very low-calorie diets, a rigid program that is nearly a complete fast (Wadden, Stunkard, & Brownell, 1983). Patients are asked not to "cheat" on the diet. Those who struggle with adherence to a moderate degree seem to do better in the long run than those who adhere perfectly from the outset. The perfect adherers seem to have trouble recovering from the inevitable slip that the early perfection merely postpones. It is possible that high motivation initially can mask strong pressures to relapse, but once internal and external pressures wear away restraint, a lapse is likely to become a relapse. Patients who struggle to a moderate degree with adherence throughout a program may do well later because they can cope with temporary setbacks.

Coping Skills

Shiffman (1984) found that both cognitive and behavioral coping responses were associated with success in smokers calling the hotline mentioned earlier. The most common behavioral responses were consumption of food and drink and other distracting activities. Several aspects of "self-talk" were the most common cognitive responses. Shiffman found positive associations between outcome and seven behavioral and five cognitive methods of coping, but the various coping strategies were about equally effective.

There is evidence in the weight control area showing the utility of a cognitive "threshold" for weight regain in persons who have lost weight (Brownell, 1984a; Wilson, 1985). Stuart and Guire (1978) examined successful maintainers in Weight Watchers and found them likely to have a personal regain threshold of three pounds or less before they instituted self-correcting actions. Bandura and Simon (1977) found that subjects who used proximal rather than distal goals were most successful at maintenance. One aspect of the proximal goals was a weight increase threshold.

Another factor that may relate to long-term success are the coping skills associated with self-efficacy (Bandura, 1977b). Self-efficacy is a person's belief that he or she can respond effectively to a situation by using available skills. This concept is at the root of the relapse prevention approach of Marlatt and Gordon (1985) and has been applied to alcoholism (Chaney, O'Leary, & Marlatt, 1978), smoking (Brown, Lichtenstein, McIntyre, & Harrington-Kostur, 1984; Hall, Rugg, Tunstall, & Jones, 1984; Killen, Maccoby, & Taylor, 1984), and obesity (Perri, McAdoo, Spevak, & Newlin, 1984; Perri, Shapiro, Ludwig, Twentyman, & McAdoo, 1984). Several studies have found measures of self-efficacy associated with positive outcome (Colletti, Supnick, & Payne, 1985; Condiotti, & Lichtenstein, 1981; Killen *et al.*, 1984; Supnick & Colletti, 1984).

Physiological Factors

Physiological factors may be a central determinant of relapse. Genetic factors appear to be important for alcoholism, smoking, and obesity (McClearn, 1981; Pomerleau, 1984; Schuckitt, 1981; Stunkard *et al.*, 1986). In the cases of alcoholism and smoking, other physiological influences are related to withdrawal, to the reinforcing properties of alcohol or nicotine, or to conditioned associations between specific cues and physiological responses (Abrams & Wilson, 1986; Hodgson, 1980; Ludwig,

Wikler, & Stark, 1974; Pomerleau, 1984; Pomerleau & Pomerleau, 1984; Poulos, Hinson, & Siegel, 1981; Siegel, 1979). A patient's use of terms like *urge* and *craving* may reflect some of these pressures.

Siegel (1979) and others (Ludwig *et al.*, 1974) proposed that alcoholics show conditioned reactions to environmental, emotional, and physiological stimuli that have ben associated with previous withdrawal. Conditioned compensatory responses are thought to elicit craving for alcohol. Poulos *et al.* (1981) suggested that treatment must deal with extinction of these cues.

Degree of physical dependency must also be considered in alcohol abuse (Hodgson, 1980; Marlatt & Gordon, 1985; Miller & Hester, 1980). Several studies by Hodgson and colleagues found that alcoholics with serious physical dependency have stronger cravings and respond differently than do mildly dependent subjects to ingestion of alcohol (Hodgson, Rankin, & Stockwell, 1979; Stockwell, Hodgson, Rankin, & Taylor, 1982). Dependency may also influence the goals and course of treatment. Because chronic alcohol use is associated with several cognitive impairments, skill acquisition may be more difficult (Wilkinson & Sanchez-Craig, 1981). If controlled drinking is a viable goal of treatment, it would be so for only a subgroup of problem drinkers: abstinence is the clear goal for severe alcohol dependence (Marlatt, 1983; Miller & Hester, 1980; Nathan & Goldman, 1979).

Similarly powerful factors may be associated with smoking (Abrams & Wilson, 1986; Pomerleau & Pomerleau, 1984). A review by McMorrow and Foxx (1983) showed that changes in smoking behavior accompany changes in blood nicotine level. Pomerleau (1984) found that nicotine stimulates release of beta-endorphin, increases heart rate, and possibly improves memory and attention; therefore he characterized nicotine as a powerful chemical reinforcer. Furthermore, the degree of physical dependence has implications for treatment. Two studies found that smokers who are highly dependent on nicotine benefit most from treatment with nicotine chewing gum (Fagerstrom, 1982; Hall, Tunstall, Rugg, Jones, & Benowitz, 1985).

Different but also influential physiological factors may be involved in obesity. Food does not seem addictive in the manner of cigarettes and alcohol, yet the physical pressures to regain lost weight may be extremely powerful (Bennett & Gurin, 1982; Bray, 1976; Brownell, 1982; Wooley, Wooley, & Dyrenforth, 1979). Such pressures could involve the lipid repletion of fat cells and alterations of several factors including body composition, metabolic rate, thermogenic response to food, and enzyme activity, each of which may be related to a body weight "set point" in which the organism defends a biological ideal against fluctuations, including weight loss. Detailed discussion of such known or suspected biological mechanisms for specific disorders is provided in preceding chapters.

Given these important physiological factors, it may be informative to examine the subjective impressions of their likely manifestations, namely, cravings, urges, and withdrawal. Studies in these areas have shown inconsistent findings. The Cummings *et al.* (1980) study found that "urges and temptations" were associated with only 6% of the relapse situations and that "negative physical states" were associated with only 7% of the situations. Mermelstein *et al.* (1983) found that craving was the major factor in only 9% of relapses in smokers. In contrast, Shiffman 1982) found that approximately half of the relapse situations in smokers occurred in conjunction with withdrawal symptoms. Even though Shiffman interpreted this result as showing that withdrawal symptoms are less important than expected, they would appear from his data to be powerful precipitating events.

Environmental and Social Factors

There is compelling evidence that enviornmental and social factors, including specific external contingencies, play an important role in the addictive disorders. These can be interactions among individuals (social support), environmental or setting events, or programs that manipulate contingencies.

Social Support

Social factors are important determinants of susceptibility to diseases, including heart disease, cancer, and psychiatric disturbances (Cobb, 1976; Cohen & Syme, 1985). They are important in a person's ability to make stressful decisions and to adhere to a therapeutic program (Janis, 1983) and have been related to success in the addictive disorders (Best, 1980; Colletti, & Brownell, 1982; Moos & Finney, 1983).

Research in this area has taken two forms: the evaluation of social support as a predictor variable and the modification of social factors to boost treatment effectiveness. Treatment will be discussed below. The work with predicting success with social variables has been fruitful.

Support from family and friends is one of the few variables that is associated with long-term success at weight reduction (Brownell, 1984a; Miller & Simms, 1981; Wilson, 1985). Studies on smoking suggest the same association (Coppotelli & Orleans, 1985; Mermelstein *et al.*, 1983). Whether a spouse is a smoker and is attempting to quit relates negatively to ability to stop smoking (Lichtenstein, 1982). Perceived general support (not specific to quitting) also relates to the maintenance of nonsmoking or reduced smoking (Mermelstein *et al.*, 1983). Moos and Finney (1983) summarized studies in the alcohol area showing that marital and family cohesion enhances response to treatment in follow-ups of as long as 2 years. In their review of the relapse area, Marlatt and Gordon (1985) and Cummings *et al.* (1980) pointed to the importance of social factors across areas of the addictions.

Interpersonal conflict can be viewed as the converse of social support, and studies have shown that it is a prognostic sign for relapse. In the study by Cummings *et al.* (1980), nearly half (48%) of the relapse episodes occurred in association with interpersonal determinants, with one-third of these coming from conflict. It appears, therefore, that stressful interpersonal relationships can hinder and that supportive relationships can help. This emerges from the literature despite inconsistent methods of measuring support. The supportive person may be helpful not only in establishing a benevolent environment but also by assisting with specific behavior changes (Coppotelli & Orleans, 1985). One challenge is to evaluate the nature of supportive behavior and the reasons why certain behaviors provide support for some people and not for others.

One possible avenue for social support is from commercial or self-help groups. Such groups abound and exist in all areas of the addictions (Gartner & Reissman, 1984). Groups like Alcoholics Anonymous, Weight Watchers, Overeaters Anonymous, and SmokEnders deliver programs to millions and reach many more people than do professional programs. Their potential is tremendous, both to teach skills and provide social support. Is this potential realized?

It is difficult to evaluate many self-help and commercial groups. They vary greatly in cost, approach, size, geographical distribution, and so forth. Different chapters of the same group sometimes differ as much from one another as they do from outside groups. It is clear that many people benefit from these approaches, both in tems of initial results and maintenance (Gartner & Reissman, 1984). Guidelines are needed to refine the active components of these groups and to determine which people are best suited for self-help approaches.

Environmental Stimuli and External Contingencies

Events in the environment can set the stage for relapse. These typically take the form of social pressure from others, exposure to the undesirable behavior during social events like parties, and cues from situations formerly associated with the addictive behavior.

Shiffman (1982) found that social events preceded one-fourth of the relapse crises of smokers and that activities previously associated with smoking (eating and drinking) were frequent antecedent events. Marlatt and Gordon (1980, 1985) also found these to be important factors. Mermelstein and Lichtenstein (1983) reported that lapses were most likely under social cues, a social celebration, or the consumption of alcohol.

Numerous progams have shown that contingency management and the systematic manipulation of environmental factors can enhance motivation. Programs using financial incentives have been useful in promoting weight loss in both adults and children (Epstein, Wing, Koeske, Andrasik, & Ossip, 1981; Jeffery, Forster, & Snell, 1985; Jeffery, Gerber, Rosenthal, & Lindquist, 1983). Reward systems have also been used with some success with smoking (Lichtenstein, 1982). The careful work of Bigelow, Stitzer, and colleagues has shown powerful effects of contingency management on drug abuse, alcohol intake, and smoking (Bigelow, Stitzer, Griffiths, & Liebson, 1981; Stitzer & Bigelow, 1984). Such work presents specific components of treatment that may help prevent relapse.

External contingencies have most often been manipulated in the alcohol area. Hunt and Azrin (1973) used an intensive community reinforcement progam in which family, social, and vocational reinforcers were altered systematically. Among the treatment components were marital and family counseling, skills training, assistance with daily needs such as obtaining a driver's license, a social club for clients, and contingency contracting. Compared to control clients, those who participated in this progam remained sober for longer periods, had better employment records, and showed seveal other tangible indications of improvement. Azrin (1976) then modified this approach using Antabuse and an early warning system for relapse. Employee assistance programs (EAP) are another example of environmental contingencies influencing alcoholics (Nathan, 1983, 1984). Participating in treatment and remaining sober may be a condition for employment. Some programs for impaired professionals require treatment for continued practice.

Individual, Environmental, and Physiological Factors: An Interaction

The risk for lapse and relapse is determined by an interaction of individual, environmental, and physiological factors. This is an area in which the distinction of lapse and relapse is particularly useful, as there may be different determinants and antecedents in each case. Mermelstein and Lichtenstein (1983) showed in their findings that lapses tended to be associated with social factors and that elapses were associated with individual factors (negative emotional states and stress events). Shiffman (1982) theorized that a situational analysis could predict increased risk for relapse but that coping skills would determine whether this risk becomes reality. Other theorists have pointed to powerful physiological cravings to help explain both addiction and relapse (Abrams & Wilson, 1986; Brownell, 1982; Pomerleau & Pomerleau, 1984).

If lapse and relapse are viewed on a time line, individual, environmental, and physiological factors may exert their influence at different stages. Physiological factors may promote lapse and may set into play a series of reactions to an initial lapse that may increase the likelihood of relapse. The environmental and social factors can provide the setting, stimuli, and pressure from others to lapse. As the choice point for the lapse approaches, coping skills can prevent the lapse. Whether the lapse recurs and ends in relapse probably results from a complex interaction of these factors, each of which may assume more or less importance depending on the individual and his or her environment.

Prevention of Lapse and Relapse

Traditional Approaches versus the Prevention Model

Traditional attempts to facilitate long-term maintenance fall into three categories. The first has been to extend treatment by adding "booster" sessions. As the name implies, patients are to be "immunized" against pressures to relapse with the initial treatment, and periodic boosters are needed to maintain the protection. Booster sessions have been used most extensively with obesity and smoking and have been consistently ineffective (Lichtenstein, 1982; Wilson, 1985).

A second approach has been to add more components to the treatment package, the most common being relaxation, contingency management, and assertion training. This has not been effective. Marlatt and Gordon (1985) stated: "All of this is heavy artillery—yet all it may do is project the cannonball a little bit further before it finally hits the ground" (p. 45). Adding new components to a package may help, but it is not enough to prevent relapse.

Adding components may also complicate a package and compromise the results of otherwise efective treatment. This result would be predicted from the literature showing that compliance is related inversely to the complexity of a regimen (Epstein & Cluss, 1982; Sackett & Haynes, 1976). There is some support for this in two obesity studies in which the combination of an appetite suppressant with behavior therapy was no more effective (Craighead, 1984) or was even less effective (Craighead, Stunkard, & O'Brien, 1981) than behavior therapy alone.

A third traditional approach to preventing relapse is to adopt a model of lifelong treatment. This model is inherent in Alcoholics Anonymous, where participants are always "recovering" and never "recovered." This same philosophy applies to Overeaters Anonymous and to some extent to the lifetime membership offered by Weight Watchers. It may be true that chronic disorders require chronic treatment. According to our mode of relapse prevention, lifelong treatment has both advantages and disadvantages. On the negative side, imparting the message that a person can control but not cure an addiction may establish a climate in which lapses create strong expectaitons of relapses. On the positive side, lifelong programs do not have the disadvantage of standard programs in which intensive treatment is followed by no treatment, the point at which relapse may be likely. These approaches must be considered viable, if for no other reason than that millions of persons have profited from their use. Program evaluation studies are difficult because of their long-term nature and the problems in doing research on commerical and self-help groups. It is, however, a pressing need for the field.

We propose that the prevention of lapse and relapse corresponds to the stages of their natural history. The approach described below is based on the three stages described earlier: motivation and commitment, initial change, and maintenance. We attempt to integrate what is known about individual, environmental, and physiological determinants of lapse and relapse.

Stage 1: Motivation and Commitment

At this stage, individuals commit themselves to change and make the first steps toward the modification of maladaptive behavior. There are two aspects of this process that are pertinent to relaps. One is the development of methods to enhance motivation. The second is screening to identify an individual's likelihood of success. Central to both is the ability to assess motivation and other factors related to prognosis. This is a pressing area for research, as good methods do not exist.

Enhancing Motivation

Many candidates for progams are motivated, but many are not. A major challenge is to enhance motivation when it is low in order to maximize readiness for change. Little systematic work has been done in this area. Education about the dangers of the addiction, support from others, matching the patient with the right therapist, and feedback about physical status are among the possible methods for increasing motivation, but even these factors have not been studied in detail. The field stands to profit from research directed toward this initial stage in the change process.

One possible approach for enhancing motivation is to use contingency-management procedures. Monetary incentives have been studied most thoroughly; the deposit–refund system is most common. In this system, patients are required to deposit money, sometimes on a sliding scale, that is then returned for attendance at meetings or for a specified behavior change (Hagen, Foreyt, & Durham, 1976; Jeffery *et al.*, 1983). This approach reduces attrition (Hagen *et al.*, 1976; Wilson & Brownell, 1980), but it is not clear whether it enhances motivation prior to treatment. The deposit–refund may simply deter people who are not motivated from entering treatment, which gives it possible utility as a screening device.

It is surprising that so little has been done on methods for enhancing motivation. The work of Prochaska and his colleagues is a move in this direction (Prochaska, 1979; Prochaska & DiClemente, 1983, 1984). These studies have helped define stages of change. The knowledge from these and similar studies may suggest methods for enhancing motivation in the early stages. Such methods could have wide application in public health programs in which the goal is to encourage attempts to change.

One important aspect of this early stage is preparing the individual for the possibility of lapse and even relapse (Lando, 1981). A fine line must be drawn between preparing a person for mistakes and giving "permission" for mistakes to occur by inferring that they are inevitable. Two analogies may be used in this context. One is that of a fire drill (Marlat & Gordon, 1985): a person must practice to escape a fire even though fires are rare. The second is that of a forest ranger whose dual tasks are to prevent and contain fires (Brownell, 1985). The best course is to prevent fires, but when they do occur, one must move swiftly before the fire consumes the entire forest.

Screening to Determine Prognosis

Screening prior to a program may have two potential benefits. First, screening may help match individuals to programs. Second, screening may focus professional efforts on those most likely to succeed.

Many potential remedies are available for the addictions. They range from no-cost effors at self-change to expensive commercial and clinical programs. In between these extremes lie community programs, the media, self-help books, self-help groups, advice from a health care provider, and many others. Each approach works for some people. Screening could be valuable if individuals could be matched to the approach with the greatest impact at lowest cost. Developing criteria for this matching is a major need for the field.

The second use of screening is to make use of predictions of who will do well and who will not. The primary implication of the search for predictors is that persons who are likely to do poorly can be identified and can receive special treatment. This idea is appealing but is not yet practical. This approach assumes that there is something beyond standard treatment. In clinical programs, standard treatment is certainly the most intensive and effective treatment known, so what else is to be done? In less intensive approaches, say self-help groups or community programs, referral to a more intensive approach may be the answer. However, there are several other tacit assumptions with this approach. One is that such people will succeed if only the right procedures are used. This assumes that the variance in outcome rests with the program rather than with the individual, which perpetuates the medial model of disease and cure. The other is that cost of such efforts is justified.

Another perspective on screening would shift the focus from those at greatest risk for failure to those with greatest chance for success. Screening might be used to direct a program to those most likely to benefit and to prevent the negative consequences of failure for those at high risk, assuming that the consequences of relapse are more negative than positive. The rationale for this has been discussed previously in the weight loss area (Brownell, 1984b). One reason is that failure, or the more likely occurrence of initial success followed by relapse, may add to a legacy of inadequacy and demoralize the patient. Second, the initial success followed by relapse may have negative physiological consequences, particularly for dieters. Third, the failure may convince the person that the problem is intractable, which may decrease the chance that treatment will be pursued later when motivation is higher. Fourth, if treatment is delivered in groups, "negative contagion" can occur when patients who are not doing well discourage those who are. Fifth, the morale of professionals suffers when a patient fails. Sixth, working with patients who are likely to fail leaves fewer resources for those who may succeed.

The object would be to screen for individual, environmental, or physiological factors that cannot be remedied easily. One factor is motivation. It is difficult to motivate a person who does not have a strong commitment to change. There are instances of programs with good success in motivating groups of people, say at a work site or in a community (Brownell, Cohen, Stunkard, Felix & Cooley, 1984; Pechacek, Mittelmark, Jeffery, Loken, & Luepker, 1985), but reliable methods for motivating individual shave not been developed. Another factor relates to a person's skills. Some skills deficits may be difficult to overcome.

Physiological factors may be among the most important objects of screening. Our earlier discussion raised some of the possible variables to be measured, including physical dependency, metabolic factors, withdrawal, and genetic loading. It is clear, therefore, that screening will be a multifaceted activity requiring assessment of many variables and specific tailoring of screening protocols to various disorders.

The concept of screening is easier to support in principle than to apply in practice. Its strength lies in the ability to separte false positives from false negatives. Using no screening increases false positives; that is, people who will eventually fail are permitted into a program. A screening procedure can produce false negatives (persons who would succeed are screened out unfairly). It is important to consider these along with the associated ethical issues (which will be discussed).

Two Methods for Screening

Little attention has been given to screening, so we can offer only preliminary ideas. One is a behavioral test of motivation, and the other is the use of predictor variables. The next few years will probably offer physiological variables for screening, but only the tentative suggestions made above are possible currently.

There are several possibilities for behavioral tests of motivation. The deposit–refund system has been effective in reducing attrition in obesity progams (Hagen *et al.*, 1976; Wilson & Brownell, 1980) and has been used in smoking programs as well (Lichtenstein, 1982). This sytem is usually conceptualized as a means for sustaining motivation during a program, but it may also serve to screen out people with low levels of motivation before a program. Another behavioral test is to institute a screening phase prior to treatment. Patients must meet established criteria prior to entrance to the program. One of us (K.D.B.) uses this in a weight control progam by requiring patients to lose 1 pound per week for 2 weeks and to complete self-monitoring diaries. These criteria, combined with the deposit–refund system, are not difficult to meet for most patients, but individuals who are not motivated may not join a program in which such a commitment is necessary. These are just examples of behavioral tests for motivation. More research may identify better methods.

The second (even less precise) method for screening is to use some combination of predictor variables to identify subjects at high risk for relapse. Marlatt *et al.* (1984) found that a motivational rating of desire to quit distinguished individuals who could not stop smoking for even a day from those who could quit for longer periods. As our discussion above shows, identifying predictors of relapse is not sufficiently advanced to warrant screening. With more research, however, this may be possible.

This discussion pertains to clinical programs wherein treatment is intensive and costly. Large-scale programs, in work sites or communities, for instance, may be inexpensive, so the aim shifts from having a strong impact on small groups to spreading lesser impact over large numbers (Brownell, 1986; Davis, Faust, & Ordentlich, 1984; Stunkard, 1986). In this case, the cost of screening may not be warranted.

The Ethics of Screening

Screening used in this fashion raises complex ethical issues. The decision of who can enter a program would no longer be based on who registers first or who can pay the fee; instead there would be a conscious effort to deliver treatment to individuals with specific characteristics. This affords the opportunity for treatment to some and denies it to others. Although such an approach has not been studied, it is likely that certain subgroups of the population would fall disproportionately into the "nonmotivated" category. These subgroups might be characterized by sex, race, religion, or ethnic background, all groups that Western society protects against discrimination.

Whether such screening can be justified ethically may depend on many factors. One is the ability to help those at high risk. In the absence of proven technology for this purpose, does screening become more important? Another issue is cost. Is the extra cost of aiding a high-risk person justifiable? Some extra cost may be justified, but how much? What allocation of these resources will have the greatest impact on society, or should society be the primary concern? A third factor will be the sensitivity and specificity of screening procedures. A screening that produces few false negatives may be warranted if the social, psychological, and health costs of false positives are high, but how many false negatives can be tolerated?

These questions are too complex to address in detail here. We do feel that screening and identification of those with high and low chances for success comprise an issue of major importance. Who receives a treatment is not currently determined by a systematic examination of the issues. It may happen in a systematic way, but for reasons that we do not understand and that may not be rational. Avoiding the questions only sidesteps the ethical issues and does not make the process of delivering treatment more ethical. We hope more research will be done in this area.

Stage 2: Initial Behavior Change

This stage of treatment is the intensive period that lies between screening and the maintenance phase. This period may be several weeks in smoking programs and 3 to 6 months in alcohol and obesity programs. This may not be the time for greatest risk of relapse, because patients are generally motivated and are gratified with their progress. However, high-risk situations do occur; therefore, this time is ideal for the acquisition and practice of skills specific to relapse (Marlatt & Gordon, 1985). Some of these have been described in detail elsewhere (Marlatt & Gordon, 1980, 1985); only the basic rationale for the use and timing of the procedures need be given here.

The choice of specific treatment procedures is important, as is the timing of their application. The tendency is to squeeze all components into the initial treatment period and to use maintenance to review material presented earlier. This can burden the subject early in a program and may focus on skills when the skills are not required. Therefore, the right mixture of relapse prevention strategies in both initial treatment and maintenance may be one key to positive outcome.

We suggest three areas to be covered in initial treatment: (a) decision-making, (b) cognitive restructuring, and (c) coping skills. These are the procedures aimed specifically at the prevention of lapse and relapse and are to be done in addition to the techniques specific to the treatment of smoking, alcoholism, or obesity. They emerge from our conceptual approach described earlier and from existing information on predictors of relapse and the success of relapse prevention programs. A fourth area, cue elimination, has preliminary support in both theory and practice and may be perceived as more important as research progresses.

The focus on these three areas does not imply that they form the sole source of treatment. We do feel that specific techniques aimed at relapse are desirable in all stages of the change process and that relapse prevention techniques may aid any treatment program. For example, treatment for a dieter might consist of a habit change program of behavior modification, a supplemented fast, or even surgery. An alcoholic may receive Antabuse, may attend Alcoholics Anonymous, or may receive a skills training program. In each case, specific approaches can be applied to the lapse and relapse processes and may improve the prognosis for long-term change.

Additional areas will undoubtedly be added to these three as knowledge on relapse expands. We do not wish to imply that these are the only targets for relapse prevention or even that they will be consistently effective. These are what the literature permits us to propose. Contingency management will probably be added to the list soon, as studies begin to apply these techniques to relapse. Physiological factors may also emerge as important targets, but specific physiological interventions aimed at relapse are not evident from current knowledge. The number of studies on relapse is increasing rapidly. Our hope is that the new work will suggest refinement of the techniques we suggest and will identify new ones for emphasis.

The first of the three areas involves decision-making skills. These prepare a person for analyzing the individual and environmental determinants of relapse. This analysis allows the person to decide which coping skills should be summoned for dealing with a particular situation. Cognitive restructuring is also central to this approach, as it teaches individuals to interpret events, attitudes, and feelings in a rational way and to respond constructively to crises. Such a scheme for analyzing the lapse and relapse sequence and of specifying methods of decision making, coping, and cognitive restructuring is shown in Figure 2, which presents examples of how an individual would use the framework described here ot prepare for high-risk situations.

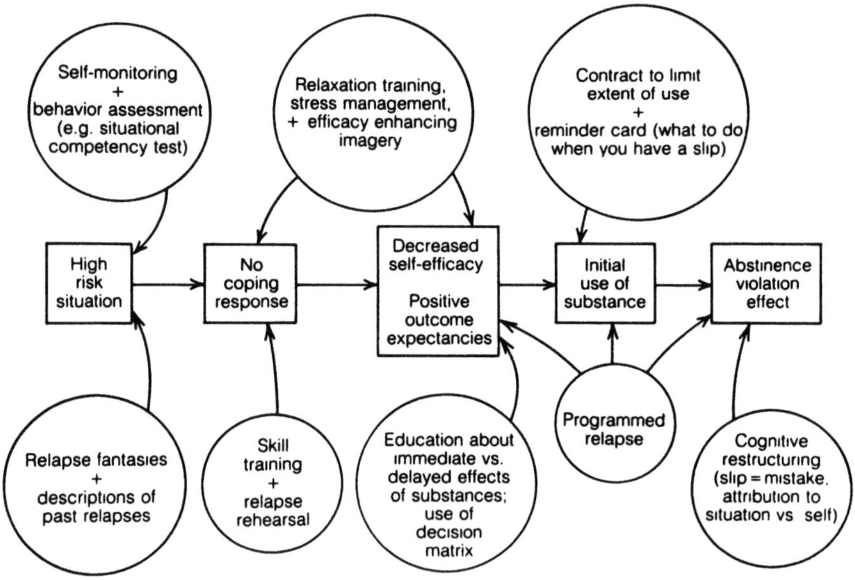

Figure 2. An example of decision making and coping skills applied to the lapse and relapse process. From *Relapse prevention: Maintenance strategies in addictive behavior change* (p. 54) by G. A. Marlatt and J. R. Gordon, 1985, New York: Guilford Press. Copyright 1985 by Guilford Press. Reprinted by permission.

Cue extinction is receiving more attention as a possible means of preventing lapse and relapse. Based on the theoretical work of Siegel (19791) and others (Ludwig *et al.*, 1974), there has been increasing emphasis on extinguishing the associations between cues and cravings (Abrams & Wilson, 1986). There may be individual, environmental, or physiological associations with substance use, and their extinction may be particularly important early in the change process when withdrawal is an issue. This is an area of potential importance, and more research is needed to test the theory and develop clinical applications.

Research is needed to refine the techniques within these categories and to determine whether these categories are most appropriate for emphasis during initial behavior change. Shiffman's (1984) study of relapse in smokers is helpful in this regard, as he discovered that a combination of cognitive and behavioral coping skills was associated with maintenance.

Stage 3: Maintenance

Most programs include some treatment during the maintenance phase, but this period has been virtually ignored as a point of intervention. With the exception of booster sessions, which are a reiteration of earlier material, few studies have used the maintenance phase as the time for targeting the lapse and relapse process. This is unfortunate, as clinical judgment would dictate emphasis in just this period. There are three areas of intervention that may be appropriate for the maintenance phase: (a) continued monitoring, (b) social support, and (c) general life-style change. Again, more areas may emerge as research continues, but these three are suggested by existing research.

It is widely believed that long-term vigilance, through either some form of self-evaluation or contact with a professional, is important in the therapeutic process. It is our impression that individuals profit from monitoring that extends beyond initial treatment. Treatment studies suggest that maintenance improves as contacts with professionals increase during follow-up, both in smoking (Colletti & Supnick, 1980) and obesity (Perri, McAdoo, *et al.*, 1984; Perri, Shapiro, *et al.*, 1984). This must be reconciled, however, with the general ineffectiveness of booster sessions. In addition, this raises the issue of when treatment ends and maintenance begins. Additional contacts may simply extend treatment and delay relapse rather than prevent it in any fundamental way. Whether these contacts actually influence relapse may depend on the nature of the contact and the type of material presented.

Marlatt and Gordon (1985) proposed social support as a component of relapse prevention. Social support is a predictor of long-term success, but attempts to intervene in a social environment have produced inconsistent results (Brownell, 1982; Brownell, Heckerman, Westlake, Hayes, & Monti 1978; Lichtenstein, 1982). We believe that social factors are crucial in the behavior change process (Cohen & Syme, 1985) but that variations in social relationships make it unlikely that any single approach will work consistently. For instance, attempts to enlist the aid of a spouse may have positive effects in some marriages and negative effects in others. It is not surprising that parametric studies with groups show no effects for such programs. This is also an area in which developmental work is needed so that the potential of social support can be exploited.

General life-style change may also be helpful (Marlatt & Gordon, 1985). The theory is that a source of gratification can be substantiated for the absence of the addictive disorder. This notion is consistent with clinical experience, but little research has been done. Likely candidates are relaxation training, meditation, and exercise. Of these, exercise has several intriguing possibilities, which we will discuss.

A controversial but thus far ineffective approach to maintenance is programmed lapse. This approach involves a planned lapse in a therapeutic setting and might include an eating binge for a dieter, smoking for an ex-smoker, or drinking for a problem drinker. This would be done only after the person has received extensive instruction in the cognitive and behavioral coping skills mentioned above. The purpose is to have the inevitable lapse occur under supervision and to demonstrate that self-management skills can be used to prevent the lapse from becoming a relapse. It may also be a useful paradoxical technique; because the therapist controls the lapse, perceptions about lack of control may change.

Coney and colleagues tested this approach with smokers (Cooney & Kopel, 1980; Cooney, Lopel, & McKeon, 1982). After 5 weeks of cessation, subjects smoked one cigarette in a controlled session. Most were surprised by how unpleasant the cigarette was and were confident they would not smoke later. These subjects had greater self-efficacy ratings than subjects receiving only the cessation program, but there were no differences in abstinence rates at a 6-month follow-up. In fact, there was a trend for programmed lapse subjects to relapse earlier.

This approach must be tested further before clinical use. The potential for harm is great, as the very cognitive patterns the procedure is designed to counter may promote uncontrolled relapse. Physiological factors may also create pressure to relapse. In addition, the studies with smokers by Cooney and colleagues did not produce favorable results. It might be a mistake, however, to dismiss the use of programmed lapse without more thorough evaluation.

A Special Role for Exercise?

The wonders of exercise have been touted to the point of provoking a backlash, but there may be a special role for physical activity in the addictive disorders. Exercise has a natural role in the weight control field, but there is increasing evidence that its generalized effects may also benefit patients in the smoking and alcoholism areas.

Exercise is emerging as one of the most important components of treatment in weight control (Brownell & Stunkard, 1980; Thompson, Jarvie, Lahey, & Cureton, 1982). It is one of the few factors correlated with long-term success (Cohen, Gelfand, Dodd, Jensen, & Turner, 1980; Graham *et al.*, 1983; Katahan, Pleas, Thackery, & Wallston, 1982; Miller & Sims, 1981; Stuart & Guire, 1978). Studies in which exercise is an independent variable show improved maintenance of weight loss (Dahlkoetter, Callahan, & Linton, 1979; Harris & Hallbauer, 1973; Stalonas, Johnson, & Christ, 1978).

Three studies suggest the benefits of exercise for smokers. Koplan, Powell, Sikes, Shirley, and Campbell (1982) sent questionnaires to 2,500 runners 1 year after they had completed the 10-kilometer Peachtree Road Race in Atlanta. Fully 81% of men and 75% of women who smoked cigarettes when they started running had stopped smoking after beginning. Having given up smoking was significantly more common among current runners than among those who had stopped running in the year following the race. In the Ontario Exercise–Heart Collaborative Study, 733 men recovering from myocardial infarction were followed for 3 years of an exercise program (Oldridge *et al.*, 1983). For the 46.5% of the men who dropped out, the two strongest predictors of dropout were smoking and blue-collar occupation. Shiffman (1984) found that exercise was used as a coping response in smokers who avoided relapse.

The only study in the alcoholism area also produced encouraging findings. Murphy, Marlatt, and Pagano (in press) trained heavy drinkers in aerobic exercise (running) or meditation. The running condition was associated with the most significant reductions in drinking rates during both treatment and follow-up.

If exercise can be used to prevent relapse, there are several possible mechanisms. It may be a general life-style activity that brings gratification, and possibly a positive addiction (Glasser, 1976), to the person who needs adaptive substitutes for the undesirable behavior (Marlatt & Gordon, 1985). It may influence self-concept or self-efficacy, which may generalize to the behavior change program. It may provide some stimulus control by removing the person to a safe setting or may provide a peer group that supports healthy behavior. There may also be physiological effects that influence the appetitive processes directly or that may change psychological functioning. These possibilities deserve further exploration.

Effects of Existing Programs

The use of relapse prevention programs is in its infancy, but many of the existing studies show positive effects. In addition to the contingency management studies mentioned above, which showed positive long-term results, several studies have used variations of the model proposed by Marlatt and Gordon (1980). Chaney *et al.* (1978) first used some elements of relapse prevention with alcoholics. They found no differences in absolute abstinence between the relapse prevention group and two control groups, but there were significant differences in favor of the relapse prevention group for duration and severity of drinking.

Hall *et al.* (1984) used a skills training program for relapse prevention in smokers. Subjects receiving the training had greater abstinence rates than subjects who did not at 6 and 52 weeks from the beginning of the study. The program had its greatest effect on light smokers. Killen *et al.* (1984) also found positive effects for relapse prevention with smokers. Brown *et al.* (1984) used a cognitive relapse prevention program with smokers and found promising results in a pilot study but no effects in a controlled study. Supnick and Colletti (1984) tested the Marlatt and gordon (1980) model with smokers and found that a problem-solving component was associated with lower relapse rates but that a relapse-coping component was not.

Several studies have tested relapse prevention with dieters. Abrams and Follick (1983) found improved long-term results by adding a relapse prevention package to a behavioral program administered in a work setting. Sternberg (1985) found similar results, in a clinical setting, but using basically the same approach. Collins, Rothblum, and Wilson (1986) found no effect. Two studies found positive effects for a relapse prevention package. Perri, McAdoo, *et al.* (1984) found better long-term results for a multicomponent maintenance program than for a control approach using booster sessions. Perri, Shapiro, *et al.* (1984) then tested various approaches to maintenance and found that relapse prevention boosted long-term results but only when mail and telephone contacts were added.

It is too early to draw specific conclusions about these studies. They vary widely in populations and in the procedures labeled "relapse prevention." Most are modeled conceptually after Marlatt and Gordon's

(1980, 1985) principles, but the application in treatment is different from setting to setting. Some studies can be faulted for small sample sizes, short follow-up periods, modest treatment effects, and so forth, so it is not surprising to find mixed results. However, the studies with results in favor of relapse prevention outnumber those with negative results; therefore, at the very least, more vigorous testing of the model is warranted.

We hope researchers will continue to test a wide range of relapse prevention procedures rather than risk the problem seen in behavioral research for obesity, in which a "package" was developed and compared to other approaches. Its statistical superiority was more important than clinical realities, and the package became standard fare (Brownell, 1982; Foreyt, *et al.*, 1982; Wilson, 1978). Instead of searching for better approaches, investigators tested small refinements in the package. We should avoid early adoption of a relapse prevention package and avoid a narrow focus only on comparative studies to the exclusion of the less rewarding but more important developmental studies that will generate useful ideas for clinical testing.

Recommendations for Research

Interest in lapse and relapse is relatively recent, and needs for additional research abound. The area is ripe for studies on issues ranging from the natural history of relapse to methods that patients might employ in high-risk situations.

Table 1 (p. 312) presents a list of research needs suggested from the various sections of this chapter. The topics include both theoretical and practical issues. We hope this will stimulate work in what is an important area of behavior change.

Conclusions

Relapse remains one of the most perplexing problems associated with the addictive disorders. Previous work has suggested that relapse rates and the shapes of relapse curves are similar across the addictions. This chapter attempts to move beyond this point by identifying commonalities in the *process* of relapse, and by pointing to the need for more information on the natural history, determinants, consequences, and prevention of lapse and relapse. We conceptualize behavior change as occurring in three stages (motivation and commitment, initial change, and maintenance of change) and propose specific methods for dealing

Table 1. Research Needs in the Areas of Lapse and Relapse

Areas	Questions to be answered
Natural History	1. Is a relapse incremental learning or a failure experience? 2. Does the chance of relapse increase or decrease with time? 3. What are the stages of the lapse and relapse processes? 4. Is there a "safe" point beyond which a person will not relapse? 5. How frequent are lapses, and do they precede relapse?
Effects of lapse and relapse	1. What are the effects on mood? 2. Do lapse and relapse influence self-efficacy? 3. Do others' reactions influence lapse and relapse? 4. What are the physiological effects of lapse and relapse? 5. How do professionals deal with relapse in their patients?
Determinants and predictors	1. Do various treatments influence probability of relapse? 2. Does early response to treatment predict relapse? 3. Is past history of success and relapse predictive? 4. What are the roles of withdrawal symptoms, cravings, and urges? 5. What are the roles of conditioning and compensatory responses? 6. What are the mechanisms of social support? 7. Do physiological factors influence risk? 8. Can relapse be predicted after treatment but before maintenance?
Prevention of lapse and relapse	1. What criteria can be used to screen patients? 2. Does screening influence false positive and false negative rates? 3. What is the role of exercise? 4. Are cue extinction procedures helpful? 5. Is there any role for programmed relapse? 6. What are the relevant coping strategies? 7. Can motivation be enhanced at various points in treatment? 8. Is lifelong treatment necessary?

with relapse at each stage. This study has strengthened our view that each area of the addictions has much to offer the others; therefore, we support more interaction among researchers and clinicians across this troublesome front.

References

Abrams, D. B., & Follick, M. J. (1983). Behavioral weight loss intervention at the worksite: Feasibility and maintenance. *Journal of Consulting and Clinical Psychology, 51,* 226–233.

Abrams, D., B., & Wilson, G. T. (1986). Habit disorders: Alcohol and tobacco dependence. In A. J. Frances & R. E. Hales (Eds.), *The American Psychiatric Association Annual Review* (Vol. 5, pp. 606–626). Washington, DC: American Psychiatric Association

Abrams, D. B., Monti, P. M., Pinto, R. P., Elder, J. P., Brown, R. A., & Jacobus, S. I. (1986). *Psychosocial stress and coping in smokers who quit.* Unpublished manuscript.

Ashley, F. W., & Kannel, W. B. (1974). Relation of weight change to change in atherogenic traits: The Framingham study. *Journal of Chronic Disease, 27,* 103–114.

Ashton, H., & Stepney, R. (1982). *Smoking: Psychology and pharmacology.* London: Tavistock.

Azrin, N. H. (1976). Improvements in the community-reinforcement approach to alcoholism. *Behaviour Research and Therapy, 14,* 339–348.

Bandura, A. (1977a). *Social learning theory.* Englewood Cliffs, NJ: Prentice-Hall.

Bandura, A. (1977b). Self-efficacy: Toward a unifying theory of behavior change. *Psychological Review, 84,* 191–215.

Bandura, A., & Simon, K. M. (1977). The role of proximal intentions in self-regulation of refractory behavior. *Cognitive Therapy and Research, 1,* 177–193.

Bennett, W., & Gurin, J. (1982). *The dieter's dilemma: Eating less and weighing more.* New York: Basic Books.

Best, J. A. (1980). Mass media, self-management, and smoking modification. In P. O. Davidson & S. M. Davidson (Eds.), *Behavioral medicine: Changing health lifestyles* (p. 371–390). New York: Bruner/Mazel.

Bigelow, G., Stitzer, M. L., Griffiths, R. R., & Liebson, I. A. (1981). Contingency management approaches to drug-self-administration and drug abuse: Efficacy and limitations. *Addictive Behaviors, 6,* 241–252.

Bray, G. A. (1976). *The obese patient.* Philadelphia: Saunders.

Brown, R. A., Lichtenstein, E., McIntyre, K. O., & Harrington-Kostur, J (1984). Effects of nicotine fading and relapse prevention on smoking cessation. *Journal of Consulting and Clinical Psychology, 52,* 307–308.

Brownell, K. D. (1982). Obesity: Understanding and treating a serious, prevalent, and refractory disorder. *Journal of Consulting and Clinical Psychology, 50,* 820–840.

Brownell, K. D. (1984a). Behavioral, psychological, and enviornmental predictors of obesity and success at weight reduction. *International Journal of Obesity, 8,* 543–550.

Brownell, K. D. (1984b). The psychology and physiology of obesity: Implications for screening and treatment. *Journal of American Dietetic Association, 84,* 406–414.

Brownell, K. D. (1985). *The LEARN Program for weight control.* Unpublished treatment manual, University of Pennsylvania.

Brownell, K. D. (1986). Public health approaches to obesity and its management. *Annual Review of Public Health, 7,* 521–533.

Brownell, K. D., Cohen, R. Y., Stunkard, A. J., Felix, M. J., & Cooley, N. B. (1984). Weight loss competitions at the work site: Impact on weight, morale, and cost-effectiveness. *American Journal of Public Health, 74,* 1283–1285.

Brownell, K. D., Greenwood, M. R. C., Shrager, E. E., & Stellar, E. (1986). The effects of repeated cycles of weight loss and regain in rats. *Physiology and Behavior, 38*, 459–464.

Brownell, K. D., Heckerman, C. L., Westlake, R. J., Hayes, S. C., & Monti, P. M. (1978). The effect of couples training and partner cooperativeness in the behavioral treatment of obesity. *Behaviour Research Therapy, 16*, 323–333.

Brownell, K. D., & Stunkard, A. J. (1980). Physical activity in the development and treatment of obesity. In A. J. Stunkard (Ed.), *Obesity* (pp. 300–324). Philadelphia: Saunders.

Brownell, K. D., & Stunkard, A. J. (1981). Couples training, pharmacotherapy, and behavior therapy in treatment of obesity. *Archives of General Psychiatry, 38*, 1223–1229.

Chaney, E. F., O'Leary, M. R., & Marlatt, G. A. (1978). Skill training with alcoholics. *Journal of Consulting and Clinical Psychology, 46*, 1092–1104. Cobb, S. (1976). Social support as a moderator of life stress. *Psychosomatic Medicine, 38*, 300–314.

Cohen, E. A., Gelfand, D. M., Dodd, D. K., Jensen, J., & Turner, C. (1980) Self-control practices associated with weight loss maintenance in children and adolescents. *Behavior Therapy, 11*, 26–37.

Cohen, S., & Syme, L. (1985). *Social support and health.* New York: Academic Press.

Colletti, G., & Brownell, K. D. (1982). The physical and emotional benefits of social support: Applications to obesity, smoking, and alcoholism. In M. Hersen, R. M. Eisler, & P. M. Miller (Eds.), *Progress in behavior modification* (Vol. 13, pp. 110–179). New York: Academic Press.

Colletti, G., & Supnick, J. A. (1980). Continued therapist contact as a maintenance strategy for smoking reduction. *Journal of Consulting and Clinical Psychology, 48*, 665–667.

Colletti, G., Supnick, J. A., & Payne, T. J. (1985). The Smoking Self-Efficacy Questionnaire: A preliminary validation. *Behavioral Assessment, 7*, 249–254.

Collins, R. L., Rothblum, E., & Wilson, G. T. (1986). Evaluation of a cognitive-behavioral program for obesity. *Cognitive Therapy and Research, 6*, 299–318.

Condiotti, M. M., & Lichtenstein, E. (1981). Self-efficacy and relapse in smoking cessation programs. *Journal of Consulting and Clinical Psychology, 49*, 648–658.

Cooney, N. L., & Kopel, S. A. (1980). *Controlled relapse: A social learning approach to preventing smoking recidivism.* Paper presented at the meeting of the American Psychological Association, Montreal.

Cooney, N. L., Kopel, S. A., & McKeon, P. (1982). *Controlled relapse training and self-efficacy in ex-smokers.* Paper presented at the meeting of the American Psychological Association, Washington, DC.

Coppotelli, H. C., & Orleans, C. T. (1985). Spouse support for smoking cessation maintenance by women. *Journal of Consulting and Clinical Psychology, 53*, 455–460.

Craighead, L. W. (1984)., Sequencing of behavior therapy and pharmacotherapy for obesity. *Journal of Consulting and Clinical Psychology, 52*, 190–199.

Craighead, L. W., Stunkard, A. J., & O'Brien, R. (1981). Behavior therapy and pharmacotherapy for obesity. *Archives of General Psychiatry, 38*, 763–768.

Cronkite, R., & Moos, R. (1980). The determinants of posttreatment functioning of alcoholic patients: A conceptual framework. *Journal of Consulting and Clinical Psychology, 48*, 305–316.

Cummings, C., Gordon, J. R., & Marlatt, G. A. (1980). Relapse: Prevention and prediciton. In W. R. Miller (Ed.), *The addictive disorders: Treatment of alcoholism, drug abuse, smoking, and obesity* (pp. 291–322). New York: Pergamon.

Dahlkoetter, J., Callahan, E. J., & Linton, J. (1979). Obesity and the unbalanced energy equation: Exercise vs. eating habit change. *Journal of Consulting and Clinical Psychology, 47*, 898–905.

Davis, A. L., Faust, R., & Ordentlich, M. (1984). Self-help smoking cessation and maintenance programs: A comparative study with 12-month follow-up by the American Lung Association. *American Journal of Public Health, 74,* 1212–1219.

DiClemente, C. C., & Prochaska, J. O. (1982). Self-change and therapy changes of smoking behavior: A comparison of processes of change in cessation and maintenance. *Addictive Behaviors, 7,* 133–142.

Dubbert, P. M., & Wilson, G. T. (1984). Goal-setting and spouse involvement in the treatment of obesity. *Behavior Research and Therapy, 22,* 227–242.

Elandt-Johnson, R. C., & Johnson, N. L. (1980). *Survival models and data analysis.* New York: Wiley.

Epstein, L. H., & Cluss, P. A. (1982). A behavioral medicine perspective on adherence to long-term medical regimens. *Journal of Consulting and Clinical Psychology, 50,* 950–971.

Epstein, L. H., Wing, R. R., Koeske, R., Andrasik, F., & Ossip, D. J. (1981). Child and parent weight loss in family-based behavior modification programs. *Journal of Consulting and Clinical Psychology, 49,* 674–685.

Fagerstrom, K. O. (1982). A comparison of psychological and pharmacological treatments in smoking cessation. *Journal of Behavioral Medicine, 5,* 343–351.

Foreyt, J. P., Mitchell, R. E., Garner, D. T., Gee, M., Scott, L. W., & Gotto, A. M. (1982). Behavioral treatment of obesity: Results and limitations. *Behavior Therapy, 13,* 153–163.

Gartner, A., & Reissman, F. (Eds.). (1984). *The self-help revolution.* New York: Human Sciences Press.

Gilbert, D. G. (1979). Paradoxical tranquilizing and emotion-reducing effects of nicotine. *Psychological Bulletin, 86,* 643–661.

Glasgow, R. E., Schafer, L., & O'Neill, H. K. (1981). Self-help books and amount of therapist contact in smoking cessation programs. *Journal of Consulting and Clinical Psychology, 49,* 659–667.

Glasser, W. (1976). *Positive addiction.* New York: Harper & Row.

Goldstein, S., Gordon, J. R., & Marlatt, G. A. (1984). *Attributional processes and relapse following smoking cessation.* Paper presented at the meeting of the American Psychological Association, Toronto.

Graham, L. E., II, Taylor, C. B., Hovell, M. F., & Siegel, W. (1983). Five-year follow-up to a behavioral weight loss program. *Journal of Consulting and Clinical Psychology, 51,* 322–323.

Grunberg, N. E. (1982). The effects of nicotine and cigarette smoking on food consumption and taste preferences. *Addictive Behaviors, 7,* 317–331.

Grunberg, N. E., & Bowen, D. J. (1985). Coping with the sequelae of smoking cessation. *Journal of Cardiopulmonary Rehabilitation, 5,* 285–289.

Grunberg, N. E., Bowen, D. J., Maycock, V. A., & Nespor, S. M. (1985). The importance of sweet taste and caloric content in the effects of nicotine on specific food consumption. *Psychopharmacology, 87,* 198–203.

Grunberg, N. E., Bowen, D. J., & Morse, D. E. (1984). Effects of nicotine on body weight and food consumption in rats. *Psychopharmacology, 83,* 98–98.

Hagen, R. L., Foreyt, J. P., & Durham, T. W. (1976). The dropout problem: Reducing attrition in obesity research. *Behavior Therapy, 7,* 463–471.

Hall, S. M., Rugg, D., Tunstall, C., & Jones, R. T. (1984). Preventing relapse to cigarette smoking by behavioral skill training. *Journal of Consulting and Clinical Psychology, 52,* 372–382.

Hall, S. M., Tunstall, C., Rugg, D., Jones, R. T. & Benowitz, N. (1985). Nicotine gum and behavioral treatment in smoking cessation. *Journal of Consulting and Clinical Psychology, 53,* 256–258.

Harris, M. G., & Hallbauer, E. S. (1973). Self-directed weight control thorugh eating and exercise. *Behaviour Research and Therapy, 11,* 523–529.

Hodgson, R. J. (1980). The alcohol dependence syndrome: A step in the wrong direction *British Journal of Addiction, 75,* 255–263.

Hodgson, R. J., Rankin, H. J., & Stockwell, T. R. (1979). Alcohol dependence and the priming effect. *Behavioral Research and Therapy, 17,* 379–387.

Horn, D. A. (1976). A model for the study of personal choice health behavior. *International Journal of Health Education, 19,* 89–98.

Hunt, G. W., & Azrin, N. H. (1973). A community-reinforcement approach to alcoholism. *Behaviour Research and Therapy, 11,* 91–104.

Hunt, W. A., Barnett, L. W., & Branch, L. G. (1971). Relapse rates in addiction programs. *Journal of Clinical Psychology, 27,* 455–456.

Hunt, W. A., & Matarazzo, J. E. (1973). Three years later: Recent developments in the experimental modification of smoking behavior. *Journal of Abnormal Psychology, 81,* 107–114.

Janis, I. L. (1983). The role of social support in adherence to stressful decisions. *American Psychologist, 38,* 143–160.

Jeffery, R. W., & Wing, R. R. (1983). Recidivism and self-cure of smoking and obesity: Data from population studies. *American Psychologist, 37,* 852.

Jeffery, R. W., Wing, R. R., & Stunkard, A. J. (1978). Behavioral treatment of obesity: State of the art in 1976. *Behavior Therapy, 6,* 189–199.

Jeffery, R. W., Gerber, W. M., Rosenthal, B. S., & Lindquist, R. A. (1983). Monetary contracts in weight control: Effects of group and individual contracts. *Journal of Consulting and Clinical Psychology, 51,* 242–248.

Jeffery, R. W., Snell, M. K., & Forster, J. L. (1984). Group composition in the treatment of obesity: Does increasing group heterogeneity improve treatment results? *Behaviour Research and Therapy, 23,* 371–373.

Jeffery, R. W., Bjornson-Benson, W. M., Rosenthal, B. S., Lindquist, R. A., Kurth, C. C., & Johnson, S. C. (1984). Correlates of weight loss and its maintenance over two years of follow-up in middle-aged men. *Preventive Medicine, 13,* 155–168.

Jeffery, R. W., Forster, J. L., & Snell, M. K. (1985). Promoting weight control at the worksite: A pilot program of self-motivation using payroll-based incentives. *Preventive Medicine, 14,* 187–194.

Katahan, M., Pleas, J., Thackery, M., & Wallston, K. A. (1982). Relationship of eating and activity self-reports to follow-up weight maintenance in the massively obese. *Behavior Therapy, 13,* 521–528.

Killen, J. D., Maccoby, N., & Taylor, C. B. (1984). Nicotine gum and self-regulation training in smoking relapse prevention. *Behavior Therapy, 15,* 234–248.

Koplan, J. P., Powell, K. E., Sikes, R. K., Shirley, R. W., & Campbell, C. C. (1982). An epidemiologic study of the benefits and risks of running. *Journal of American Medical Association, 248,* 3118–3121.

Lando, H. (1981). Effects of preparation, experimenter contact, and a maintained reduction alternative on a broad-spectrum program for eliminating smoking. *Addictive Behaviors, 6,* 361–366.

Lando, H., & McGovern, P. (1982). Three-year data on a behavioral treatment for smoking: A follow-up note. *Addictive Behaviors, 7,* 177–181.

Levison, P. K., Gerstein, D. R., & Maloff, D. R. (Eds.). (1983). *Commonalities in substance abuse and habitual behaviors.* Lexington, MA: Lexington.

Lichtenstein, E. (1982). The smoking problem: A behavioral perspective. *Journal of Consulting and Clinical Psychology, 50,* 804–819.

Lichtenstein, E. (1984). *Systematic follow-up of slips and relapses after smoking cessation.* Manuscript in preparation.

Lichtenstein, E., Antonuccio, D. O., & Rainwater, G. (1977). *Unkicking the habit: The resumption of cigarette smoking*. Paper presented at the meeting of the Western Psychological Association, Seattle.

Lichtenstein, E., & Rodrigues, M-R. P. (1977). Long-term effects of rapid smoking treatment for dependent cigarette smokers. *Addictive Behaviors, 2*, 109–112.

Ludwig, A. M., Wikler, A., & Stark, L. H. (1974). The first drink: Psychobiological aspects of craving. *Archives of General Psychiatry, 30*, 539–547.

Marlatt, G. A. (1978). Craving for alcohol, loss of control, and relapse: A cognitive-behavioral analysis. In P. E. Nathan, G. A. Marlatt, & T. Loberg (Eds.), *Alcoholism: New directions in behavioral research and treatment* (pp. 271–314). New York: Plenum Press.

Marlatt, G. A. (1983). The controlled-drinking controversy: A commentary. *American Psychologist, 38*, 1097–1110.

Marlatt, G. A., Goldstein, S., & Gordon, J. R. (1984). *Unaided smoking cessation: A prospective analysis*. Manuscript in preparation.

Marlatt, G. A., & Gordon, J. R. (1980). Determinants of relapse: Implications for the maintenance of behavior change. In P. O. Davidson & S. M. Davidson (Eds.), *Behavioral medicine: Changing health lifestyles* (pp. 410–452). Elmsford, NY: Pergamon.

Marlatt, G. A., & Gordon, J. R. (Eds.). (1985). *Relapse prevention: Maintenance strategies in addictive behavior change*. New York: Guilford. McClearn, G. (1981). Genetic studies in animals. *Alcoholism: Clinical and Experimental Research, 5*, 447–448.

McClearn, G. (1981). Genetic studies in animals. *Alcoholism: Clinical and Experimental Research, 5*, 447–448.

McMorrow, J. J., & Foxx, R. M. (1983). Nicotine's role in smoking: An analysis of nicotine regulation. *Psychological Bulletin, 2*, 302–327.

Mermelstein, R. J., & Lichtenstein, E. (1983). *Skips versus relapses in smoking cessation: A situational analysis*. Paper presented at the meeting of the Western Psychological Association, San Francisco.

Mermelstein, R., Cohen, S., & Lichtenstein, E. (1983). *Psychosocial stress, social support, and smoking cessation maintenance*. Paper presetned at the annual meeting of the American Psychological Association, Anaheim, CA.

Miller, P. M. (1980). Theoretical and practical issues in substance abuse and treatment. In W. R. Miller (Ed.), *The addictive behaviors: Treatment of alcoholism, drug abuse, smoking, and obesity* (pp. 265–290). New York: Pergamon.

Miller, P. M., & Sims, K. L. (1981). Evaluation and component analysis of a comprehensive weight control program. *International Journal of Obesity, 5*, 57–66.

Miller, W. R., & Hester, R. K. (1980). Treating the problem drinker: Modern approaches. In W. R. Miller (Ed.), *The addictive behaviors: Treatment of alcoholism, drug abuse, smoking, and obesity* (pp. 11–142). New York: Pergamon.

Moos, R. H., & Finney, J. W. (1983). The expanding scope of alcoholism treatment evaluation. *American Psychologist, 38*, 1036–1044.

Murphy, T., Marlatt, G. A., & Pagano, R. (In press). The effect of aerobic exercise and meditation on alcohol consumption in male heavy drinkers. *Addictive Behaviors*.

Myers, R. D. (1978). Psychopharmacology of alcohol. *Annual Review of Pharmacology and Toxicology, 18*, 125–144.

Nathan, P. E. (1980). Etiology and process in the addictive behaviors. In W. R. Miller (Ed.), *The addictive behaviors: Treatment of alcoholism, drug abuse, smoking and obesity* (pp. 241–264). New York: Pergamon.

Nathan, P. E. (1983). Failures in prevention: Why we can't prevent the devastating effect of alcoholism and drug abuse. *American Psychologist, 38*, 459–467.

Nathan, P. E. (1984). Alcoholism prevention in the work place: Three examples. In P. M. Miller & T. E. Nirenberg (Eds.), *Prevention of alcohol abuse* (pp. 235–261). New York:

Plenum Press.

Nathan, P. E., & Goldman, M. S. (1979). Problem drinking and alcoholism. In O. F. Pomerleau & J. P. Brady (Eds.), *Behavioral medicine: Theory and practice* (pp. 255–278). Baltimore, MD: Williams & Wilkins.

Nathan, P. E., & Wiens, A. N. (1983). Alcoholism: Introduction and overview. *American Psychologist, 38,* 1035.

National Institute on Drug Abuse. (1979). *Behavioral analysis and treatment of substance abuse.* NIDA Research Monograph 25, Washington, DC: U.S. Department of Health, Education, and Welfare.

Ockene, J. K. (1984). Toward a smoke-free society. *American Journal of Public Health, 74,* 1198–1200.

Ockene, J. K., Hymowitz, N., Sexton, M., & Broste, S. K. (1982). Comparison of patterns of smoking behavior change among smokers in the Multiple Risk Factor Intervention Trial (MRFIT). *Preventive Medicine, 11,* 621–638.

Oldridge, N. B., Donner, A. P., Buck, C. W., Jones, N. L., Andrew, G. M., Parker, J. O., Cunningham, D. A., Kavanaugh, T., Rechnitzer, P. A., & Sutton, J. R. (1983). Predictors of dropout from cardiac exercise rehabilitation: Ontario exercise–heart collaborative study. *American Journal of Cardiology, 51,* 70–74.

Ossip-Klein, D. J., Shapiro, R. M., & Stiggins, J. (1984). Freedom Line: Increasing utilization of a telephone support service for ex-smokers. *Addictive Behaviors, 9,* 227–230.

Pechacek, T. P. (1979). Modification of smoking behavior. In *Smoking and health: A report of the Surgeon General.* DHEW Pub. No. PHS 19-50066. Washington, DC: U.S. Government Printing Office.

Pechacek, T. P., Mittelmark, M., Jeffery, R. W., Loken, B., & Luepker, R. (1985). *Quit and win: Direct incentives for smoking cessation.* Manuscript submitted for publication.

Perri, M. G., McAdoo, W. G., Spevak, P. A., & Newlin, D. B. (1984). Effect of a multicomponent maintenance program on long-term weight loss. *Journal of Consulting and Clinical Psychology, 52,* 480–481.

Perri, M. G., Shapiro, R. M., Ludwig, W. W., Twentyman, C. T., & McAdoo, W. G. (1984). Maintenance strategies for the treatment of obesity: An evaluation of relapse prevention training and posttreatment contact by mail and telephone. *Journal of Consulting and Clinical Psychology, 52,* 404–413.

Pomerleau, O. F. (1984). Reinforcing properties of nicotine: Smoking and induced vasopressin and beta-endorphin release, antioception and anxiety reduction. *Pavlovian Journal of Biological Science, 19,* 107.

Pomerleau, O. F., & Pomerleau, C. S. (1984). Neuroregulators and the reinforcement of smoking: Towards a biobehavioral explanation. *Neuroscience and Biobehavioral Reviews, 8,* 503–513.

Pomerleau, O. F., Adkins, D., & Pertschuk, M. (1978). Predictors of outcome and recidivism in smoking cessation treatment. *Addictive Behaviors, 3,* 65–70.

Poulos, C. X., Hinson, R. E., & Siegel, S. (1981). The role of Pavlovian processes in drug tolerance and dependence: Implications for treatment. *Addictive Behaviors, 6,* 205–212.

Prochaska, J. O. (1979). *Systems of psychotherapy: A transtheoretical analysis.* Homewood, IL: Dorsey.

Prochaska, J. O. (1983). Self-changers versus therapy changers versus Schachter. *American Psychologist, 37,* 853–854.

Prochaska, J. O., & DiClemente, C. C. (1982). Transtheoretical therapy: Toward a more integrated model of change. *Psychotherapy: Theory, Research, and Practice, 19,* 276–288.

Prochaska, J. O., & DiClemente, C. C. (1983). Stages and processes of self-change of smoking: Toward an integrative model of change. *Journal of Consulting and Clinical Psychology, 52,* 390–395.

Prochaska, J. O., & DiClemente, C. C. (1984). *The transtheoretical approach: Crossing traditional boundaries of therapy*. Homewood, IL: Down Jones/Irwin.

Rodin, J. (1981). Current status of the internal-external hypothesis for obesity: What went wrong? *American Psychologist, 36*, 361–372.

Rosen, T. J., & Shipley, R. H. (1983). A strange analysis of self-initiated smoking reductions. *Addictive Behaviors, 8*, 263–272.

Sackett, D. L., & Haynes, R. B. (Eds.). (1976). *Compliance with therapeutic regimens*. Baltimore, MD: Johns Hopkins University Press.

Schachter, S. (1982). Recidivism and self-cure of smoking and obesity. *American Psychologist, 37*, 436–444.

Schuckitt, M. A. (1981). The genetics of alcoholism. *Alcoholism: Clinical and Experimental Research, 5*, 439–440.

Shiffman, S. (1982). Relapse following smoking cessation: A situational analysis. *Journal of Consulting and Clinical Psychology, 50*, 71–86.

Shiffman, S. (1984). Coping with temptations to smoke. *Journal of Consulting and Clinical Psychology, 52*, 261–267.

Siegel, S. (1979). The role of conditioning in drug tolerance and addiction. In J. D. Keehen (Ed.), *Psychopathology in animals: Research and treatment implications*. New York: Academic Press.

Simopoulos, A. P., & Van Itallie, T. B. (1984). Body weight, health, and longevity. *Annals of Internal Medicine, 100*, 285–295.

Stalonas, P. M., Johnson, W. G., & Christ, M. (1978). Behavior modification for obesity: The valuation of exercise, contingency management, and program adherence. *Journal of Consulting and Clinical Psychology, 2*, 225–235.

Sternberg, B. S. (1985). Relapse in weight control: Definitions, processes, and prevention strategies. In G. A. Marlatt & J. R. Gordon (Eds.), *Relapse prevention: Maintenance strategies in addictive behavior change* (pp. 521–545). New York: Guilford.

Stitzer, M. L., & Bigelow, G. E. (1984). Contingent reinforcement for carbon monoxide reduction: Within-subject effects of pay amount. *Journal of Applied Behavior Analysis, 17*, 477–484.

Stockwell, T. R. Hodgson, R. J., Rankin, H. J., & Taylor, C. (1982). Alcohol dependence, beliefs, and the priming effect. *Behaviour Research and Therapy, 20*, 513–522.

Stuart, R. B., & Guire, K. (1978). Some correlates of the maintenance of weight loss through behavior modification. *International Journal of Obesity, 2*, 225–235.

Stunkard, A. J. (1986). The control of obesity: Social and community perspectives. In K. D. Brownell& J. P. Foreyt (Eds.), *The physiology, psychology, and treatment of the eating disorders*. New York: Basic Books.

Stunkard, A. J., & Penick, S. B. (1979). Behavior modification in the treatment of obesity: The problem of maintaining weight loss. *Archives of General Psychiatry, 36*, 810–816.

Stunkard, A. J., Sorenson, T. I. A., Hanis, C., Teasdale, T. W., Chakraborty, R., Schull, W. J., & Schulsinger, F. (1986). An adoption study of human obesity. *New England Journal of Medicine, 314*, 193–198.

Supnick, J. A., & Colletti, G. (1984). Relapse coping and problem solving training following treatment for smoking. *Addictive Behaviors, 9*, 401–404.

Sutton, S. R. (1979). Interpreting relapse curves. *Journal of Consulting and Clinical Psychology, 47*, 96–98.

Thompson, J. K., Jarvie, G. J., Lahey, B. B., & Cureton, K. J. (1982). Exercise and obesity: Etiology, physiology, and intervention. *Psychological Bulletin, 91*, 55–79.

U.S. Department of Health and Human Serivces. (1983). *The health consequences of smoking: Cardiovascular disease: A report of the Surgeon General*. Washington, DC: Author.

Vaillant, G. E. (1983). *The natural history of alcoholism: Causes, patterns, and paths to recovery.*

Cambridge, MA: Harvard University Press.

Vaillant, G. E., & Milofsky, E. S. (1982). The etiology of alcoholism: A prospective viewpoint. *American Psychologist, 37,* 494–503.

Wadden, T. A., Stunkard, A. J., & Brownell, K. D. (1983). Very low calorie diets: Their efficacy, safety, and future. *Annals of International Medicine, 99,* 675–684.

Wilkinson, D. A., & Sanchez-Craig, M. (1981). Relevance of brain dysfunction to treatment of objectives: Should alcohol-related cognitive deficits influence the way we think about treatment? *Addictive Behaviors, 6,* 253–260.

Wilson, G. T. (1978). Methodological considerations in treatment outcome research on obesity. *Journal of Consulting and Clinical Psycholgy, 46,* 687–702.

Wilson, G. T. (1980). Behavior therapy for obesity. In A. J. Stunkard (Ed.), *Obesity* (pp. 325–344). Philadelphia: Saunders.

Wilson, G. T. (1985). Psychological prognostic factors in the treatment of obesity. In J. Hirsch & T. B. Van Itallie (Eds.), *Recent advances in obesity research* (Vol. 4, pp. 301–311). London: Libbey.

Wilson, G. T., & Brownell, K. D. (1980). Behavior therapy for obesity: An evaluation of treatment outcome. *Advances in Behaviour Research and Therapy, 3,* 49–86.

Wooley, S. C., Wooley, O. W., & Dyrenforth, S. R. (1979). Theoretical, practical, and social issues in behavioral treatments of obesity. *Journal of Applied Behavior Analysis, 12,* 3–26.

Index

MIX
Papier aus verantwortungsvollen Quellen
Paper from responsible sources
FSC® C105338
FSC
www.fsc.org

If you have any concerns about our products,
you can contact us on
ProductSafety@springernature.com

In case Publisher is established outside the EU,
the EU authorized representative is:
Springer Nature Customer Service Center GmbH
Europaplatz 3, 69115 Heidelberg, Germany

Printed by Libri Plureos GmbH
in Hamburg, Germany